HANDBOOK OF

ANALYTICAL METHOD VALIDATION

FOR PHARMACEUTICALS

A Practical Guide to Validating Assay, Impurities, Dissolution & Residual Solvents Using HPLC and GC

To all pharmaceutical professionals,
This book is dedicated to you, with utmost respect and gratitude.

BHASKAR NAPTE

BlueRose ONE.com DIY
Stories Matter
NewDelhi • London

BLUEROSE PUBLISHERS
India | U.K.

For permissions requests or inquiries regarding this publication, please contact:

BLUEROSE PUBLISHERS
www.BlueRoseONE.com
info@bluerosepublishers.com
+91 8882 898 898
+4407342408967

ISBN: 978-93-7310-805-6

First Edition: September 2025

PREFACE

It is with great gratitude and a deep sense of purpose that I present to you Handbook of Analytical Method Validation for Pharmaceuticals. Thank you for choosing this book as your guide in understanding the practical aspects of method validation. In writing this book, my foremost aim was to make the subject accessible and actionable avoiding heavy jargon and instead adopting a clear, practical approach. From selecting appropriate performance characteristics to designing concentration mapping, this book is structured to help you confidently implement validation processes in the pharmaceutical setting. It is built upon my personal experiences and the real-world challenges encountered during method validation projects.

This work has been greatly enriched by the invaluable support of **Dr. Rajendra Chavan,** whose technical insights, detailed reviews, and thoughtful discussions have strengthened the quality and depth of the content. I am sincerely grateful for his contribution, which has truly enhanced the overall impact of this book.

I would also like to express my heartfelt thanks to my wife, **Manisha,** my daughter, **Anushka,** and my son, **Yash,** for their unwavering support, patience, and encouragement throughout this journey. Their understanding and the comfort they provided were essential in giving me the space and time needed to complete this endeavour.

A special note of thanks goes to the **"Pharma Growth Hub"** community a vibrant group of passionate professionals whose continuous encouragement and enthusiasm have been a tremendous source of motivation for me.

Lastly, I extend my sincere appreciation to every pharmaceutical professional who works tirelessly to uphold the quality, safety, and integrity of medicines. Your dedication continues to inspire, and it is my hope that this book serves as a valuable companion in your professional journey.

- Bhaskar Napte

—INDEX—

—INDEX—

—INDEX—

—INDEX—

CHAPTER: 01

INTRODUCTION TO PERFORMANCE CHARACTERISTICS

★ Why is Method Validation Important?

Let's begin with a simple example. Imagine you're at a busy traffic signal, and suddenly the lights stop working. Chaos, right? Now think of analytical methods as those traffic lights when they function properly, everything flows smoothly. But when they are not working or validated correctly, it can lead to confusion and errors.

Just as each traffic signal follows a predefined program to control traffic effectively, an analytical method must function as intended under defined conditions. Analytical Method Validation (AMV) is the documented process to ensure that an analytical method performs reliably, accurately, and consistently for its intended purpose.

Understanding the Intended Purpose

Before we get into validation parameters, let's understand what we mean by "intended purpose." This refers to what the method is designed to do:

- **Assay:** To quantify the amount of drug substance in a sample.
- **Impurity analysis:** To identify and quantify known and unknown impurities.
- **Residual solvent analysis:** To quantify trace amounts of solvents remaining after manufacturing.

Each of these purposes comes with specific expectations and performance criteria. That's where method validation comes in it ensures the method meets these expectations.

Challenges in Choosing the Right Parameters

With a wide range of analytical techniques available like chromatography, spectroscopy, potentiometry, and more - selecting the right validation parameters and their acceptance criteria can feel complex. Different techniques require different considerations.

Guidelines like ICH Q2(R2), and others help simplify this process by defining what needs to be validated and suggesting how to do it.

Every validation parameter comes with a predefined limit, known as the acceptance criteria. For instance:

- **Precision** is often evaluated using SD or %RSD.
- **Accuracy** may be expressed as % recovery.
- **Linearity** is assessed using correlation coefficient.

We will explore all these parameters and their criteria in detail in the following chapters.

Why New Analytical Methods Are Constantly Needed

With growing regulatory demands and the evolving complexity of pharmaceutical products, there is a continuous need for new analytical methods. These range from simple routine assays to highly sensitive techniques for detecting nitrosamines and other genotoxic impurities.

This evolving landscape makes it even more important to know how to select the right validation parameters and ensure that each method serves its purpose efficiently and accurately.

Key Validation Parameters

To ensure an analytical method is suitable for its intended use, it must be evaluated against a specific set of parameters. These are outlined in regulatory guidelines such as ICH Q2(R2) and form the core of method validation.

Here are the key parameters typically studied:

1. **Specificity / Selectivity**
2. **Precision**
3. **Detection Limit (DL / LOD)**
4. **Quantitation Limit (QL / LOQ)**
5. **Response / Linearity**
6. **Accuracy**
7. **Range**
8. **Robustness**

Let's begin with the first one:

1. Specificity/Selectivity

According to ICH Q2(R2)

"Specificity and selectivity are both terms to describe the extent to which other substances interfere with the determination of an analyte according to a given analytical procedure. Specificity is typically used to describe the ultimate state, measuring unequivocally a desired analyte. Selectivity is a relative term to describe the extent to which particular analytes in mixtures or matrices can be measured without interferences from other components with similar behaviour."

Specificity/selectivity can be shown by demonstrating that the identification and/or quantitation of an analyte is not impacted by the presence of other substances (e.g., impurities, sample matrix, or other components likely to be present).

In simpler term, specificity/selectivity means your method should be able to clearly identify and if applicable quantify the analyte of interest without being affected by other substances that might be present in the sample.

Why is this important?

Imagine you're analyzing a drug product using HPLC. In the case of an API, related impurities could interfere with your measurement. For drug formulations like tablets, placebo components or degradation products might become potential interferences. Such interference may result in inaccurate measurement.

But it's not just about sample components, instrumental factors like detector noise and baseline fluctuations (especially in chromatographic methods like HPLC or GC) can also affect selectivity.

How do we evaluate specificity/selectivity?

Below are the various ways to evaluate specificity/selectivity.

i. Absence of Interference:

Specificity/selectivity can be shown by demonstrating that the identification and/or quantitation of an analyte is not impacted by the presence of other substances (e.g., impurities, degradation products, related substances, placebo, or other components likely to be present).

ii. Orthogonal Procedure Comparison:

Specificity/selectivity can be verified by demonstrating that the measured result of an analyte is comparable to the measured result of a second, well characterised analytical procedure that ideally applies a different measurement principle.

iii. Technology Inherent Justification:

In some cases where the specificity of the analytical technology can be ensured and predicted by technical parameters (e.g., resolution of isotopes in mass spectrometry, chemical shifts in NMR spectroscopy), additional experimental studies may not be required, if justified.

iv. Forced degradation:

A common way to assess specificity/selectivity is through forced degradation studies. This involves subjecting the sample to stress conditions such as:

- **Acid/base/water hydrolysis**
- **Oxidation**
- **Thermal degradation**
- **Photolytic degradation**

You then examine whether the method can still identify and if necessary, quantify the analyte accurately in the presence of its degradation products.

2. Precision

According to ICH guideline Q2(R2), "The precision of an analytical procedure expresses the closeness of agreement (degree of scatter) between a series of measurements obtained from multiple samplings of the same homogeneous sample under the prescribed conditions. Precision can be considered at three levels: repeatability, intermediate precision and reproducibility."

The precision of an analytical procedure is usually expressed as the variance, standard deviation or coefficient of variation of a series of measurement

In simple terms, precision tells us how consistent our results are when we repeat the same test under the same conditions.

For example, imagine you and your colleague, Avinash, are both performing the assay for Paracetamol tablets. You're using tablets from the same batch and following the same test procedure. Each of you prepares six individual test solutions and carries out the analysis as per the method.

The results obtained by both of you for the Paracetamol assay are shown in the table below:

Table-1: Assay results obtained by two analysts

Paracetamol Assay Value						
Analyst Name	Prep #1	Prep #2	Prep #3	Prep #4	Prep #5	Prep #6
You	99.5%	100.2%	98.9%	101.2%	99.7%	100.8%
Avinash	99.0%	103.9%	103.8%	97.5%	100.6%	104.0%

When we look at the data, we can observe that your assay values are quite consistent and fall within a narrower range. In contrast, Avinash's results show a wider spread. This difference suggests that your method execution was more precise, as the closeness of agreement among your six values is better.

It's important to note that for evaluating precision, the sample must be homogeneous. If the sample itself varies, it becomes difficult to conclude whether the variation is due to the method or the sample. A homogeneous sample ensures that any observed differences are a result of the analytical procedure alone and not because of sample variability. This is a fundamental requirement for a meaningful precision study.

Levels of Precision

Precision can be evaluated at different levels to understand the consistency of results under varying conditions. As per ICH guidelines, precision is typically considered at three levels:

i. Repeatability

As per ICH Q2(R2), "Repeatability expresses the precision under the same operating conditions over a short interval of time.

It involves the same analyst, same equipment, same laboratory, and is often performed in a single analytical run. This is also known as intra-assay precision, and it gives an idea of how consistent the method is when repeated immediately under identical conditions.

How repeatability should be assessed?

Repeatability should be assessed using:

A minimum of 9 determinations covering the reportable range for the procedure (e.g., 3 concentrations/3 replicates each) or a minimum of 6 determinations at 100% of the test concentration.

ii. Intermediate Precision

As per ICH Q2(R2) "The extent to which intermediate precision should be established depends on the circumstances under which the procedure is intended to be used. The applicant should establish the effects of random events on the precision of the analytical procedure. Typical variations to be studied include different days, environmental conditions, analysts and equipment, as relevant. Ideally, the variations tested should be based on and justified by using analytical procedure understanding from development and risk assessment (ICH Q14). Studying these effects individually is not necessary. The use of design of experiments studies is encouraged."

Intermediate precision assesses how well the method performs when small, deliberate variations are introduced within the same laboratory. These variations help simulate real-world conditions where different people and equipment might be involved in routine testing. It includes factors such as:

•**Different Analysts:** For example, one analyst performs the Paracetamol assay in the morning, and another analyst repeats the same test in the afternoon, following the same method and using the same batch of sample.

•**Different Instruments:** Suppose the assay is performed first using an Agilent HPLC system and then repeated using a Waters HPLC system both systems must be qualified and operated as per SOPs.

•**Different Days or Times:** One set of test results may be generated on Monday morning and then repeated on Wednesday afternoon to check for day-to-day consistency.

•**Different Environmental Conditions (if applicable):** Although labs are controlled, minor fluctuations can still occur. For example, the lab temperature might be 22°C on Day 1 and 25°C on Day 2. The method should still deliver consistent results.

Intermediate precision helps assess the robustness and reliability of the analytical method under typical variations encountered in daily lab operations.

iii. Reproducibility

As per ICH Q2(R2), "Reproducibility is assessed by means of an inter-laboratory trial. Investigation of reproducibility is usually not required for regulatory submission but should be considered in cases of standardisation of an analytical procedure, for instance, for inclusion of procedures in pharmacopoeias and in cases where analytical procedures are conducted at multiple sites."

Reproducibility takes it one step further by evaluating the method's performance across different laboratories. This is usually done during collaborative studies or when a method is being standardized or transferred between locations. It includes variations such as different lab environments, different instruments, and analysts from separate facilities.

This level is especially important when a method is intended for use across multiple sites, such as in global pharmaceutical operations or regulatory submissions.

3. Detection Limit (DL/LOD)

As per ICH Q2(R2), "The detection limit is the lowest amount of an analyte in a sample which can be detected but not necessarily quantitated as an exact value." Different approaches can be used to determine the detection limit, depending on whether the method is instrumental or non-instrumental:

i. Based on Visual Evaluation:

This is often used for non-instrumental methods, but it can also apply to instrumental ones. The process involves analyzing samples with known concentrations and identifying the lowest level at which the analyte is clearly visible or detectable.

Example: In Thin Layer Chromatography (TLC), a series of standard solutions of the analyte are spotted on a TLC plate at concentrations of 5 ppm, 10 ppm, 20 ppm, and 30 ppm. After development and visualization, spots are clearly visible for the 10, 20, and 30 ppm concentrations but no spot is observed at 5 ppm. In this case, the detection limit of the method can be considered as 10 ppm, since it is the lowest concentration at which the analyte is visibly detectable.

ii. Based on Signal-to-Noise Ratio (S/N):

Applicable to instrumental methods that exhibit baseline noise (e.g., HPLC, GC). The DL is estimated by comparing the signal from a low-concentration sample with the baseline noise from a blank.
A signal-to-noise ratio of 2:1 or 3:1 is typically accepted as the minimum for reliable detection.

Example: During an HPLC analysis of 4-aminophenol, a known impurity in Paracetamol tablets, a standard solution containing 0.02% of 4-aminophenol is injected. The chromatogram shows a signal-to-noise ratio of 3.3:1 for this concentration. Based on this observation, 0.02% is qualified as the detection limit (DL) of the method for this impurity.

iii. Based on the Standard Deviation of a Linear Response and a Slope:

This is a statistical approach that uses the calibration curve. The detection limit is calculated using the formula:

$DL = 3.3\sigma/S$

- σ = Standard deviation of the response
- **S** = Slope of the calibration curve

You can estimate σ in two ways:

a. Estimation of standard deviation from blank responses:

Analyze several blank samples and calculate the standard deviation of their signals.

Example: Determination of Detection Limit (DL) for Sodium by AAS:
In this example, the detection limit is established for sodium content analysis using Atomic Absorption Spectroscopy (AAS). The approach used is based on the standard deviation of the blank response and the slope of the calibration curve. Ten blank measurements were recorded to evaluate the background noise of the system. Based on the blank response variability and the slope of the calibration

curve, the detection limit of the method for sodium content by AAS is estimated to be 0.92 ppm.

Table 2: Blank measurements for calculation of standard deviation

Blank Measurement	
Measurement No.	Background Absorbance
1	0.010
2	0.020
3	0.005
4	0.015
5	0.000
6	0.010
7	0.012
8	0.014
9	0.009
10	0.008
Standard Deviation (σ)	0.0055

Calibration curve preparation for calculation of slope: A calibration curve was generated using sodium standard solutions at five concentrations:

Table 3: Calibration curve for sodium standard for calculation of slope (S)

Calibration Curve		
Level	Conc. Of Sodium (ppm)	Absorbance
1	10	0.20
2	20	0.40
3	30	0.59
4	40	0.81
5	50	0.98
	Slope (S)	0.0197

Calculation of Detection Limit (DL)

Using the formula from ICH Q2(R2):
$DL = 3.3x\ 0.0055/0.0197 = 0.92$ ppm

It is important to note that while the ICH Q2(R2) guideline does not specify the number of blank measurements required, the EURACHEM ("The Fitness for Purpose of Analytical Methods: A Laboratory Guide to Method Validation and Related Topics", 2014) recommends the number of replicates sufficient to obtain an adequate estimate of the standard deviation. Typically between 6 and 15 replicates are considered necessary; 10 replicates are often recommended for calculation of slope.

b. Estimation of standard deviation from the calibration curve:

Use the standard deviation of y-intercepts or the residual standard deviation of the regression line from low-level analyte samples. To estimate the standard deviation (σ) using a calibration curve, prepare a series of samples containing the analyte at concentrations close to the expected detection limit. Construct a calibration curve by plotting the response against concentration. Then, calculate either the residual standard deviation of the regression line or the standard deviation of the y-intercept. These values can serve as estimates of σ for calculating the detection limit.

Example: Determination of Detection Limit (DL) for 4-Aminophenol in Paracetamol Tablets by HPLC: In this example, the Detection Limit (DL/LOD) for 4-Aminophenol, a known impurity in Paracetamol tablets, is determined using the calibration curve approach based on ICH Q2(R2).

A calibration curve was prepared using standard solutions of 4-Aminophenol ranging from 0.05 ppm to 5 ppm, and the corresponding detector responses were recorded. The residuals were calculated to assess the fit of the data.

Table 4: Low-level analyte sample measurements for calculation of standard deviation

Calibration Curve with Analyte at Expected DL Concentration			
Level	Conc. Of 4-Aminophenol (ppm)	Response	Residuals = [Actual Response - (S*x + c)]
1	0.05	650	433.8928489
2	1.0	1200	61.12516287
3	1.5	1400	-224.54204
4	2	1600	-510.209244
5	2.5	2600	4.123553307
6	3.0	3100	18.45635012
7	3.5	3500	-67.2108531
8	4.0	4100	47.12194374
9	4.5	4400	-138.545259
10	5.0	5400	375.7875374
Slope (S)		971.3344064	
Y-Intercept (C)		167.5404308	
Residual Standard Deviation (σ)			272.8936238

Preparation of Calibration Curve (Linearity Range):

To determine the slope (S) accurately, a calibration curve was established using five concentrations of 4-Aminophenol ranging from 10 to 50 ppm, which fall within the linear response range of the method. This satisfies the ICH recommendation of using a minimum of five concentrations.

Table 5: Calibration curve for 4 -Aminophenol standard for calculation of slope (S)

Calibration Curve		
Level	Conc. Of 4-Aminophenol (ppm)	Response
1	10	10000
2	20	20000
3	30	28000
4	40	42000
5	50	51000
Slope (S)		1040
Y-intercept (c)		-1000

Calculation of Detection Limit (DL):

Using the formula from ICH Q2(R2):
DL = 3.3x 272.8936238/1040 = 0.87 ppm

✦ **Instrument Detection Limit vs. Method Detection Limit:** It is also essential to understand the difference between the instrument detection limit and the method detection limit, as outlined in the guide "The Fitness for Purpose of Analytical Methods: A Laboratory Guide to Method Validation and Related Topics" (Eurachem, 2014):

- The instrument detection limit is typically determined by introducing a simple sample (like a reagent blank) directly into the instrument excluding sample preparation steps. It often relies on the signal-to-noise ratio observed in the instrument output, such as a chromatogram.

- In contrast, the method detection limit is determined using samples that undergo the complete analytical process, including sample preparation and all procedural steps. The results are calculated in the same manner as actual test samples.

✦ **Why this matters:** For method validation, it is the method detection limit that provides the most realistic and practical measure of a method's capability. Therefore, it should be the primary focus during validation studies.

4. Quantitation Limit (QL/LOQ):

As per ICH Q2(R2), "The quantitation limit is the lowest amount of analyte in a sample which can be quantitatively determined with suitable precision and accuracy."

This parameter is particularly important for the quantification of impurities, degradation products, and residues (after cleaning) at low levels, and it plays a key role in the validation of methods used for stability studies, impurity profiling, and residual analysis.
Just like the detection limit, the quantitation limit can be determined through various approaches, depending on whether the method is instrumental or non-instrumental:

i. Based on Visual Evaluation:

This approach is mostly used for non-instrumental methods but may also apply to some instrumental methods. The quantitation limit is established by analyzing samples with known low concentrations of analyte and determining the lowest concentration at which the analyte can be measured with acceptable precision and accuracy.

Example: In titrimetric analysis, this might be the smallest titrant volume that consistently gives reproducible endpoint.

ii. Based on Signal-to-Noise Ratio (S/N):

This method applies to instrumental techniques that exhibit baseline noise (e.g., HPLC, GC). The analyst compares signals from low-concentration analyte samples to those of blank samples.

A signal-to-noise ratio of about 10:1 is generally accepted for estimating the quantitation limit.

iii. Based on the Standard Deviation of a Linear Response and a Slope:

This statistical approach is widely used and provides a reliable estimate for QL using the formula:

$QL = 10 \times \sigma / S$

Where:

- σ = standard deviation of the response
- S= slope of the calibration curve

The slope (S) is a measure of how much the detector response changes with concentration. It can be estimated from a calibration curve prepared using the analyte at known concentrations within the method's linear range.

To ensure accuracy, prepare a minimum of five different concentrations of the analyte within the linearity range. Plot the responses against concentrations and calculate the slope from the resulting regression line.

To estimate σ, two common methods are used:

a. Estimation of standard deviation from blank responses:

Analyze multiple blank samples and calculate the standard deviation of their responses to determine σ.

b. From the Calibration Curve

Prepare a calibration curve using analyte concentrations close to the expected quantitation limit. Then, determine the residual standard deviation of the regression line, or calculate the standard deviation of the y-intercept. Either value may be used as the estimate of σ.

✈ Why Quantitation Limit Matters

The quantitation limit is not just a number—it reflects your method's sensitivity and reliability in detecting small quantities of substances that could impact product quality or patient safety. Establishing a realistic and well-supported QL ensures the method is fit for purpose, especially when dealing with regulatory limlit for imputitis.

5. Response:

One of the noteworthy updates in ICH Q2(R2), 2023 is the explicit inclusion of the term "response". While earlier versions of the guideline implied the idea, the revised version brings it to the forefront making the concept clearer and more aligned with actual analytical practice.

What is "Response"?

In the context of analytical method validation, response refers to the measured signal obtained from an instrument such as peak area, peak height, absorbance, or intensity that corresponds to the concentration or amount of an analyte in a sample.

This output is what analysts use to quantify how much of a substance is present. For example, in HPLC, it could be the peak area detected by a UV detector. In a UV spectrophotometer, it might be the absorbance at a particular wavelength.

Why is it important?

The inclusion of "response" in ICH Q2(R2) serves several important purposes:

i.Clarity in Method Validation:

It formalizes the link between the analyte concentration and the observed signal, especially when assessing parameters like:

- **Linearity:** Checking if response increases proportionally with concentration.
- **Range:** Determining the interval over which the response is accurate and precise.
- **Accuracy and Precision:** Ensuring the response consistently reflects the actual analyte amount.

ii.Better Representation of Real-World Practices:

Analytical methods, whether traditional or modern, revolve around how reliably a response can be used to calculate an analyte's quantity. By highlighting "response," the guideline mirrors what analysts do in everyday lab settings.

iii.Applicability to Advanced Techniques:

Modern analytical tools like mass spectrometry or spectroscopic methods often rely heavily on signal-based measurements. A clear definition of "response" helps standardize how these technologies are validated across different labs and regulatory submissions.

6. Accuracy

As per ICH Q2(R2), "The accuracy of an analytical procedure expresses the closeness of agreement between the value which is accepted either as a conventional true value or as an accepted reference value and the value or set of values measured."

Accuracy is one of the most critical parameters in method validation, as it directly reflects how well the method can measure the actual content of an analyte.

The most common way to assess accuracy is by spiking that is, adding a known amount of analyte into the sample matrix. This spiked sample is then analyzed, and the found value is compared to the true (added) value. Accuracy is usually expressed as percent recovery (%Recovery).

Example:

Let's say you are evaluating the accuracy of a method for measuring Impurity A in a drug product. You spike 16 µg/mL of Impurity A into the sample. Upon analysis, the instrument reports 14 µg/mL as the found value.

The %Recovery can be calculated using the formula:

%Recovery = (Found Value / True Value) × 100

%Recovery = (14 µg/mL ÷ 16 µg/mL) × 100 = 87.5%

Note: In this example, it is assumed that the unspiked drug product does not contain Impurity A.

Accuracy testing is typically done at multiple concentration levels, often ranging from QL (reporting threshold), 50% to 120% of the target concentration, depending on the regulatory requirement and the purpose of the method.

How is accuracy assessed?

Accuracy should be assessed using an appropriate number of determinations and concentration levels covering the reportable range (e.g., 3 concentrations/3 replicates each of the full analytical procedure).

Accuracy is typically verified through one of the studies described below. In certain cases, accuracy can be inferred once precision, response within the range and specificity have been established.

i. Reference Material Comparison:

The analytical procedure is applied to an analyte of known purity (e.g., a reference material, a well characterised impurity or a related substance) and the measured versus theoretically expected results are evaluated.

ii. Spiking Study:

The analytical procedure is applied to a matrix of all components except the analyte where a known amount of the analyte of interest has been added. In cases where all the expected components are impossible to reproduce, the analyte can be added to or enriched in the test sample. The results from measurements on unspiked and spiked/enriched samples are evaluated.

iii. Orthogonal Procedure Comparison:

The results of the proposed analytical procedure are compared with those of an orthogonal procedure. The accuracy of the orthogonal procedure should be reported. Orthogonal procedures can be used with quantitative impurity measurements to verify primary measurement values in cases where obtaining samples of all relevant components needed to mimic the matrix for spiking studies is not possible.

✦ Accuracy, Trueness, Bias, and Recovery: Are They the Same or Different?

In the world of analytical method validation, terms like accuracy, trueness, bias, and recovery are often used interchangeably. However, they each carry distinct meanings and implications, especially when it comes to method validation as per regulatory standards such as ICH Q2(R2), ANVISA RDC 166, AOAC guidelines, and EURACHEM.

What is Accuracy?

As per ICH Q2(R2), "The accuracy of an analytical procedure expresses the closeness of agreement between the value which is accepted either as a conventional true value or as an accepted reference value and the value or set of values measured."

In simple terms:

Accuracy = Closeness of test result to the true value

Different regulatory and scientific bodies define accuracy in slightly varying ways, but the core idea remains consistent.

EURACHEM provides a deeper perspective by breaking down accuracy into two key components:

- **Trueness** – how close the average value is to the true value.
- **Precision** – how reproducible the values are when repeated.

So, as per EURACHEM:

Accuracy = Trueness + Precision

Bias is defined as the difference between the reported average value and the true or accepted value. It is a quantitative measure that directly reflects trueness.
In short:

Bias = Reported Mean Value – True Value

If the bias is minimal, it indicates good trueness. High bias signifies systematic error in the method.

Recovery: Another way to express accuracy, especially in quantitative analysis, is through % Recovery. This is particularly relevant in impurity testing, residual solvent analysis, and trace element quantification.

% Recovery = (Measured Value / True Value) × 100

A recovery close to 100% indicates that the method is accurate. Most guidelines accept recovery in a range depending on the analyte and matrix.

Perspectives from Regulatory Guidelines:

Here's how different regulatory and scientific bodies present the concept of accuracy:

- ICH Q2(R2): Accuracy = closeness to the true value
- EURACHEM: Accuracy = trueness + precision
- ANVISA (RDC #166/2017): Accuracy can be expressed by % recovery

• AOAC: Accuracy = bias = trueness, when averaged over multiple results

These definitions reflect both qualitative and quantitative interpretations of the term.

Conclusion:

Let us summarize the key takeaways:

• Accuracy and trueness are qualitative descriptors, they describe the nature of closeness.
• Bias and recovery are quantitative expressions, they give measurable numbers.
• Trueness focuses on how close your average result is to the true value, while accuracy combines this with reproducibility.
• Bias and recovery help us express how accurate or true our results are in numeric terms.

In essence:

Accuracy & Trueness = Qualitative

Bias & Recovery = Quantitative

Understanding the subtle differences between these terms is vital for method validation and regulatory compliance.

7. Range:

As per ICH Q2(R2), "The range of an analytical procedure is the interval between the lowest and the highest results in which the analytical procedure has a suitable level of precision, accuracy and response"

To establish the method's range, it is important to demonstrate:

• Acceptable precision at both the lowest and highest levels
• Linearity across the entire range
• Accuracy at the selected levels within that range

In practical terms, this means validating the method's performance from the lowest spiked level to the highest, using consistent concentrations for all three parameters precision, linearity, and accuracy. This harmonized approach helps ensure reliability and reduces variability across validation studies.

Example: Range for Telmisartan Assay

The table below illustrates how different concentrations were selected and studied for Telmisartan during method validation. It shows where each validation parameter precision, linearity, and accuracy was evaluated to support the defined range.

Table 6: Range for Telmisartan Tablet assay

Conc. of Telmisartan	Precision	Linearity	Accuracy
40ppm	√	√	√
60ppm		√	
80ppm		√	√
100ppm		√	
120ppm	√	√	√

√: Indicates concentration studied

From this data, we can see that the method demonstrated suitable performance characteristics across 40 ppm to 120 ppm, making this the validated range for the assay of Telmisartan tablets.

Table 7: Examples of reportable ranges for common uses of analytical procedures (Reference: ICH Q2(R2)

Use of analytical procedure	Low end of reportable range	High end of reportable range
Assay of a product (1)	80% of declared content or 80% of lower specification acceptance criterion	120% of declared content or 120% of the upper specification acceptance criterion
Potency	Lowest specification acceptance criterion -20%	Highest specification acceptance criterion +20%
Content uniformity	70% of declared content	130% of declared content
Dissolution: Immediate release • one point specification	Q - 45% of the lowest strength	130% of declared content
• multiple point specification	Lower limit of reportable range (as justified by the specification) or QL, as appropriate.	
Modified release	Lower limit of reportable range (as justified by the specification) or QL, as appropriate.	
Impurity (1)	Reporting threshold	120% of specification acceptance criterion
Purity (as area %)	80% of lower specification acceptance criterion	Upper specification acceptance criterion or 100%

(1) Where assay and impurity are performed as a single test and only one standard is used, linearity should be demonstrated for both the reporting level of the impurities and up to 120% of the specification acceptance criterion for assay.

Understanding the Reportable Range for Each Analytical Procedure – with Example:

Let's take an example to understand how to define the low end of the reportable range for assay of a product using Paracetamol 500 mg tablets. Specification for assay is 90% to 110%. Concentration of paracetamol in test solution is 250ppm.

I. Assay of a Product:

a. Understanding the Low End of the Reportable Range – with Example:

According to guidelines, the low end of the reportable range can be either:

• 80% of declared content, or
• 80% of the lower specification acceptance criterion

Let's break this down with an example:
• Declared content = 500 mg
• Test solution concentration at 100% assay (with declared content of 500mg) = 250 ppm

Option 1: 80% of declared content

• 80% of 500 mg = 400 mg
• 400 mg is 80% of the declared content, so test solution = 80% of 250 ppm =200 ppm

Option 2: 80% of lower specification acceptance criterion

• Lower limit of spec = 90%
• 90% of 250 ppm = 225 ppm
• 80% of lower spec. (i.e., 225ppm) = 180 ppm

Now, we have two possible values:

• 200 ppm (from Option 1)
• 180 ppm (from Option 2)

Which one should we choose?

180 ppm is the better choice because it covers a wider range, including 200 ppm. But if you only validate at 200 ppm, you won't be covering 180 ppm.

In Percentage Terms:

• 80% of declared content = 80%
• 80% of lower spec (i.e., 80% of 90%) = 72%

So, whether you look at it in ppm or percentage, 72% (or 180 ppm) gives you the more conservative and appropriate low end of the reportable range.

b. Understanding the High End of the Reportable Range – with Example

According to the guideline, the high end of the reportable range can be defined by either:
• 120% of the declared content, or
• 120% of the upper specification acceptance criterion

We'll evaluate both options using this example:
• Declared content = 500 mg
• Test concentration at 100% assay (with declared content of 500mg) = 250 ppm
• Specification = 90.0% to 110.0%

Option 1: 120% of declared content

• 120% of 500 mg = 600 mg
• That's 120% of the declared label claim
• So, test concentration = 120% of 250 ppm = 300 ppm

Option 2: 120% of upper specification acceptance criterion

• Upper spec limit = 110%

• 110% of 250 ppm = 275 ppm
• 120% of 275 ppm = 330 ppm

So now we have two values:

• 300 ppm (from Option 1)
• 330 ppm (from Option 2)

Which one should we select?

330 ppm is the more conservative (higher) value. If you only validate up to 300 ppm, you are not covering up to 330 ppm—which may be required based on the broader interpretation of the specification range.
So, selecting 330 ppm ensures that the method is robust enough to quantify up to this upper level.

In Percentage Terms:

• 120% of declared content = 120%
• 120% of upper spec (i.e., 120% of 110%) = 132%

So again, whether in ppm or %, 132% (or 330 ppm) gives a broader and safer validation window.

Conclusion:

• High end of reportable range = 330 ppm or 132%
• It's preferred over 300 ppm (120%) because it covers a wider range, including potential overages

Summary:

Choose 180 ppm (or 72%) as the low end of reportable range for Paracetamol assay validation.
Choose 330 ppm (or 132%) as the high end of reportable range for Paracetamol assay validation.

II. Potency:

According to the guideline, the reportable range for potency is defined as:
• Low end: Lowest specification acceptance criterion – 20%
• High end: Highest specification acceptance criterion + 20%

Let's Take an Example:

Suppose you are evaluating the potency of an API with the following details:
• Specification range: 90.0% to 110.0%
• Declared potency/label claim: 500 mg
• Test solution at 100% potency = 250 ppm

a. Understanding Low End of Reportable Range

Low end = Lowest specification – 20%
= 90.0% – 20%
= 70.0%

Let's convert this to ppm:
• 70% of 250 ppm = 175 ppm
So, 175 ppm becomes the low end of the reportable range for potency.
This means during validation; the method should be able to accurately and

precisely measure the drug even if its potency is as low as 70%.

b. Understanding High End of Reportable Range

High end = Highest specification + 20%
= 110.0% + 20%
= 130.0%

Let's convert this to ppm:
• 130% of 250 ppm = 325 ppm
So, 325 ppm becomes the high end of the reportable range for potency.

Summary:

Choose 175 ppm (or 70%) as the low end of reportable range for potency validation.
Choose 325 ppm (or 130%) as the high end of reportable range for potency validation

III. Content uniformity:

According to the guideline, the reportable range for content uniformity is:
• Low end = 70% of declared content
• High end = 130% of declared content

Product Details:

• Declared paracetamol content = 500 mg per tablet
• Test concentration at 100% = 250 ppm

a. Understanding Low End of Reportable Range:

Low end = 70% of declared content
• 70% of 500 mg = 350 mg
• In ppm terms: 70% of 250 ppm = 175 ppm
So, 175 ppm is the low end of reportable range for content uniformity.

b. Understanding High End of Reportable Range:

High end = 130% of declared content
• 130% of 500 mg = 650 mg
• In ppm terms: 130% of 250 ppm = 325 ppm
So, 325 ppm is the high end of reportable range for content uniformity.

Summary:

Choose 175 ppm (or 70%) as the low end of reportable range for potency validation.
Choose 325 ppm (or 130%) as the high end of reportable range for potency validation

IV. Dissolution:

i. Dissolution: Immediate release product with one point specification

Using the Paracetamol Tablets example with three strengths: 250 mg, 500 mg, and 1000 mg

Assumptions:

- Q value = 75% (at 30 minutes)
- Strengths = 250 mg, 500 mg, 1000 mg
- Dissolution volume = 1000 mL
- Dose per vessel = 1 unit

This gives the following concentrations at 100% release:
- 250 mg → 250 ppm
- 500 mg → 500 ppm
- 1000 mg → 1000 ppm

a. Understanding Low End of Reportable Range

As per guideline:
Low end = Q – 45% of the lowest strength
1. Q = 75%
2. Q – 45% = 30%

Now apply 30% to the lowest strength (250 mg):
- 30% of 250 mg = 75 mg
- In 1000 mL, this equals 75 ppm

So, the low end of the reportable range is 75 ppm

b. Understanding High End of Reportable Range

As per guideline:
High end = 130% of declared content of the highest strength
- Highest strength = 1000 mg
- 130% of 1000 mg = 1300 mg
- In 1000 mL = 1300 ppm

So, the high end of the reportable range is 1300 ppm

Summary:

Choose 75 ppm (30% of 250 mg) as the low end of reportable range for dissolution validation.

Choose 1300 ppm (130% of 1000 mg) as the high end of reportable range for dissolution validation

ii. Dissolution: Immediate release product with multiple point specification

Product Specification:

- NLT 60% in 15 minutes
- NLT 75% in 30 minutes

Product Strengths:

- 250 mg → 250 ppm at 100% release
- 500 mg → 500 ppm at 100% release
- 1000 mg → 1000 ppm at 100% release

One tablet per 1000 mL dissolution medium for all strengths.

a. Understanding Low End of Reportable Range (Using USP <711> Stage S3 Criteria)

Acceptance Table-1

Stage	Number Tested	Acceptance Criteria
S_1	6	Each unit is not less than Q + 5%.
S_2	6	Average of 12 units ($S_1 + S_2$) is equal to or greater than Q, and no unit is less than Q-15%
S_3	12	Average of 24 units (S1 + S2 +S3) is equal to or greater than Q, not more than 2 units are less than Q-15%, and no unit is less than Q-25%.

Regulatory Reference:

As per Stage S3 of USP <711>, no individual unit should be less than Q – 25%. To ensure the method is suitable to detect the lowest acceptable individual unit, a conservative multiplier (commonly 80%) is applied to this threshold to define the minimum reportable level.

Let's use Q = 60% (from the 15-minute specification):

Step-by-Step Calculation:

- Q – 25% = 60% – 25% = 35%
- 80% of 35% = 28%
- Apply this to the lowest strength (250 mg):
  - o 28% of 250 mg = 70 mg
  - o 70 mg in 1000 mL = 70 ppm

Therefore, the lower end of the reportable range is 70 ppm.

As per ICH Q2(R2), the lower end of reportable range for IR product with multiple points is "Lower limit of reportable range (as justified by the specification) or QL, as appropriate". In the given example, if the method's QL is lower than 70 ppm (e.g., 60 ppm), it is perfectly acceptable and in fact desirable as it shows higher sensitivity. In such cases, QL becomes the lower end of the reportable range, not the 70 ppm. On the other hand, if the method's QL is higher than 70 ppm, the method would not be suitable, as it cannot reliably quantify the lowest expected concentrations based on regulatory criteria.

b. Understanding High End of Reportable Range

As per regulatory guidance, the upper limit is typically set as 130% of the declared content of the highest strength.

- 1000 mg × 130% = 1300 mg
- In 1000 mL = 1300 ppm

Summary

- Low End of Reportable Range: 70 ppm (based on 80% of Q – 25% of 60% for 250 mg strength) or QL whichever is lower.
- High End of Reportable Range: 1300 ppm (130% of 1000 mg strength)

• Method QL must be ≤ 70 ppm to ensure suitability and compliance

iii. Dissolution: Modified release product

Example of Paracetamol 250 mg, 500 mg, and 1000 mg tablets with a 3-point dissolution specification.

Product Strengths:

• 250 mg → 250 ppm at 100% release
• 500 mg → 500 ppm at 100% release
• 1000 mg → 1000 ppm at 100% release

Each tablet is dissolved in 1000 mL dissolution medium.

Specification: 3 Time Points

1. 2 hours: Between 30% to 50%
2. 8 hours: Between 50% to 70%
3. 12 hours: NLT 80%

a.Understanding Low End of Reportable Range (Using USP <711> Stage L3 Criteria)

Level	Number Tested	Acceptance Criteria
L_1	6	No individual value lies outside each of the stated ranges and no individual value is less than the stated amount at the final test time.
L_2	6	The average value of the 12 units (L1+L2) lies within each of the stated ranges and is not less than the stated amount at the final test time; none is more than 10% of labeled content outside each of the stated ranges; and none is more than 10% of labeled content below the stated amount at the final test time.
L_3	12	The average value of the 24 units (L1 + L2 + L3) lies within each of the stated ranges, and is not less than the stated amount at the final test time; not more than 2 of the 24 units are more than 10% of labeled content outside each of the stated ranges; not more than 2 of the 24 units are more than 10% of labeled content below the stated amount at the final test time; and none of the units is more than, 20% of labeled content outside each of the stated ranges or more than 20% of labeled con-tent below the stated amount at the final test time.

Regulatory Reference:

As per Stage L3 of USP <711>, none of the units is more than 20% of labeled content outside each of the stated ranges or more than 20% of labeled content below the stated amount at the final test time.

Let's use 2 hr.'s specification: 30% to 50%
Step-by-Step Calculation:
- 30% – 20% = 10%
- 80% of 10% = 8% (80% is the commonly used conservative factor)
- Apply this to the lowest strength (250 mg):
  - o 8% of 250 mg = 20 mg
  - o 20 mg in 1000 mL = 20 ppm

Therefore, the lower end of the reportable range is 20 ppm.

As per ICH Q2(R2), the lower end of reportable range for Modified release products is "Lower limit of reportable range (as justified by the specification) or QL, as appropriate". In the given example, if the method's QL is lower than 20 ppm (e.g., 15 ppm), it is perfectly acceptable and in fact desirable as it shows higher sensitivity. In such cases, QL becomes the lower end of the reportable range, not the 20 ppm. On the other hand, if the method's QL is higher than 20 ppm, the method would not be suitable, as it cannot reliably quantify the lowest expected concentrations based on regulatory criteria.

b. Understanding High End of Reportable Range

As per regulatory guidance, the upper limit is typically set as 130% of the declared content of the highest strength.
- 1000 mg × 130% = 1300 mg
- In 1000 mL = 1300 ppm

Summary

- Low End of Reportable Range: 20 ppm or QL whichever is lower.
- High End of Reportable Range: 1300 ppm (130% of 1000 mg strength)
- Method QL must be ≤ 20 ppm to ensure suitability and compliance

V. Impurity:

Case: Impurity (4-Aminophenol) in Paracetamol Tablets

Product Details:

- Analyte: Paracetamol
- Test sample concentration: 500 ppm
- Impurity: 4-Aminophenol
- Impurity specification: NMT 1.0%
- Reporting threshold (ICH Q3B): 0.05% (MDD > 1 g/day)

a. Understanding Low End of Reportable Range

Guideline: "Low end = Reporting threshold"
The reporting threshold is the minimum level at which an impurity must be reported. For Paracetamol (MDD > 1 g/day), ICH Q3B sets this at:
- 0.05% of the test concentration

Let's calculate 0.05% of 500 ppm:
- 500 ppm x 0.05%/100 = 0.25 ppm

So, the low end of reportable range is 0.25 ppm

b. Understanding High End of Reportable Range

Guideline: "High end = 120% of the specification acceptance criterion"
The specification limit for 4-aminophenol = 1.0%

Let's calculate 120% of this:

- 120% of 1.0% = 1.2%
- 500 ppm x 1.2%/100 = 6.0 ppm

So, the high end of reportable range is 6.0 ppm

Summary:

Choose 0.25 ppm (0.05% of 500 ppm) or QL (if less than 0.25 ppm) as the low end of reportable range for 4 aminophenol.
Choose 6.0 ppm (1.2% of 500 ppm) as the high end of reportable range for 4-Aminophenol.

VI. Purity (as % area):

Case: Purity (as Area %) in Paracetamol Tablets

Purity is evaluated using chromatographic techniques like HPLC and is expressed as area % of the main peak (API) compared to total peak area (API + impurities).

Assumptions:

- Specification for purity = NLT 98.0% (area %)
  (i.e., the main peak should be ≥ 98.0% of the total area)
- No degradation or additional peaks should exceed certain levels

a. Understanding Low End of Reportable Range

Guideline: "80% of the lower specification acceptance criterion"

Here, the lower specification limit is 98.0%
→ 80% of 98.0 = 78.4%

Now apply this to 500 ppm total sample concentration:
•78.4% of 500 ppm = 392 ppm

So, the low end of the reportable range is 392 ppm of paracetamol

b. Understanding High End of Reportable Range

Guideline: "Upper specification acceptance criterion or 100%"

In this case:

- Upper spec is not always defined explicitly for purity, so we take the default maximum = 100%

So, the high end of the reportable range is 100% or 500 ppm.

Summary:

Choose 392 ppm (78.4% of 500 ppm) as the low end of reportable range for purity (as % area) validation.
Choose 500 ppm (100% of 500 ppm) as the high end of reportable range for purity (as % area) validation

8. Robustness:

How do you assess the strengths and weaknesses of your analytical method? The answer lies in a critical validation parameter known as robustness.

As per ICH Q2(R2), "The robustness of an analytical procedure is a measure of its capacity to meet the expected performance criteria during normal use. Robustness is tested by deliberate variations of analytical procedure parameters."

Robustness refers to the ability of an analytical procedure to remain unaffected by small, deliberate variations in method parameters. It provides a measure of the method's reliability under routine usage conditions.

To design a meaningful robustness study, one must have a deep understanding of the analytical technique and the critical steps involved in the method. The purpose is not to test method failure, but to identify areas where the method might be sensitive and ensure those variations don't impact results significantly.

a. Example – Robustness in HPLC:

If you're using HPLC as your technique, ask yourself:

- What are the potential weak points in HPLC?
  - o Flow rate fluctuations
  - o Column oven temperature changes
  - o Mobile phase composition variation

Similarly, in the sample preparation stage, consider:

- Sonication time
- Solution stability
- Filtration step (e.g., different filter types or pore sizes)

b. Example – Robustness in GC:

If you're using GC as your technique, ask yourself:

- What are the potential weak points in GC?
  - o Flow rate fluctuations
  - o Column oven temperature changes
  - o Head space parameter changes (such as vial eq. time, eq. temperature, etc.)

Similarly, in the sample preparation stage, consider:

- Sonication time
- Solution stability
- Filtration step (e.g., different filter types or pore sizes)

c. Example – Spectrophotometry:

If you're using spectrophotometry (UV, FTIR) as your technique, ask yourself:

- What are the potential weak points in spectrophotometry?
  - o pH variation of the solution
  - o Different solvent batches or manufacturer

Based on scientific rationale, these parameters should be selected for robustness evaluation. The idea is to simulate small, real-world changes that may occur in day-to-day lab operations and ensure the method continues to produce reliable results.

✦ System Suitability

As described in ICH Q14, the system suitability test (SST) is an integral part of analytical procedures and is generally established during development as a regular check of performance.

System suitability tests are developed and used to verify that the measurement system and the analytical operations associated with the analytical procedure are fit for the intended purpose and increase the detectability of unacceptable perfor mance. (ICH Q14)

System Suitability Test (SST) is a critical part of any analytical method validation. It is performed to verify that the analytical system is working correctly before analyzing the actual samples. SST provides assurance about the performance of the analytical system (such as chromatographic system) and ensures reproducibility of results during routine testing.

Performing SST during validation is essential to:

- Demonstrate that the chromatographic system is suitable for the intended analysis
- Ensure consistent and reproducible performance of the instrument
- Detect any potential system malfunctions or variability before testing actual samples
- Confirm that the method can reliably separate and quantify the analyte under the specified conditions
- Support regulatory compliance, as per ICH Q2 and pharmacopeial expectations

Without satisfactory SST results, any subsequent analytical data may be deemed invalid, which can impact the credibility and outcome of the entire validation exercise.

Execute the SST before performing any validation parameter. Confirm that the system complies with the acceptance criteria specified in the standard test procedure (STP). Only after successful SST performance should you proceed with the analysis of validation samples.

CHAPTER: 02

UNDERSTANDING PERFORMANCE CHARACTERISTICS FOR TEST PROCEDURE

★ What Are Performance Characteristics?

In the context of analytical method validation, performance characteristics refer to specific parameters used to evaluate how well an analytical method performs. These parameters are essential for ensuring that the method is suitable for its intended purpose whether that's identifying, quantifying, or evaluating the quality of a pharmaceutical substance or product.

Here are the key parameters typically studied:

1.Specificity/Selectivity

2.Precision

3.Detection Limit (DL/LOD)

4.Quantitation Limit (QL/LOQ)

5.Response / Linearity

6.Accuracy

7.Range

8.Robustness

But here's the key: not all these characteristics apply to every analytical procedure. The choice depends on the type of method being validated.

Categorizing Analytical Procedures

Let's categorize different analytical methods, as per USP (General Chapter 1225: Validation of compendial procedures) and ICH guidelines. Each category requires a specific set of validation parameters.

1.**Assay of API or Key Components** (Category I as per USP General Chapter 1225): Quantifies active pharmaceutical ingredient (API) or major functional excipients like preservatives or antioxidants.

2.**Quantitative Test for Impurities** (Category II as per USP General Chapter 1225): Determines the amount of individual or total impurities (e.g., related substances test).

3.**Limit Test for Control of Impurities** (Category II as per USP General Chapter 1225): Verifies that impurities are below a certain threshold (e.g., TLC method to show impurity A is less than 100 ppm).

4.**Performance Testing** (Category III as per USP General Chapter 1225): Measures product performance e.g., dissolution, particle size, viscosity, or drug release.

5.**Identification Test** (Category IV as per USP General Chapter 1225): Used to confirm the identity of a compound (e.g., confirming the presence of Metformin in tablets).

Deciding Parameters as per Type of Analytical Method:

1. Performance Characteristics for Identification Test (Category IV)

Let us logically and scientifically identify the performance characteristics for validating identification test.

i. Specificity / Selectivity

Specificity is all about checking whether the method can clearly identify the target analyte, even when other substances like excipients, impurities, or diluent are present. Let's take the example of identifying Metformin using UV spectrophotometry. In this case, we compare the UV spectrum of the Metformin test sample with that of a Metformin standard. The acceptance criteria would typically state that both spectra should be concordant or match well.

In practice, excipients, impurities, or diluents might also absorb UV light and interfere with the spectral pattern. This can lead to inaccurate conclusions, and hence, identifying their interference is highly important. But is it possible to study the extent of interference from these potential interfering components? The answer is yes. It is very much feasible to record the UV spectra of these components and assess their interference. So, specificity can be performed for identification methods.

More importantly, is specificity required? Absolutely. Imagine a situation where the sample truly contains Metformin, but due to interference from excipients, the spectra do not match the standard. This may lead to a false negative result, where you wrongly conclude that the sample doesn't contain Metformin. To avoid such misleading outcomes, confirming specificity is essential. Hence, for identification tests, specificity is both possible and required.

ii. Precision

Precision is generally used to evaluate the consistency of repeated measurements, usually expressed in terms like SD or %RSD. But in an identity test, especially using UV, we aren't recording numerical values such as absorbance for calculation we are simply comparing the spectral patterns of the test and standard.

To define precision or degree of scatter, we need numerical values. Since there is no numerical measurable value involved, it's not possible to calculate the scatter or variability among readings. Therefore, while precision is a required validation parameter, it is technically not feasible for qualitative methods like identification tests.

However, many laboratories still perform repeat tests during identification not to establish variability, but just to check if all measurements are consistently meeting the acceptance criteria (e.g., matching spectra). This approach is useful because it gives analysts hands-on experience with the method and ensures procedural consistency.

iii. Accuracy

Accuracy is about how close your result is to the true value. Accuracy is expressed in terms of recovery with the help of 'amount found' and 'amount added'. Accuracy is the ratio of the amount found to the amount added.

A recovery experiment typically involves spiking a known amount of the analyte and checking how much is recovered or found. Even though, in an identity test, you may prepare a solution with a known concentration (by spiking a known amount of analyte in a sample matrix), you don't record the numerical response. If the response is not measured, then you can't calculate the amount found. And if you don't know the 'amount found', you can't calculate recovery.

So, while accuracy is a required parameter in general validation practices, in the case of identification tests, it is not practically possible because there's no quantitative measurement involved.

iv. Response / Linearity

Linearity is used to show that the response of the analyte is directly proportional to the concentration of the analyte. This is relevant for quantitative tests where responses such as peak area or absorbance are plotted against concentration.

In identification tests, even if you prepare samples at different concentrations, you are not measuring the numerical response. And in the absence of a response, you can't study linearity. Therefore, since no numerical data is generated, linearity is not applicable to identification methods.

v. Detection Limit (DL) and Quantification Limit (QL)

DL and QL are important parameters when you need to detect or measure a component that is expected to be present "as low as possible," such as impurities, residual solvents, residues after cleaning, etc. In the case of an identification test, you are expected to confirm the presence of the analyte at a desired concentration, and hence, logically, performing DL or QL does not make any sense.

vi. Range

Range is not applicable as precision, accuracy, and linearity is not possible.

vii. Robustness

Robustness checks whether the method continues to work reliably when small, deliberate changes are made to testing conditions such as changes in pH, solvent composition, sample preparation time, or instrument settings like wavelength.

If your identification method includes multiple preparation steps or depends on certain critical conditions, even minor changes can affect the result. In such cases, robustness testing is highly recommended. However, for simple identification methods, where conditions are straightforward and stable, robustness may not be necessary.

Still, it is considered good practice to evaluate robustness especially when the method is expected to be used across different labs, analysts, or equipment.

Summary Table: Performance Characteristics for Identification Test

Parameter	Is it Possible?	Is it Required?	Key Scientific Rationale
Specificity	Yes	Yes	Confirms the analyte is identified without interference from sample matrix (e.g. excipients, diluents, impurities)
Precision	No (Not Possible)	No	No numerical values are generated; only visual analysis (e.g. spectral matching), provides qualitative response and hence repeatability cannot be statistically assessed.
Accuracy	No (Not Possible)	No	No quantification is involved; amount found cannot be calculated.
Response / Linearity	No (Not Possible)	No	No measurable response; response vs. concentration cannot be plotted.
Detection Limit (DL)	No (Not Possible)	No	Test is to confirm presence, not detect trace levels; DL is not relevant.
Quantitation Limit (QL)	No (Not Possible)	No	Test is to confirm presence, not quantify trace levels; QL is not relevant.
Robustness	Yes	Optional (Recommended)	Confirms the analyte is identified without interference from sample matrix (e.g. excipients, diluents, impurities)

2. Performance Characteristics for Limit Test for Control of Impurities (Category II)

What is a Limit Test for Control of Impurities?

A limit test for control of impurities is used to check whether an impurity is present below a specified limit, it does not quantify the exact amount. A good example is Thin Layer Chromatography (TLC), where the impurity spot from sample solution is visually compared to an impurity reference standard solution (e.g. 100 ppm) spot. If the sample spot is lighter or smaller, it indicates that the impurity is present at a lower concentration than the standard (e.g., 100 ppm). This kind of test gives a qualitative or semi-quantitative result, not an exact numerical value.

Let us now discuss about the performance characteristics for Limit test for control of impurities. We will consider TLC technique for explaining.

i. Specificity / Selectivity

In the case of TLC, specificity ensures that the spot you're observing on the TLC plate truly represents the target impurity and not something else, such as an excipient, active substance, other impurities, or the mobile phase/diluent.

Is it possible to identify interference from these potential components in the sample matrix? The answer to this question is yes! To confirm this, you can apply a placebo (excipients without the drug substance), a blank (only diluent), other likely impurities present in the sample, and the active substance onto the TLC plate, and then compare their spots with that of the standard impurity.

If no spots from the excipients, diluent, other impurities, or the active substance appear at the same Rf value as the impurity, then there is no interference, and the method can be considered specific. This step is important to avoid reporting false positives due to other components appearing at the same position.

Hence, specificity is both possible and required in the case of a limit test for the control of impurities.

ii. Precision

Precision usually involves calculating the variability among repeated measurements for example, %RSD from several readings. However, in a limit test using TLC, you're not generating any numerical data to calculate variability. You simply observe the spot and decide whether it is darker or lighter than the standard. Since there is no measurable value like "ppm" or "peak area," you cannot assess repeatability in the traditional sense.

Therefore, while precision is a required validation parameter, it is technically not possible for qualitative or semi-quantitative methods like the limit test.
That said, many laboratories still perform repeat tests during a limit test not to establish statistical variability, but to check whether all observations consistently meet the acceptance criteria (e.g., intensity of the test spot is less than that of the standard spot). This approach is useful as it gives analysts hands-on experience with the method and helps ensure procedural consistency.

Note: In some cases, such as identification by NIR, FTIR, or HPLC, where a specific wavenumber or retention time is specified, precision can be evaluated by calculating the standard deviation (SD) or %RSD of the numerical values obtained from repeated measurements.

iii. Accuracy

Accuracy is about checking how close your found value is to the true amount, often using recovery studies by spiking known quantities. However, in a limit test, you're not trying to find out "how much" impurity is present, only whether it is less than a certain limit. So, there's no scope to calculate recovery or accuracy.
Therefore, while accuracy is a required validation parameter, it is technically not possible for qualitative or semi-quantitative methods like the limit test.

iv. Response (Linearity)

Linearity involves measuring the response at different concentrations and checking if it follows a straight line or predictable pattern. In TLC, the response is visual (how dark a spot looks), not numeric. Since you're not plotting any values against concentration, there's no way to assess linearity.

v. Detection Limit (DL)

Detection Limit (DL) refers to the lowest amount of impurity that can be detected, though not necessarily quantified.

Is it possible to identify the lowest concentration of an impurity that can be detected through a limit test such as TLC? The answer is yes! In TLC, this is quite relevant because you can visually determine the smallest concentration that still produces a visible spot.

To establish the DL, you can prepare standards at lower concentrations for example, 30 ppm, 40 ppm, 50 ppm, 60 ppm, and 70 ppm and observe at which level the spot just becomes visible. That concentration is considered the detection limit.

Since impurities are typically expected to be present at "as low as possible", defining the DL is both logical and meaningful in the context of impurity control. Hence, DL is both possible and required in the case of limit tests for the control of impurities.

vi. Quantitation Limit (QL)

The Quantitation Limit (QL) is used when to quantify a substance with acceptable accuracy and precision present to be "as low as possible". However, since TLC limit tests are semi quantitative and do not provide exact numerical measurements, it is not possible to calculate or apply QL in this context (as precision and accuracy won't be proved at the proposed QL value).

So, while QL is generally required for impurity measurement, in the case of a limit test, it cannot be practically determined or applied.

vii . Range

Range is not applicable as precision, accuracy, and linearity is not possible.

viii . Robustness

Robustness checks whether the method still performs well even when small, deliberate changes are made to conditions such as the solvent mix, plate drying e slightly.

To test robustness, you can vary one parameter at a time and see if the results still meet the acceptance criteria (for example, the sample spot remains lighter than the standard). While robustness is not mandatory, it's a good idea to evaluate it specially if the method is to be used by different analysts or in different labs. Therefore, robustness is optional but recommended for better method reliability.

Summary Table: Performance Characteristics for Limit Test for Control of Impurities

Parameter	Is it Possible?	Is it Required?	Key Scientific Rationale
Specificity	Yes	Yes	Confirms that the impurity is not interfered with by sample matrix (e.g. excipients, diluent, API, or other impurities (e.g. Rf-based check in case of TLC).
Precision	No (Not Possible)	No	No numerical values available; comparison is visual and semi quantitative, so %RSD or SD cannot be calculated.
Accuracy	No (Not Possible)	No	No measurable response: cannot determine amount found, so recovery cannot be calculated.
Linearity	No (Not Possible)	No	No measurable response; response vs. concentration cannot be plotted.
Detection Limit (DL)	Yes	Yes (Highly Recommended)	Impurities are expected "as low as possible"; DL confirms the minimum detectable level visually (e.g., spot visibility in case of TLC).
Quantitation Limit (QL)	No (Not Possible)	No	Cannot quantify; response is qualitative, so acceptable accuracy and precision cannot be demonstrated at low levels.
Robustness	Yes	Optional (Recommended)	Useful to confirm visual results are not affected by small changes

3. Performance Characteristics for Quantitative Test for Impurities (Category II):

What is a Quantitative Method?

Quantitative methods are designed to measure how much of a compound such as an impurity is present in a sample. These methods provide numerical results, which makes them suitable for evaluating the full range of method validation parameters.

A common example is the estimation of related substances in a drug product using HPLC.

i. Specificity / Selectivity

Is specificity possible and is it required for impurity quantification methods?
Yes, it is not only possible but absolutely necessary. Specificity ensures that the impurity response (such as a peak in the case of HPLC or absorbance in the case of UV) is not affected by any interference from other sample components such as the active substance, excipients, diluent, residual solvents, other impurities, or degradation products.

To establish specificity, you need to analyze the above-mentioned potential interfering components and forced degradation samples (wherever applicable, e.g., in

chromatographic techniques). You then verify that the peak of interest (e.g., Impurity A) is well resolved and does not overlap with any other peaks.
To conclude, specificity is both possible and required. It is a core validation requirement for impurity quantification methods.

ii. Precision

Is precision possible and is it required in impurity quantification methods?
Yes, precision is both possible and required. Since impurity quantification methods generate numerical data such as peak area or calculated concentration—it is fully possible to assess the consistency of the method. Precision helps determine how reproducible the results are when the test is repeated under the same conditions.

In conclusion, precision is not only feasible to measure but also an essential validation parameter especially for impurity testing, where even minor variations can significantly affect product quality, patient safety, and regulatory compliance.

iii. Accuracy

Is accuracy possible, and is it required for impurity quantification methods?
Yes, accuracy is both possible and required. In quantitative impurity methods, we aim to confirm that the method can correctly measure the true amount of impurity present in the sample.

Accuracy is evaluated through recovery studies, which involve spiking known amounts of impurity into the sample matrix at different levels of the impurity specification limit. Since these are quantitative methods, solutions with known concentrations can be easily prepared, so the amount added is clearly known. Likewise, the method provides a numerical result for the impurity level—referred to as the amount found.

With both values available, accuracy can be expressed in terms of %Recovery, using the formula:

%Recovery = (Amount Found / Amount Added) × 100

This calculation shows how close the test results are to the actual values, helping ensure the reliability of impurity measurement.

To conclude, accuracy is scientifically valid, practically possible, and regulatory required in impurity quantification. It confirms that the method can reliably recover and measure impurities across the expected range.

iv. Linearity (Response)

Is linearity possible, and is it required for quantitative impurity methods?
Yes, linearity is both possible and required. Linearity demonstrates whether the method's analytical response is directly proportional to the concentration of the impurity across a specified range. Linearity demonstrates that the detection technique provides a proportional response to the concentration of the analyte and is not a limiting factor in measuring its response.

To establish linearity, two key pieces of information are needed:
1.The concentration of the analyte (in this case, the impurity), and
2.The response from the instrument (such as peak area in HPLC or absorbance in UV).

In quantitative methods for impurities, both of these requirements are met. It is scientifically feasible to prepare impurity solutions with known concentrations, and the analytical method provides a measurable numerical response for each concentration. This makes it fully possible to evaluate the relationship between concentration and response.

To conclude, Linearity is clearly possible and mandatory for impurity quantification methods. It provides confidence that the method will deliver reliable and proportional results across the entire range of expected impurity levels.

v. Detection Limit (DL)

Is it possible, and is it required to determine the detection limit for quantitative tests for impurities?

Yes. The detection limit (DL) represents the lowest concentration of an impurity that can be detected, although not necessarily quantified. It is a key parameter that reflects the sensitivity of the analytical method.

DL becomes particularly important in impurity testing because impurities are usually expected to be present "as low as possible." Detecting them at such low levels is critical to ensure patient safety, meet regulatory expectations, and assess product quality especially during early development or when testing for trace-level impurities.

To conclude, DL is both possible and, in many cases, necessary. It helps confirm that the method is sufficiently sensitive to detect impurities at levels that may be well below the specification limit, depending on the purpose and stage of the analysis.

vi. Quantitation Limit (QL)

Is it possible, and is it required to determine the quantitation limit for quantitative tests for impurities?

Yes. The Quantitation Limit (QL) also referred to as LOQ (Limit of Quantification) is the lowest concentration of an impurity that can be quantified with acceptable accuracy and precision.

While the Detection Limit (DL) confirms that an impurity can be detected, QL takes it a step further by ensuring that the impurity can be measured reliably at low concentrations. This is especially important in impurity testing, as impurities are generally expected to be present "as low as possible." Therefore, being able to quantify them accurately and reproducibly at such levels is critical.

To conclude, QL is both possible and essential. It defines the method's ability to accurately and precisely quantify trace-level impurities, ensuring confidence in regulatory compliance and product safety.

vii. Range

Is it possible, and is it required to define a working range for impurity quantification methods?

Yes. The range refers to the span of concentrations over which the method has been demonstrated to be accurate, precise, and linear. It defines the boundaries within which the method consistently performs as intended.

In impurity testing, the range is typically established using the same concentration levels selected for linearity, accuracy, and precision studies. It should adequately cover the expected impurity levels—starting from the LOQ (the lowest quantifiable concentration) up to around 120% to 150% of the impurity specification limit.

Establishing an appropriate range ensures that the method is suitable not only for detecting and quantifying impurities at trace levels but also for handling slightly elevated concentrations that may arise during product development, manufacturing variations, or stability study.

To conclude, defining the range is both possible and required. It confirms that the method can perform reliably across the entire concentration window relevant to regulatory and product specifications.

viii. Robustness

Is it possible, and is it required to evaluate robustness for quantitative impurity methods?

Yes. Robustness is the ability of an analytical method to remain unaffected by small, deliberate variations in analytical parameters, and still deliver reliable results. It ensures that the method performs consistently under typical conditions encountered during routine analysis.

Robustness is particularly important for impurity quantification, where even minor deviations in parameters like mobile phase pH, organic solvent composition, column temperature, flow rate, or sample preparation conditions can impact impurity separation, detection, or quantitation.

Robustness testing is especially valuable when a method is to be transferred across different laboratories, used by multiple analysts, or run on different instruments, where slight variations are inevitable.

To conclude, robustness is both possible and strongly recommended. Using DoE enhances the reliability of the robustness study, ensuring the method remains dependable under routine operating conditions.

Summary Table: Performance Characteristics for Quantitative Impurity Methods

Parameter	Is it Possible?	Is it Required?	Key Scientific Rationale
Specificity	Yes	Yes	Ensures impurity response is free from interference (placebo, diluent, active, degradants, etc.).
Precision	Yes	Yes	Numerical data (e.g., peak area/concentration) allows %RSD/SD calculation to confirm method consistency.
Accuracy	Yes	Yes	Known impurity amounts can be spiked; recovery (%Recovery = Amount Found / Amount Added × 100) can be calculated.
Linearity	Yes	Yes	Both concentration and response are measurable; confirms proportionality and range suitability.
Detection Limit (DL)	Yes	Yes (as applicable)	Impurities expected "as low as possible"; DL confirms method sensitivity at trace levels ($S/N \geq 3$).
Quantitation Limit (QL)	Yes	Yes	Defines lowest concentration that can be quantified with acceptable accuracy and precision ($S/N \geq 10$).
Range	Yes	Yes	Confirms method validity across expected impurity levels, from LOQ to 120–150% of the limit.
Robustness	Yes	Strongly Recommended	Confirms method reliability under small changes; DoE approach preferred for identifying critical method variables.

4. Performance Characteristics for Assay Method (USP Category I)

An assay method under USP Category I is a quantitative analytical procedure used to determine the amount of active pharmaceutical ingredient (API) or other key components (such as preservatives) present in a drug product.

Examples include:

• HPLC assay of Paracetamol tablets

• Assay of Benzyl Alcohol (preservative) in a multi-dose injection

Let's evaluate the applicability of each validation parameter:

i. Specificity / Selectivity

Is specificity possible, and is it required for assay methods?

Yes, specificity is both scientifically possible and regulatorily required. In quantitative assay methods, it is feasible to measure the individual response of interfering components such as excipients, solvents, degradation products, or other actives and confirm they do not interfere with the quantification of the API or key component. This is done by analyzing blank, placebo, impurity, API/preservative standards, and spiked samples.

Specificity is required because regulatory bodies like USP, ICH demand assurance that only the analyte of interest is being measured. Without specificity, misidentification or inaccurate quantification can occur,

compromising product safety and efficacy.
To conclude, specificity is both possible and essential. It ensures the assay measures only the target compound, free from interference.

ii. Precision

Is precision possible, and is it required for assay methods?
Yes, precision is fully measurable in assay methods since they produce quantitative data such as peak areas or calculated concentrations. By preparing multiple individual sample solutions, degree of scatter can be expressed in terms of SD or %RSD.

Precision is required because pharmaceutical assays must demonstrate consistency under identical conditions. This ensures batch-to-batch reliability and compliance with quality control standards.
To conclude, precision is both possible and required. It confirms the method provides consistent results under the same conditions.

iii. Accuracy

Is accuracy possible, and is it required for assay methods?
Yes. Accuracy is scientifically possible because you can prepare known concentrations by spiking the API or preservative into placebo. Since the method provides a numerical result, both the amount added and amount found can be measured allowing %Recovery to be calculated.

Accuracy is required because it determines how close the test result is to the true value. Regulatory authorities expect assay methods to prove they measure the actual amount of the analyte accurately.

To conclude, accuracy is both possible and required. It verifies that the method reflects the true content of the API or key component.

iv. Response (Linearity)

Is linearity possible, and is it required for assay methods?
Yes. Linearity is possible because you can prepare standard solutions at known concentrations and measure the method's response (e.g., peak area or absorbance). Plotting concentration vs. response and calculating parameters like correlation coefficient (r^2) allows a clear assessment of linearity.

Linearity is required because it proves that the method can be used confidently across a range of concentrations. This is essential in manufacturing, where slight over- or under-filling can occur, and the method must still perform reliably.
To conclude, linearity is both possible and required. It ensures the method provides proportional and valid results across a defined concentration range.

v. Detection Limit (DL) and Quantitation Limit (QL)

Is DL and QL possible, and is it required for assay methods?
Yes, DL and QL is technically possible you can calculate it using the signal-to-noise ratio or other means. However, DL and QL is not required for assay methods because these are designed to measure content at specified levels, not trace amounts.

To conclude, DL and QL is possible but not required for routine assay validation.

vi. Range

Is range possible, and is it required for assay methods?
Yes. Range is scientifically possible because assay methods can be tested across different known concentrations. These levels are already used for accuracy, precision, and linearity validation.

Range is required because it demonstrates that the method performs reliably within the concentration span likely to be encountered during routine product analysis, formulation variability, or batch release.

To conclude, range is both possible and required. It confirms the method is valid across the expected working range of the analyte.

vii. Robustness

Is robustness possible, and is it required for assay methods?
Yes. Robustness is entirely possible because assay methods involve several operational parameters mobile phase pH, organic content, flow rate, column temperature, wavelength, and sample preparation steps (e.g., filtration, sonication). These can be varied individually or assessed using Design of Experiments (DoE) to identify critical method parameters.

Robustness is required (or at least strongly recommended) because it ensures the method remains stable and reliable under typical variations, which are common during routine use, method transfer, or analyst-to-analyst variability.

To conclude, robustness is both possible and highly recommended. It ensures the method continues to perform as expected under practical laboratory conditions.

Summary Table: Performance Characteristics for Assay Methods (USP Category I)

(For API and Key Components such as Preservatives)

Parameter	Is it Possible?	Is it Required?	Key Scientific Rationale
Specificity	Yes	Yes	The method allows measurement of individual responses; confirms no interference from excipients or degradants.
Precision	Yes	Yes	Quantitative data enables calculation of %RSD; confirms consistency across repeated measurements.
Accuracy	Yes	Yes	Known concentrations can be spiked and recovered; %Recovery confirms closeness to the true value.
Linearity	Yes	Yes	Known concentrations and responses can be plotted; r^2 value confirms proportionality.
Detection Limit (DL)	Yes	No	Can be calculated, but not relevant since assay targets specified levels, not trace detection.
Quantitation Limit (QL)	Yes	No	Technically possible, but unnecessary; low-level quantification is not the goal of assay methods.
Range	Yes	Yes	Can be defined using linearity, accuracy, and precision data; ensures performance across expected concentrations.
Robustness	Yes	Strongly Recommended	Possible through variation of method parameters; ensures reliability under routine conditions and minor changes.

5. Performance Testing (USP Category III)

Performance testing methods under USP Category III are designed to evaluate the overall behaviour or performance of the drug product rather than the content of a specific ingredient. These are often functional tests and simulate how the product is expected to perform in actual use.

Common examples include:

- Dissolution testing of tablets or capsules
- Disintegration testing
- Aerosol spray pattern or dose uniformity for inhalers
- Pump delivery for nasal sprays

The goal is to assess whether the product releases the active ingredient(s) in a way that supports therapeutic effectiveness.

Let's evaluate each validation parameter:

i. Specificity / Selectivity

Is specificity possible, and is it required for performance tests?

Yes, specificity is possible and generally required when a detection technique (e.g., UV, HPLC) is used to monitor drug performance test like release. The test must ensure that the measured response corresponds only to the API, and not to excipients, degradation products, or dissolution media components.

In performance testing like dissolution, if a detection method is involved, specificity must be established by analyzing blank, media, placebo, and API to confirm no interference occurs at the detection point.

To conclude, specificity is possible and required, especially when instrumental detection is used.

ii. Precision

Is precision possible, and is it required for performance tests?
Yes. Precision is both possible and required. Performance tests like dissolution often involve multiple dosage units (e.g., 6 or 12 units), and the results (e.g., % drug released) can be used to calculate %RSD.

Precision ensures that the method provides consistent results across units of the same batch, reflecting uniform product performance.

To conclude, precision is possible and required to ensure uniformity in drug release or product performance.

iii. Accuracy

Is accuracy possible, and is it required for performance tests?
Yes, but with context. In many cases, performance tests measure the amount of drug released (e.g., % dissolved), which can be compared against a known reference value or theoretical amount. Accuracy can be established by spiking the drug into the dissolution medium and measuring recovery.

It is required when the performance test is designed to quantify drug release, not just observe physical behavior.
To conclude, acuracy is possible and required when the performance test involves quantitative measurement (e.g., in dissolution or delivered dose uniformity).

iv. Linearity

Is linearity possible, and is it required for performance tests?
Yes. If the test involves instrumental detection (like UV or HPLC), linearity must be demonstrated between the concentration of analyte in the media and the detector response.

Linearity is required to ensure that the measurement system provides valid results over the expected range of drug release during the test.

v. Detection Limit (DL)

Is DL possible, and is it required for performance tests?
DL can be calculated, but it is generally not required, as performance tests typically involve measurable quantities of drug (not trace levels). However, if trace release or low-dose testing is involved (e.g., inhalation products), DL might become relevant.

To conclude, DL is possible but not routinely required, unless the performance test is for low-dose or trace delivery products.

vi. Quantitation Limit (QL)

Is QL possible, and is it required for performance tests?
QL is similar to DL it's possible to calculate using standard methods (e.g., 10 × SD/Slope), but it is not typically required for most performance tests. If the performance measurement involves very low analyte levels, QL may be justified. According to ICH Q2(R2)- QL may require for modified release dosage forms and for IR product with multiple point specification.

To conclude, QL is possible but usually not required, unless quantifying low levels of API is part of the test.

vii. Range

Is range possible, and is it required for performance tests?
Yes. The range of the method must encompass the expected release levels or delivered doses. For example, in dissolution testing, the range typically spans from Q-45 % of the lowest strength to 130% of declared content of the highest strength for IR product.

Range is required to demonstrate that the method can measure performance accurately throughout the expected release profile or delivery span.

To conclude, range is possible and required, to confirm the method is suitable across expected product performance.

viii. Robustness

Is robustness possible, and is it required for performance tests?
Yes. Robustness is important for performance tests, particularly those involving dissolution media, agitation speed, temperature, or delivery mechanisms. Minor changes in these parameters can impact test results.

Robustness can be evaluated by varying one factor at a time, or more efficiently, using Design of Experiments (DoE).

To conclude, robustness is possible and strongly recommended, to ensure the test is reliable under normal laboratory variations.

Summary Table: Performance Characteristics for Performance Testing (USP Category III)

(e.g., Dissolution, Disintegration, Inhalation Delivery Tests)

Parameter	Is it Possible?	Is it Required?	Key Scientific Rationale
Specificity	Yes	Yes	If detection is involved, interference from media, excipients, or placebo must be ruled out.
Precision	Yes	Yes	Quantitative results (e.g., % release) across units allow calculation of %RSD to confirm uniformity.
Accuracy	Yes	Yes	Spike recovery or theoretical comparison can verify if the test measures the true performance of the product.
Linearity	Yes	Yes	Instrumental response must be proportional to analyte concentration in the media; required for valid measurements.
Detection Limit (DL)	Yes	No (context-based)	Can be calculated but not needed unless testing very low-dose or trace-level delivery.
Quantitation Limit (QL)	Yes	No (context-based)	Possible but not required unless very low analyte levels are measured. (may be required for dissolution)
Range	Yes	Yes	Must cover expected product performance window
Robustness	Yes	Strongly Recommended	Ensures test reliability under variations.

NOTE: As per ICH Q2(R2), QL is required for dissolution testing for immediate release product with multiple point specification and modified release dosage form.

Observations:

- Only specificity / selectivity is universally applicable across all method types.
- LOD and LOQ are relevant only for impurity methods, limit tests, dissolution (with multiple point specification, and modified release) not for assays or identification.
- Assay and impurity methods require nearly all parameters due to their quantitative nature.
- Precision and accuracy go hand-in-hand and are only needed where results are numerical and measurable.
- Robustness, while not always mandated, adds great value, especially in routine use scenarios.

CHAPTER: 03

PREREQUISITES FOR ANALYTICAL METHOD VALIDATION

★ Introduction

Before diving into the actual validation of an analytical method, it's essential to ensure that all foundational elements are in place. These prerequisites not only lay the groundwork for a successful validation but also help avoid delays, repeat efforts, and non-compliance issues later on. A well-prepared validation exercise reflects scientific discipline and a commitment to data integrity.

In simple terms, having clear prerequisites ensures that the method being validated is appropriate, that all resources are ready, and that the team is aligned with regulatory expectations. Skipping or underestimating this stage often leads to avoidable challenges, impacting the credibility of the method and, more importantly, the quality of the product.

Below are the pre-requisites of analytical method validation:

1. Specification (Release and Shelf Life)

Specifications describe the set of quality parameters that define product acceptability like assay, impurities, dissolution, and appearance. These specifications must be finalized and approved before validation begins. Both release and shelf-life specifications are essential as they influence the design of experiments and selection of test parameters.

Having these helps build an accurate concentration matrix and ensures that the method is evaluated against its real-world application.

2. Well-Defined Method

A method cannot be validated unless it is finalized and clearly documented. This means the method must have completed its development phase and should include all necessary details like the procedure, system suitability, preparation of solutions, chromatographic conditions (if applicable), and calculations. Without a stable and repeatable method in place, validation becomes meaningless.

Moreover, the method document should be version-controlled and approved as per the internal quality system. Any ambiguity in the procedure can cause variability in results and misinterpretation during validation. Therefore, this is one of the most fundamental prerequisites that sets the tone for the entire validation process.

3. Understanding of the Product and Process

A solid understanding of the product being tested, including its physical and chemical properties, is crucial before starting method validation. This includes knowledge of potential degradation pathways, excipient interactions, and impurity profiles. Such insights help in anticipating challenges like interference, matrix effects, or peak merging during chromatographic analysis.

In addition, understanding the manufacturing process offers a holistic view of where and how the method will be applied. This enables better planning for method robustness and ensures the method is suitable for its intended purpose whether it's for release testing, stability studies, or in-process controls.

4. Proper Equipment and Instruments

Reliable analytical results depend not only on the method but also on the condition and readiness of the instruments used. For method validation to proceed smoothly, all required instruments and equipment must be available, qualified, and calibrated.

Key instruments such as HPLCs, balances, pH meters, and spectrophotometers must have current calibration status and should be qualified through Installation Qualification (IQ), Operational Qualification (OQ), and Performance Qualification (PQ). These qualifications confirm that the equipment performs as expected within defined operating limits.

In addition to qualification, it's important to verify that the instruments are in good working condition, have undergone routine maintenance, and are suitable for the method's analytical requirements. Checking the operating range and readiness of each instrument in advance helps prevent unexpected delays or errors during validation execution.

5. Well Qualified Reference/Working Standards

Reference and working standards play a vital role in analytical method validation, as they are used for calibration, system suitability testing, spiking, and identification. The reliability of validation data heavily depends on the quality and consistency of these standards.

There are two primary types:

- Reference Standards: These are highly pure, certified substances, typically sourced from official pharmacopeias (e.g., USP, EP) or prepared in-house if a compendial source is unavailable. They act as the benchmark for evaluating accuracy and should be well-characterized in terms of identity, purity, potency, and stability.
- Working Standards: These are secondary standards qualified against reference standards. The potency of working standards should be established using a validated method, preferably calculated on an "as is" basis using the formula:

Potency = (% Assay on dried basis) × (100 – F) / 100,

where F represents the percentage of water and residual solvents.

It is important to note that, for ease of storage and improved stability, suppliers may sometimes provide reference standards in a different salt form (e.g., hydrochloride, sulfate). In such cases, make sure to apply the correct conversion factor when calculating potency and weighing the material. Using the wrong form without proper adjustment can lead to significant analytical errors.

To ensure integrity, standards must be stored under controlled conditions typically in amber containers, protected from light, heat, and moisture. Dried standards should not be returned to the original container. Also, verify their availability in sufficient quantity and ensure that expiry or retest dates align with the expected validation timeline. Proper qualification and documentation including certificates of analysis (CoA) and defined storage conditions are essential for generating reliable, reproducible results and maintaining confidence in the method's performance.

6. Suitable Samples

Ensuring the availability of appropriate samples is a critical prerequisite for method validation. The samples used must closely represent actual production batches to accurately assess the method's performance under real-world conditions. These typically include finished product samples, placebos, blank matrices, and, where applicable, spiked or degraded samples.

The samples selected for validation must be homogeneous, within specification, and available in sufficient quantity to support the full range of validation experiments. Consistency in sample type and composition is key, as variability can lead to misleading conclusions and compromise the reliability of results.

In cases where actual product samples are not readily available, it is acceptable to prepare simulated samples using the active pharmaceutical ingredient (API) and excipients in the same proportion as the intended formulation. Additionally, stress or stability samples should be prepared according to protocol to effectively evaluate parameters such as specificity.

7. Placebo (for Finished Products)

A placebo is a formulation that contains all the excipients of a drug product but excludes the active pharmaceutical ingredient (API). It plays a crucial role in analytical method validation, particularly in specificity and interference studies, where it helps to identify any response from the excipients.

Placebos can be prepared in two ways:

1. Handmade Placebo – This involves weighing and manually blending all excipients in the same proportion as in the finished product, typically done in a laboratory setting.
2. Processed Placebo – This is prepared by following the actual manufacturing process, including steps like granulation, blending, compression, or coating (as applicable).

While both approaches are acceptable, it is strongly advisable to use processed placebo whenever possible. This is because processed placebo more accurately reflects the physical and chemical characteristics of the final drug product. In contrast, a handmade placebo may not replicate the same particle size distribution, flow properties, or homogeneity, potentially leading to differences in analytical response.

Regardless of the approach used, placebo preparation must be performed in a clean, controlled environment to prevent cross-contamination and to ensure the placebo accurately simulates the matrix of the actual product.

8. Reagents and Chemicals

The accuracy and consistency of method validation largely depend on the quality and availability of reagents and chemicals. Every solvent, reagent, and standard used must be of suitable analytical grade such as HPLC grade or AR grade based on the specific method requirements.

Before validation begins, it's essential to prepare a complete list of required chemicals and confirm their availability in the laboratory. This proactive step helps avoid unnecessary delays due to missing or unsuitable reagents. Each item should be verified for quality, with documented lot numbers, expiry dates, and certificates of analysis (where applicable).

Far from being a routine formality, ensuring the suitability and traceability of reagents reflects a genuine commitment to generating accurate and reliable analytical data.

9. Environmental Conditions

Environmental factors like temperature, humidity, and cleanliness can significantly affect the performance of certain analytical methodsespecially those involving chromatography, weighing, or moisture-sensitive materials. Hence, maintaining a controlled lab environment is essential.

Before initiating validation, the lab should be monitored and maintained as per SOPs, and the working conditions should be logged. This ensures that the data generated reflects true method performance and is not skewed by uncontrolled external variables.

10. Concentration Matrix

A concentration matrix is a detailed plan listing the concentrations of standard and sample solutions for each validation parameter—accuracy, linearity, robustness, etc. This matrix ensures accuracy in preparation and consistency during execution.

It also helps in protocol development, minimizing chances of error in solution preparation or test planning.

11. Pre-Approved Protocol

A method validation exercise must be guided by a well-defined, pre-approved protocol. This document should outline the scope of the validation, the parameters to be evaluated, acceptance criteria, responsibilities, and a clear plan of execution. Approval by the Quality Assurance (QA) department ensures that all regulatory and quality expectations are met before execution begins.

Having a protocol in place avoids ambiguity and provides a structured roadmap for the validation process. It helps align all stakeholders and ensures consistency in data generation, review, and reporting.

12. Validated Calculation Sheets

Manual calculations are prone to human error. Hence, it's advisable to use pre-validated Excel sheets or customized software tools (like Empower, Chromeleon,

LabSolutions) for calculations. These should be validated beforehand and reviewed for formula accuracy.

Automating calculations ensures speed, reduces errors, and builds confidence in results during audits or regulatory review.

13. Validation Report

The final step is preparing a comprehensive validation report, which captures all observations, results, calculations, and conclusions. It must follow the protocol closely, comparing each result against its acceptance criteria and documenting any deviations with justification.

The report must reflect the scientific integrity of the process and serve as a reliable record for audits, inspections, and submissions.

14. Validation Execution Plan (Team & Timeline)

Having all resources in place is important, but successful method validation ultimately depends on how well the execution is planned and carried out. A clear execution plan defining team responsibilities, timelines, and sequencing of activities is essential to ensure the process is smooth, controlled, and error-free.

Each team member should be briefed thoroughly, and roles must be clearly assigned to avoid confusion or duplication of efforts. Establishing checkpoints for review and oversight helps identify any deviations early and allows timely corrective action. Avoiding overconfidence or rushing is crucial; a calm and methodical approach with proper documentation ensures accuracy and regulatory compliance.

Equally important is the competence of the personnel involved. All analysts participating in validation must be adequately trained in both the analytical method and applicable good laboratory practices (GLP). Their training records should be up to date, and their qualifications should include hands-on experience as per internal procedures. When skilled professionals lead the execution, the outcome is not only efficient but also inspires confidence in the validity and reliability of the data generated.

15. Compliance with Regulatory Guidelines

Finally, all preparations must be aligned with current regulatory expectations, such as those outlined by ICH Q2(R2), USP, FDA, EMA, and local authorities. Keeping up with these guidelines ensures that the validation will stand up to regulatory scrutiny and support submissions and audits confidently.
This also includes ensuring alignment with internal quality systems and any client-specific requirements, particularly in contract research or manufacturing setups. Regulatory alignment at the preparation stage saves time and prevents major compliance risks later.

Conclusion

Preparing for method validation is just as important as the validation itself. These prerequisites ensure that the method is mature, the tools are ready, and the people are trained. They help set the stage for a smooth, effective, and compliant validation process that not only generates trustworthy data but also reflects the scientific integrity of the organization.

By following these steps carefully, teams can avoid costly errors, ensure regulatory compliance, and contribute to the broader mission of delivering safe and effective pharmaceutical products to patients.

CHAPTER: 04

CONCENTRATION MATRIX FOR ASSAY BY HPLC METHOD

★ Objective

Before you start preparing a protocol, I suggest preparing a concentration matrix or concentration mapping for the validation parameters to be performed. This will help you to identify the concentration of test and standard solution across various performance characteristics in advance. I call this as "concentration matrix" preparation. This will help to avoid errors and make your protocol ready to execute. You can use simple excel sheet to prepare concentration matrix.

This chapter is designed as a workbook, where you will fill in the blanks, calculate concentrations, and build your own validation concentration matrix.

To help you understand and calculate concentrations of standard and sample solutions, I am going to take a practical case study where we are going to prepare a concentration matrix for assay of Paracetamol in paracetamol 500 mg tablets by HPLC. I hope you are ready and excited!

For preparing concentration matrix, you need the key information below.

1. Product composition
2. Standard Test Procedure (STP)
3. Specification

1. Product Composition:

The excipients used in paracetamol tablets are maize starch, potassium sorbate, purified talc, hydroxypropyl methylcellulose.

Table 1: Composition of a drug product

Name	Quantity
Paracetamol	500 mg
Maize starch	100 mg
Potassium sorbate	20 mg
Hydroxypropyl methylcellulose	50 mg
Purified talc	30 mg
Total Weight	700 mg

2. Standard Test Procedure (STP) for Assay of Paracetamol in Paracetamol Tablets 500 mg by HPLC:

Chemicals / Reagents:
Triethylamine: HPLC Grade
Orthophosphoric acid: AR Grade
Acetonitrile: HPLC Grade
Water: Milli-Q / HPLC Grade

Preparation of Buffer: Dissolve 2.0 mL of Triethylamine in 1000 mL of water and adjust the pH to 2.5 (± 0.05) with diluted orthophosphoric acid. Filter through 0.45 um Nylon filter paper.

Mobile phase preparation: Mix buffer and acetonitrile in 68: 32 v/v ratio, sonicate and degas for 10 min.

Diluent: Mix Acetonitrile and Water in 50: 50 v/v ratio.

Preparation of Standard stock solution: Weigh accurately 25.0 mg of Paracetamol working standard and transfer into 100 mL of volumetric flask, add 70 mL of diluent and sonicate it for 10 minutes and dilute it up to the mark with diluents.

Preparation of Standard solution: Dilute 10 mL of standard stock solution to 50 mL with diluent and mix well.

Preparation of test solution: Weigh accurately 20 tablets of Paracetamol. Determine average weight and crush tablets to fine powder. Weigh accurately a tablet powder equivalent to 250mg of Paracetamol and transfer it to 1000 mL volumetric flask. Add 500 ml of diluent, sonicate it for 10 minutes and make up to volume with Diluent. Mix well and centrifuge a portion of solution at 5000 rpm for 10 minutes. Dilute 10 mL of centrifuged portion of above sample solution to 50 mL with diluents and mix well.

Chromatographic conditions:
Column : 250X4.6mmX4µm, Phenomenex Synergi 4µm Polar RP-80A0 or equivalent
Column temperature: 35°C
Flow rate: 1.5 mL/min
Detection: 225 nm
Injection volume: 50µL
Run time: 15 min

Procedure: Inject 50 µL portion of the diluents for blank (one injection), standard preparation (five injections), test preparation (one injection) into the chromatographic system, record the chromatograms and measure the responses for major peak.

System suitability:

(a) Tailing factor from standard chromatogram should be within 0.8 to 1.5.

(b) The relative standard deviation for five replicate injections of standard preparation should not be more than 2.0 %

(c) Theoretical plates should be not less than 2000.

Calculations:

$$\text{Quantity of Paracetamol Present in the portion of the Tablets as \% of labeled amount} = \frac{A}{B} \times \frac{Ws}{100} \times \frac{10}{50} \times \frac{1000}{Tw} \times \frac{50}{10} \times \frac{Aw}{L} \times \frac{P}{100} \times 100$$

Where,

A = Peak area of Paracetamol for test preparation

B = Average peak area of Paracetamol for standard preparation

Ws = Weight of Paracetamol standard taken, in mg

Tw = Weight of Test taken, in mg

P = % Potency of Paracetamol standard on as is basis.

L = Labeled amount of Paracetamol, in mg, per tablet.

Aw = Average weight in mg.

3. Specification:

Let us assume that the specification for assay and related substances for paracetamol tablet is below.

- Paracetamol assay: Between 95.0 % to 105.0 % against Labelled Claim
- Impurity A: NMT 1.0 %
- Impurity B: NMT 0.5 %

Note: Purposefully I have not considered other tests from the specification as they are not relevant.

We will convert the impurity specification from percentage (%) to ppm, since all the solutions being prepared for various method validation parameters such as linearity, accuracy, and precision will have their concentrations expressed in ppm. This ensures consistency in units and helps in accurate calculation, comparison, and interpretation of results during validation.

$$\text{Impurity conc. in ppm present in test as per the limit} = \frac{(\text{Impurity limit in \%}) \times (\text{Test conc. in ppm})}{100}$$

Let us calculate impurity A and impurity B conc. in ppm present in test as per the limit

$$\text{Impurity A conc. in ppm present in test as per the limit} = \frac{1.0\,\% \times 50\text{ ppm}}{100} = 0.50\text{ ppm}$$

Where:

-Impurity A specification = 1.0 % (Refer point number 3: specification)

-Test conc. in ppm = 50 ppm (Refer sample preparation under STP (point No. 2))

Now, you can calculate the Impurity B conc. in ppm present in test as per the limit

Impurity B conc. in ppm present in test as per the limit = ------------------------------ = ppm

Let us now tabulate the impurity A and impurity B specification both in % and in ppm

Table 2: Specification of known impurities in percentage (%) and ppm

Impurity Name	Specification in %	Specification in ppm
Impurity A	1.0%	--------------------
Impurity B	0.5%	--------------------

PREPARATION OF CONCENTRATION MATRIX:

For assay test procedure specificity, precision, linearity, and accuracy needs a concentration matrix.

The following points are covered as part of the concentration matrix for assay:

1. General information about product
2. Standard and Test concentration
2.1. Standard concentration
2.2. Test concentration
3. Concentration mapping for validation parameters
3.1. Specificity/Selectivity
3.2. System suitability
3.3. Precision
3.4. Response/Linearity
3.5. Accuracy

1. General information about the product:

At the beginning of concentration matrix, provide general information such as the product name, label claim, placebo weight, etc. Also, include the release and shelf-life specifications for the test for which the concentration matrix is being prepared.

Fig. 1: Excel sheet screenshot for product details.

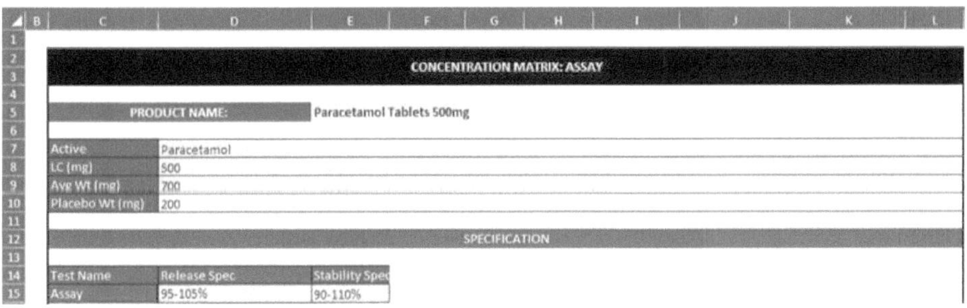

2. Standard and Test Concentration:

It is also a good idea to map the concentration of standard and test solution preparation. This will help to prepare linearity, accuracy and specificity related solutions.

2.1 Standard Concentration

- Weigh 25 mg of paracetamol and dilute to 100 mL → Standard stock solution
- Take 10 mL of this standard stock and dilute to 50 mL → Standard solution

$$\text{Resulting conc (ppm)} = \frac{\text{Standard Weight (mg)}}{\text{Dilution Volume (mL)}} \times \frac{\text{Pipetted Volume (mL)}}{\text{Dilution Volume (mL)}} \times 1000$$

Please refer to the following details for test preparation as per the Excel sheet:

- Standard weight: 25 mg *(Refer cell D20, Fig. 2)*
- Standard stock dilution: 100 mL *(Refer cell D21, Fig. 2)*
- Pipetted standard volume (mL): 10 mL *(Refer cell E20, Fig. 2)*
- Further standard dilution volume (mL): 50 mL *(Refer cell E21, Fig. 2)*

Table 3: Standard solution preparation steps

Weight/Volume	Description	Resulting Concentration (ppm)
25 mg / 100 mL	Standard stock solution	
10 mL / 50 mL	Standard solution	

Note: The potency of the API standard is generally close to 100%, and for simplification, it has been excluded from the initial concentration matrix calculations. However, please remember that while calculating actual results after performing validation experiments, the standard potency must be considered wherever applicable.

2.2 Test Concentration:

- Weigh and crush 20 paracetamol tablets and weigh powder equivalent to 250 mg of paracetamol and dilute to 1000 mL→ Test stock solution
- Take 10 mL of test stock solution and dilute to 50 mL → Test solution

The weight of paracetamol in test sample can be calculated using the formula below

$$\textit{Weight of drug product eq. to target API wt. (mg)} = \frac{\textit{Average Tablet wt. (mg)} \times \textit{Target API wt. (mg)}}{\textit{LC (mg)}}$$

Let us calculate the weight of drug product (paracetamol tablet) equivalent to 250 mg of paracetamol using above formula

$$\textit{Weight of drug product eq. to 250mg paracetamol (mg)} = \frac{700\ mg \times 250\ mg}{500\ mg} = 350\ mg$$

Where:

- Average wt. of paracetamol tablet = 700 mg *(Refer cell D9, Fig. 1)*
- Target paracetamol weight in mg = 250 mg *(Refer test preparation)*
- LC of paracetamol = 500 mg *(Refer cell D8, Fig. 1)*

Please refer to the following details for test preparation as per the Excel sheet:

- Sample/Test weight: 250 mg of paracetamol *(Refer cell D24, Fig. 2)*
- Sample/Test stock dilution volume: 1000 mL *(Refer cell D25, Fig. 2)*

- Volume pipetted from test stock: 10 mL *(Refer cell E24, Fig. 2)*
- Final dilution volume for test solution: 50 mL *(Refer cell E25, Fig. 2)*

Table 4: Test solution preparation steps

Step	API weight / Volume	Description	Resulting Concentration (ppm)
1	250 mg / 1000 mL	Test stock solution	--------------------
2	10 mL / 50 mL	Test solution	--------------------

Please check excel sheet screenshot.

Fig. 2: Excel sheet screenshot for standard and sample concentration.

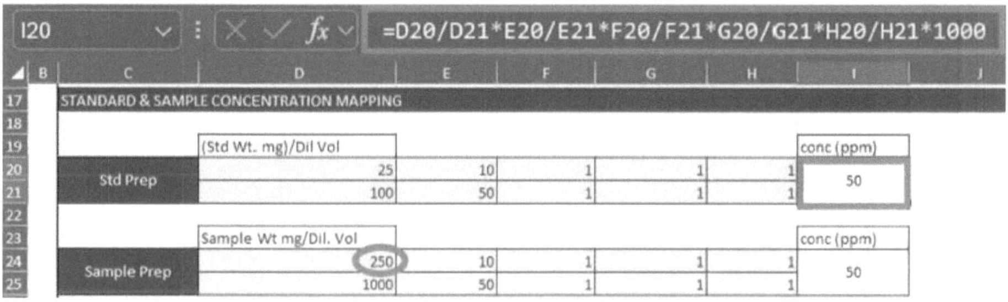

Please note, here 250mg is not the sample weight, but it is the weight of paracetamol present in test.

3. CONCENTRATION MAPPING FOR VALIDATION PARAMETERS

3.1. Specificity/Selectivity:

Specificity/Selectivity is all about checking whether the method can clearly identify the target analyte, even when other substances like excipients, impurities, or diluent are present. We are going to prepare standard solution, test solution, placebo solution, blank, individual impurity identification solution, and impurity spiked test solution for specificity of assay by HPLC. Forced degradation solutions preparation are not considered here, we will discuss it in a separate chapter.

a. Standard solution

b. Test solution

c. Blank / Dilucnt

d. Placebo solution

e. Individual known impurity solutions

f. Impurity spiked test solution

Table 5: Specificity/Selectivity solutions preparation

Solution Name	Discussion	Weight in mg	Dilution 1	Dilution 2	Conc. (ppm)
Standard Solution	Follow the test procedure	------------------	100mL	10mL → 50mL	---------------
Test Solution	Follow the test procedure. Weight equivalent to paracetamol shall be considered	------------------	1000mL	10mL → 50mL	---------------
Blank/ diluent	Follow the test preparation procedure by omitting sample				
Placebo solution	Follow the test preparation procedure by replacing sample by placebo. To determine the placebo content in the test solution, it is important to note that 500 mg of paracetamol contains 200 mg of placebo. Therefore, for a test solution using 250 mg of paracetamol, the placebo content will be (200/500)×250=100 mg of placebo.	------------------	1000mL	10mL → 50mL	---------------
Impurity A Identification Solution	Prepare impurity A identification solution at its specification level, which is 1.0% or 0.50 ppm	5mg	50mL (Imp A stock Sol)	1mL → 100mL Further dilute 2.5mL → 5mL	0.50 ppm
Impurity B Identification Solution	Prepare impurity B identification solution at its specification level, which is ______% or ______ ppm	------------------	------------- (Imp B stock Sol)	___mL → ___mL Further dilute ___mL → ___mL	________ppm
Impurity spiked test solution	Test solution shall be spiked with or added with impurity A and impurity B at their respective specification.	Weight of a sample eq. 250 mg of paracetamol + ________ mL of impurity A] stock + ________ mL of impurity B stock	1000mL	10mL → 50mL	Paracetamol is ________ ppm Impurity A is ________ ppm Impurity B is ________ ppm

Follow the test preparation procedures outlined in the STP while preparing for the spiked test, and placebo solutions. However, you can adjust the weight and dilution of the impurity to achieve the desired concentration. Another important point is the dilution process. Ensure that impurity is soluble in the diluent used (especially while making impurity stock solution). If Impurity is not soluble in the test diluent, you may use another diluent in which the impurity is soluble when preparing the stock solution. However, the final solution, which will be analyzed, should preferably be prepared in the diluent used for the test solution.

Note: The test solution and impurity-spiked test solution can alternatively be prepared using the API and placebo, in case the test sample is unsuitable or unavailable. In above case, use 100 mg of placebo and 250 mg of Paracetamol API to prepare the test solution. Similarly, for the impurity-spiked test solution, use 100 mg of placebo, 250 mg of Paracetamol API, and the respective impurity stock solutions.

a. Standard Solution: Follow the STP

b. Test solution: Follow the STP

c. Diluent: Follow the test solution preparation by omitting test sample.

d. Placebo solution preparation: Follow the test solution preparation by replacing test sample by placebo.

e. Individual impurity solution preparation: For preparation of individual impurity solutions, below two steps are involved.

i. Preparation of the Impurity Identification Stock Solution, and
ii. Preparation of the Impurity Identification Solution

Let us prepare these solutions

i.Preparation for Impurity identification Stock Solution:

The screenshot below (Fig. 3) guides the preparation of individual impurity stock solutions. These stock solutions are primarily used for impurity identification and impurity spiked sample preparation during specificity testing.

Now, let's understand how to prepare the impurity identification solution. In the current example, the impurity stock solution has been prepared at a concentration of 100 ppm for both Impurity A and Impurity B

$$\text{Stock sol. conc (ppm)} = \frac{\text{Weight (mg)}}{\text{Dilution Volume (mL)}} \times 1000$$

Let us calculate the concentration of Impurity A identification stock solution

$$\text{Impurity A identification stock sol. conc (ppm)} = \frac{5\ mg}{50\ mL} \times 1000 = 100\ ppm$$

Weight of impurity A: 5 mg *(Refer cell D42, Fig. 3)*
Impurity A dilution: 50 mL *(Refer cell D43, Fig. 3)*

Similarly calculate the concentration of impurity B identification stock solution

$$\text{Impurity B identification stock sol. conc (ppm)} = \frac{\quad}{\quad} \times 1000 = \ldots\ldots\ldots\ldots\ ppm$$

ii.Preparation for Individual Impurity Identification Solution:

After preparing the impurity stock solution (as described above), the next step is to calculate the required volume of stock to achieve the desired impurity concentration through dilution.

In this example, we've selected a dilution volume of 100 mL for both Impurity A and Impurity B. You are free to choose the dilution volume as per requirement. The target concentrations are:

- **Impurity A:** 0.50 ppm *(release specification conc., Table 2)*
- **Impurity B:** 0.25 ppm *(release specification conc., Table 2)*

Impurity identification solution concentration can be calculated by using below formula

$$\text{Conc. of Impurity in ppm} = \text{Impurity stock conc (ppm)} \times \frac{\text{Impurity stock vol (mL)}}{\text{Dilution vol (mL)}} \times \frac{\text{Pipetted Vol (mL)}}{\text{Dilution vol (mL)}}$$

Let us calculate the impurity A identification solution concentration by using above formula

$$\text{Conc. of Impurity A identification solution in ppm} = 100\ ppm \times \frac{1\ mL}{100\ mL} \times \frac{2.5\ mL}{5\ mL} = 0.50\ ppm$$

Where:

- Impurity A stock conc. (ppm)= 100 ppm *(Refer cell I42, Fig. 3)*
- Volume of Impurity A stock taken (mL) = 1 mL *(Refer cell D53, Fig. 3)*
- Impurity A stock volume dilution (mL)= 100 mL *(Refer cell D54, Fig. 3)*
- Pipetted volume (mL) = 2.5 mL *(Refer cell E53, Fig. 3)*
- Further solution dilution (mL) = 5 mL *(Refer cell E54, Fig. 3)*

Expected conc. (ppm) of impurity can be calculated as per below formula

$$\text{Expected conc. (ppm) of impurity at its release spec} = \frac{\text{Sample conc (ppm)} \times \text{Impurity release spec (\%)}}{100}$$

The cell K53 from Fig. 3 calculates the expected concentration of impurity A (0.50 ppm) as below

$$\text{Expected conc. (ppm) of impurity A at its release spec} = \frac{50\ ppm \times 1.0\ \%}{100} = 0.50\ ppm$$

Where:

- Sample concentration (ppm) = 50 ppm *(Refer cell I24, Fig. 2)*
- Impurity A limit in % = 1.0 % *(Refer cell J53, Fig. 3)*

Conclusion: The calculated concentration of Impurity A (cell I53, Fig. 3) matches the expected concentration (cell K53, Fig. 3).

Similarly calculate the expected concentration of impurity B

$$\text{Expected conc. (ppm) of impurity B at its release spec} = \frac{\_\_\_\_\ ppm \times \_\_\_\_}{100} = \_\_\_\_\ ppm$$

f. Impurity spiked test solution for specificity:

In specificity (or selectivity) testing, known impurities must be spiked into the test solution to demonstrate that they do not interfere with the analyte of interest (such as API). In this example, the impurities will be spiked at their release specification concentrations.

You can calculate the concentration of impurity in spiked sample with below formula

$$\text{Conc. of Impurity in ppm} = \text{Impurity stock conc (ppm)} \times \frac{\text{Impurity stock vol (mL)}}{\text{Dilution vol (mL)}} \times \frac{\text{Pipetted Vol (mL)}}{\text{Dilution vol (mL)}}$$

Let us calculate the impurity A concentration in spiked sample by using above formula

$$\text{Conc. of Impurity A (in ppm) in spiked solution} = 100\ ppm \times \frac{25\ mL}{1000\ mL} \times \frac{10\ mL}{50\ mL} = 0.50\ ppm$$

Where:

- Impurity A stock conc. (ppm)= 100ppm *(Refer cell I42, Fig 3)*
- Volume of Impurity A stock taken (mL) = 25 mL *(Refer cell E64, Fig. 3)*
- Impurity A stock volume dilution (mL)= 1000 mL *(Refer cell D65, Fig. 3)*
- Pipetted volume (mL) = 10 mL *(Refer cell G64, Fig. 3)*
- Further solution dilution (mL) = 50 mL *(Refer cell G65, Fig.3)*

Similarly calculate the concentration of impurity B in spiked solution

$$\textit{Conc. of Impurity B (in ppm) in spiked solution} = .\text{----------}\ ppm \times \frac{\_\_\_\_\_\_\ mL}{\_\_\_\_\_\_\ mL} \times \frac{\_\_\_\_\_\_\ mL}{\_\_\_\_\_\_\ mL} = \_\_\_\_\_\_\ ppm$$

Fig. 3: Excel sheet screenshot for specificity.

	B	C	D	E	F	G	H	I	J	K
30		1. SPECIFICITY								
31										
32			Placebo Wt (mg)/Dil. Vol							
33		Placebo	100	10	1	1	1			
34		Preparation	1000	50	1	1	1			
35										
36										
37		**Preparation of Impurity Identification Solution:**								
38										
39		**Impurity stock solution**								
40										
41			Impurity Wt. (mg)					conc (ppm)		
42		Imp-A stock	5	1	1	1	1	100		
43		Preparation	50	1	1	1	1			
44										
45		Imp-B stock	5	1	1	1	1	100		
46		Preparation	50	1	1	1	1			
47										
48										
49		**Preparation of Impurity Identification Solution:**								
50										
51										
52			Imp Stock Vol (ml)					Resulted conc (ppm)	Imp Spec (%)	Imp Spec (ppm)
53		Imp A sol	1	2.5	1	1	1	0.5	1%	0.5
54		Preparation	100	5	1	1	1			
55										
56		Imp B sol	1	12.5	1	1	1	0.25	0.5%	0.25
57		Preparation	100	50	1	1	1			
58										
59										
60		**Preparation of Impurity spiked test Solution:**								
61										
62										
63			Sample Wt. (mg)	Imp A stock	Imp B stock				Imp A conc (ppm)	Imp B conc (ppm)
64		Impurity Spiked	350	25	12.5	10	1	1	0.5	0.25
65		Test Sol.	1000			50	1	1		

3.2. System Suitability

Prepare the standard solution or system suitability solutions as per STP

Please check excel sheet screenshot for system suitability solution preparation

67	2. SYSTEM SUITABILITY
68	
69	Just Prepare stdandard solution as above

3.3. Precision:

The precision of an analytical procedure expresses the closeness of agreement (degree of scatter) between a series of measurements obtained from multiple samplings of the same homogeneous sample under the prescribed conditions. Precision can be considered at three levels: repeatability, intermediate precision and reproducibility. For all three levels you can use the same concentration matrix as concentration of standard, test, or method of preparation remains one and the same.

Repeatability should be assessed using a minimum of 9 determinations covering the reportable range for the procedure (e.g., 3 concentrations/3 replicates each) or a minimum of 6 determinations at 100% of the test concentration. Below table provides the concentration matrix for preparation of test at 100% of the test concentration.
We are going to prepare the concentration matrix for the solutions below

3.3.1 Preparation of repeatability solutions using finished product
3.3.2 Preparation of repeatability solutions using (API + Placebo)

Table 6: Repeatability solution preparation

Solution Name	Discussion	Weight in mg	Dilution 1	Dilution 2	Conc. of API (ppm)
Test Solution	Follow the test procedure	------------------	1000mL	10mL → 50mL	----------------
Test solution using placebo + API	Placebo Weight + Paracetamol Weight	Placebo Wt. .... API Wt.	1000mL	10mL → 50mL	----------------

Follow the accuracy section to understand the concentration matrix for precision with 9 determinations covering the reportable range for the procedure (e.g., 3 concentrations/3 replicates each)

3.3.1 Preparation of repeatability solutions using finished product:

The repeatability using finished product can be studied by analyzing test solutions as per STP.

3.3.2 Preparation of repeatability solutions using (API + Placebo):

If the test sample is unavailable or unsuitable, you can use a combination of placebo and API based on the product's composition. The first step involves accurately weighing the required quantities of placebo and API to prepare the sample. From there, the procedure follows the same steps as described earlier for "Repeatability Using Finished Product."

Note: The amount of API present in sample is 250 mg. The test sample contains 100 mg of placebo. (Refer to 'Placebo Solution' preparation in Table 5 under Specificity to verify the placebo content in the test sample.)"

Fig. 5: Excel sheet screenshot for precision covering preparation of repeatability solution at 100%

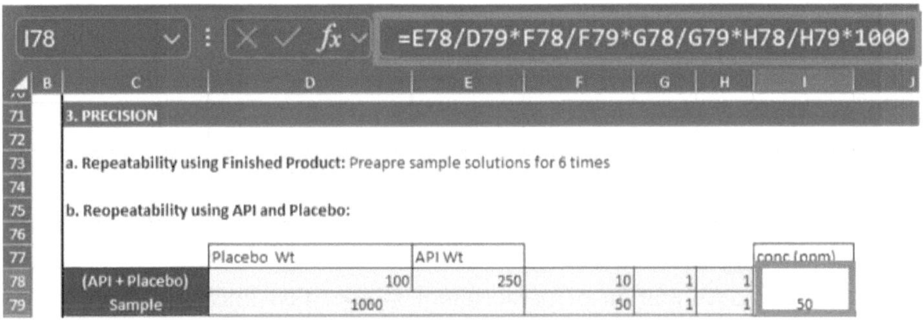

3.4 Response/Linearity:

The response of an analytical procedure is its ability (within a given range) to obtain a signal which is effectively related to the concentration (amount) or activity of analyte in the sample by some known mathematical function. (ICH Q2)

To systematically design the linearity concentration matrix, follow these key steps:

Step 1: Deciding linearity levels

Step 2: Preparation of linearity stock solutions

Step 3: Calculation of expected concentration across various linearity levels

Step 4: Required volume of linearity stock solution for the preparation of linearity solutions

Step 5: Verification of resulted linearity solution at various linearity levels

Step 1: Deciding linearity levels

From the above stock solution, we will be preparing 5 linearity levels as below (50%, 75%, 100%, 125%, and 150%)

Step 2: Preparation of linearity stock solutions

Prepare a stock solution from which further linearity solutions at different levels can be prepared. This approach helps in avoid multiple weighing errors.
The concentration of linearity stock solution can be calculated using below formula

$$\text{Linearity tock conc. (ppm)} = \frac{\text{Weight of compound (mg)}}{\text{Dilution volume (mL)}} \times 1000$$

Where:

-Weight pf Paracetamol for linearity stock preparation = 50 *mg (Refer cell D85, Fig. 6)*

-Dilution volume (mL)= 100 mL *(Refer cell D86, Fig. 6)*

Table 7: Linearity stock preparation

Solution Name	Discussion	Weight in mg	Dilution 1	Conc. (ppm)
Linearity stock	Paracetamol	50mg	100mL	---------------

Fig. 6: Excel sheet screenshot for linearity stock solution preparation

I85 | fx =D85/D86*E85/E86*F85/F86*G85/G86*H85/H86*1000

	C	D	E	F	G	H	I
82	4. RESPONSE/LINEARITY						
84		Wt. in mg/Dil vol					conc (ppm)
85	Lin Stock	50	1	1	1	1	500
86		100	1	1	1	1	

Step 3: Calculation of expected concentration across various linearity levels

The expected concentration of paracetamol at specified linearity level can be calculated as below

Expected conc. in ppm = [Linearity level (%) x Test conc (ppm)]/100

The expected concentration in ppm at 50% = (50% x 50 ppm)/100 = 25 ppm

Where:

- Linearity level = 50% *(Refer cell C89, Fig. 7)*
- Test conc. (ppm) = 50 ppm *(Refer cell I24, Fig. 2)*

Fig. 7: Excel sheet screenshot for expected concentration of a paracetamol at various linearity levels

D89 | fx =C89*$I$24

	C	D	E	F	G	H	I
82	4. RESPONSE/LINEARITY						
84		Wt. in mg/Dil vol					conc (ppm)
85	Lin Stock	50	1	1	1	1	500
86		100	1	1	1	1	
88	Lin level	Exp conc (ppm)	Lin Stock Vol (ml)	Dil to (ml)	Resulted conc (ppm)		
89	50%	25.00	5	100	25.00		
90	75%	37.50	7.5	100	37.50		
91	100%	50.00	10	100	50.00		
92	125%	62.50	12.5	100	62.50		
93	150%	75.00	15	100	75.00		

Step 4: Required volume of linearity stock solution for the preparation of linearity solutions

The required volume of linearity stock solution for the preparation of linearity solutions is calculated as below

$$\text{Required Vol. of Linearity stock solution (in mL)} = \frac{A \times B}{C}$$

Where:

- A = Expected concentration of API at a specified linearity level (in ppm)
- B = Dilution of 'linearity stock' to prepare a specified linearity level solution (in mL)

- C = Conc. of linearity stock solution (in ppm)

Let us calculate the required volume of linearity stock for 50% linearity level by using the above formula

Required volume of Linearity stock solution for 50% level= (25 ppm x 100 mL)/500 ppm = 5 mL

Where:

- Expected concentration in ppm = 25 ppm *(Refer cell D89, Fig. 8)*
- Diluted volume = 100 mL *(Refer cell F89, Fig. 8)*
- Concentration of linearity stock solution = 500 ppm *(Refer cel I85, Fig. 7)*

Fig. 8: Excel sheet screenshot for required volume of the linearity stock to achieve expected concentration of a paracetamol at various linearity levels

E89 =D89*F89/$I$85

4. RESPONSE/LINEARITY

	Wt. in mg/Dil vol					conc (ppm)
Lin Stock	50	1	1	1	1	500
	100	1	1	1	1	

Lin level	Exp conc (ppm)	Lin Stock Vol (ml)	Dil to (ml)	Resulted conc (ppm)
50%	25.00	5	100	25.00
75%	37.50	7.5	100	37.50
100%	50.00	10	100	50.00
125%	62.50	12.5	100	62.50
150%	75.00	15	100	75.00

Step 5: Verification of resulted linearity solution at various linearity levels

The resulting concentration of API at specified linearity level can be calculated as below

$$\text{Resulted conc. in ppm} = \frac{\text{Conc. of linearity stock (ppm) x Linearity stock volume (mL)}}{\text{Dilution Volume (mL)}}$$

Let us calculate the resulted conc. in ppm for paracetamol at 50% linearity level by using the above formula

The resulted conc. of paracetamol in ppm at 50% level = 500 ppm x 5 mL/100 mL = 25 ppm

Where:

- Conc. of linearity stock (in ppm) = 500 ppm (Refer cell I85, Fig. 9)
- Linearity stock volume (mL) = 5 mL (Refer cell E89, Fig. 9)
- Dilution Volume (mL) = 100 mL (Refer cell F89, Fig. 9)

Conclusion: The resulting solution, prepared using the above details, achieves the expected concentration of paracetamol at the 50% linearity level *(see cell D89, Fig. 7)*.

Fig. 9: Excel sheet screenshot for resulted concentration of paracetamol at various linearity levels

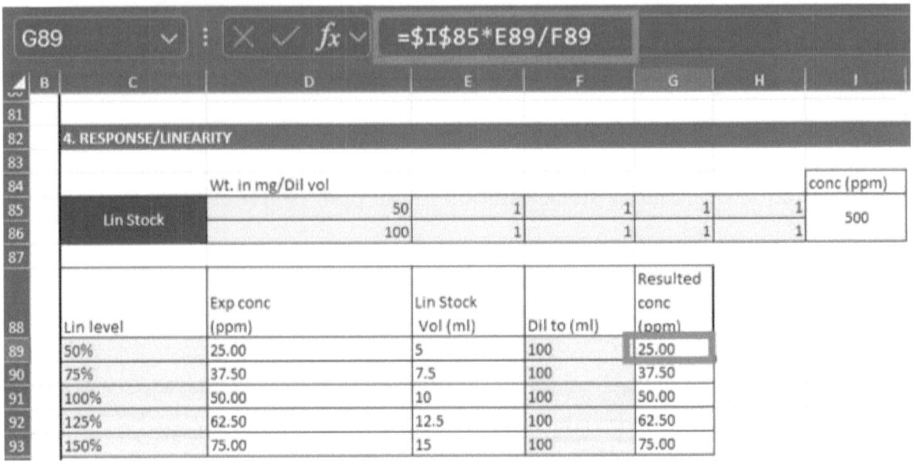

G89 f_x =$I$85*E89/F89

4. RESPONSE/LINEARITY

	Wt. in mg/Dil vol					conc (ppm)
Lin Stock	50	1	1	1	1	500
	100	1	1	1	1	

Lin level	Exp conc (ppm)	Lin Stock Vol (ml)	Dil to (ml)	Resulted conc (ppm)
50%	25.00	5	100	25.00
75%	37.50	7.5	100	37.50
100%	50.00	10	100	50.00
125%	62.50	12.5	100	62.50
150%	75.00	15	100	75.00

Based on the above information, calculate the expected concentrations, the required volume of linearity stock, and the resulting concentrations for the remaining linearity levels. Enter the values in the table below.

Table 8: Linearity solution preparation

Linearity Level	Expected conc. of paracetamol in ppm	Lin Stock Vol (ml)	Dil to (ml)	Resulted conc (ppm)
50%	25 ppm	5 mL	100mL	25 ppm
75%	------------------	------------------	------------------	------------------
100%	------------------	------------------	------------------	------------------
125%	------------------	------------------	------------------	------------------
150%	------------------	------------------	------------------	------------------

3.5. Accuracy:

The accuracy of an analytical procedure expresses the closeness of agreement between the value which is accepted either as a conventional true value or an accepted reference value and the value found. This is sometimes termed trueness. We are going to prepare concentration matrix for below accuracy solutions

3.5.1 Accuracy using drug product/test sample

3.5.2 Accuracy using (API + Placebo)

3.5.1 Accuracy using drug product/test sample

To systematically design the accuracy concentration matrix using drug product, follow these key steps:

Step 1: Deciding accuracy levels

Step 2: Calculation of expected concentration across various accuracy levels

Step 3: Calculating the required weight of API at various accuracy levels

Step 4: Preparation of accuracy solutions

Step 5: Verification of concentration of resulted solution at various accuracy levels

Step 1: Deciding accuracy levels

We can prepare 5 accuracy levels such as 50%, 75%, 100%, 125%, and 150%

Step 2: Calculation of expected concentration across various accuracy levels

The expected concentration of paracetamol at specified accuracy level can be calculated as below

Expected conc. in ppm = [Accuracy level (%) x Test conc (ppm)]/100

The expected concentration in ppm at 50% accuracy level = (50 % x 50 ppm)/100 = 25 ppm

Where:

- Accuracy level in percentage (%) = 50% (Refer cell C99, Fig. 10)
- Test conc. in ppm = 50 ppm (Refer cell I24, Fig. 2)

Fig. 10: Excel sheet screenshot for the expected concentration of paracetamol at various accuracy levels

D99 =C99*$I$20

5. ACCURACY

Acc. level	Exp conc (ppm)	Placebo Wt.(mg)	API Wt. (mg)	Dil to ml)	Pipetted (ml)	Dil to (ml)	Pipetted (ml)	Dil to (ml)	Resulted conc (ppm)
50%	25	100	125	1000	10	50	1	1	25
75%	37.5	100	187.5	1000	10	50	1	1	37.5
100%	50	100	250	1000	10	50	1	1	50
125%	62.5	100	312.5	1000	10	50	1	1	62.5
150%	75	100	375	1000	10	50	1	1	75

Step 3: Calculating the required weight of API at various accuracy levels

The required weight of API for various accuracy levels is calculated by using the formula below

Required weight of API in mg = [Accuracy level (%) x Weight of API in test preparation]/100

Required weight of API in mg at 50% accuracy level = [50% x 250 mg]/100 = 125 mg

Note: Although the target concentrations for paracetamol at various accuracy levels are 25 ppm, 37.5 ppm, 50 ppm, 62.5 ppm, and 75 ppm, it is essential to understand a critical concept- the concentration of the accuracy stock solution plays a pivotal role in simulating realistic and challenging recovery scenarios at each level.

Let me explain this more precisely.

To evaluate the accuracy of a method effectively, each spiking level should replicate the actual recovery challenge that would be encountered in routine analysis. This requires a clear understanding of the test preparation concentration as defined in the Standard Test Procedure (STP).

According to the STP, the test stock solution is prepared by dissolving 250 mg of paracetamol in 1000 mL, resulting in a test concentration of 250 ppm in test stock.

To create a 50% accuracy level solution, we must simulate a scenario where the analyte is present at 50% of the test stock level. This means spiking 125 mg of paracetamol (i.e., 50% of 250 mg) along with the corresponding placebo amount (100 mg in this case) and diluting the mixture to 1000 mL. This results in a stock solution of 125 ppm, which mimics a 50% challenge level in terms of recovery.

From this 125 ppm accuracy stock solution, you would then follow the standard dilution procedure taking 10 mL of stock and diluting to 50 mL, resulting in a final solution of 25 ppm, which is your 50% accuracy test level.

This approach ensures that each accuracy level is constructed based on a proportional challenge against the actual test concentration. It is important to reflect this logic while calculating and preparing accuracy solutions.

Please refer to the table below to identify the appropriate accuracy stock concentrations required for each level. Do note that while this approach may not be reflected in the default accuracy Excel sheet, it is scientifically recommended and has been applied in Figure 11, which illustrates the correct preparation strategy.

Table 9: Concentration of accuracy stock solutions

Accuracy level	Paracetamol Weight (mg)	Placebo Weight (mg)	Diluted to (mL)	Concentration of Paracetamol in ppm
50%	125 mg	100 mg	1000mL	125 ppm
75%	187.5 mg	100 mg	1000mL	187.5 ppm
100%	250 mg	100 mg	1000mL	250 ppm
125%	312.5 mg	100 mg	1000mL	312.5 ppm
150%	375 mg	100 mg	1000mL	375 ppm

Step 4: Preparation of accuracy solutions

The accuracy solutions at various accuracy levels can be prepared by using the API (as calculated in step 3), and the amount of placebo present in test sample. The amount of placebo must be kept the same across all accuracy levels. The 100 mg of the placebo is present in test sample (Refer "Placebo solution" preparation as per Table 5 (specificity) to know the placebo present in test sample). Follow the sample preparation procedure as per STP by using calculated amount of API required at specified accuracy level and 100 mg of placebo.

In below Fig. 11 (cell F99, F100, F101, F102, and F103) you will find the required API weight for various accuracy levels.

Fig. 11: Excel sheet screenshot for the paracetamol weight at various accuracy levels

F99 — fx =$D$24*C99

5. ACCURACY

Acc. level	Exp conc (ppm)	Placebo Wt.(mg)	API Wt. (mg)	Dil to ml)	Pipetted (ml)	Dil to (ml)	Pipetted (ml)	Dil to (ml)	Resulted conc (ppm)
50%	25	100	125	1000	10	50	1	1	25
75%	37.5	100	187.5	1000	10	50	1	1	37.5
100%	50	100	250	1000	10	50	1	1	50
125%	62.5	100	312.5	1000	10	50	1	1	62.5
150%	75	100	375	1000	10	50	1	1	75

Step 5: Verification of concentration of resulted solution at various accuracy levels

The resulted concentration of paracetamol at specified accuracy level can be calculated as below (refer cell L99, Fig. 12)

$$\textit{Resulted conc. in ppm} = \frac{\textit{Weight of API in mg}}{\textit{Dilution Volume (mL)}} \times \frac{\textit{Pipetted vol (mL)}}{\textit{Dilution vol (mL)}} \times 1000$$

$$\textit{The Resulted concentration in ppm at 50\%} = \frac{125\ mg}{1000\ mL} \times \frac{10\ mL}{50\ mL} \times 1000 = 25\ ppm$$

Where:

- Weight of API at 50% Accuracy level = 125 mg *(Refer cell F99, Fig. 12)*
- Dilution volume = 1000 mL *(Refer cell G99, Fig. 12)*
- Pipetted volume = 10 mL *(Refer cell H99, Fig. 12)*
- Further dilution volume = 50 mL *(Refer cell I99, Fig. 12)*

Conclusion: The resulted concentration of paracetamol at 50% accuracy level (refer cell L99, Fig. 12) meets the expected concentration at the same level (refer cell D99, Fig. 10)

Fig. 12: Excel sheet screenshot for the resulted concentration of paracetamol at various accuracy levels

L99 — fx =F99/G99*H99/I99*J99/K99*1000

5. ACCURACY

Acc. level	Exp conc (ppm)	Placebo Wt.(mg)	API Wt. (mg)	Dil to ml)	Pipetted (ml)	Dil to (ml)	Pipetted (ml)	Dil to (ml)	Resulted conc (ppm)
50%	25	100	125	1000	10	50	1	1	25
75%	37.5	100	187.5	1000	10	50	1	1	37.5
100%	50	100	250	1000	10	50	1	1	50
125%	62.5	100	312.5	1000	10	50	1	1	62.5
150%	75	100	375	1000	10	50	1	1	75

Using the information provided above, complete the table below by entering the appropriate values. This will help ensure that the calculations and preparations are aligned with the required concentrations and procedures.

Table 10: Accuracy solution preparation

Accuracy level	Exp conc (ppm)	Placebo Wt.(mg)	API Wt. (mg)	Dil to (mL)	Pipetted (ml)	Dil to (ml)	Resulted conc. (ppm)
50%	25 ppm	100 mg	125mg	1000 mL	10 mL	50 mL	25 ppm
75%	.... ppm	100 mg	.... mg	.... mL	.... mL	.... mL	.... ppm
100%	.... ppm	100 mg	.... mg	.... mL	.... mL	.... mL	.... ppm
125%	.... ppm	100 mg	.... mg	.... mL	.... mL	.... mL	.... ppm
150%	.... ppm	100 mg	.... mg	.... mL	.... mL	.... mL	.... ppm

CHAPTER: 05

CONCENTRATION MATRIX FOR RELATED SUBSTANCES BY HPLC

★ Objective

This chapter is designed as a workbook, where you will fill in the blanks, calculate concentrations, and build your own validation concentration matrix.

Let us prepare a concentration matrix for related substances of Paracetamol in paracetamol 500 mg tablets by HPLC.

For preparing concentration matrix, you need the key information below.

1. Product composition
2. Standard Test Procedure (STP)
3. Specification

1. Product Composition:

The excipients used in paracetamol tablets are maize starch, potassium sorbate, purified talc, hydroxypropyl methylcellulose.

Table 1: Composition of a drug product

Name	Conc. Of Telmisartan
Paracetamol	500 mg
Maize starch	100 mg
Potassium sorbate	20 mg
hydroxypropyl methylcellulose	50 mg
Purified talc	30 mg
Total Weight	700 mg

2. Standard Test Procedure (STP) for Related substances of Paracetamol Tablets 500 mg by HPLC:

Chemical / Reagents:

Potassium dihydrogen phosphate	:	HPLC Grade
Methanol	:	HPLC Grade (J.T.Baker) or equivalent
Water	:	Milli-Q / HPLC Grade
Orthophosphoric acid	:	HPLC Grade

Buffer pH 2.0: Weigh and transfer 1.36 gm of potassium dihydrogen phosphate in 1000 mL of water, adjust pH to 2.0 with diluted orthophosphoric acid and Filter through 0.45µm Nylon membrane filters.

Mobile phase preparation: Mix buffer pH 2.0 and methanol in ratio 60:40 v/v respectively, sonicate to degas.

Diluent: Mobile phase

Preparation of standard stock solution: Weigh accurately 50 mg of Paracetamol working standard and transfer into 100 mL volumetric flask, add 70 mL of diluent and sonicate it to dissolve and dilute it up to the mark with diluent.

Preparation of standard solution: Pipette out 5 ml of standard stock solution into 50 mL volumetric flask and dilute to volume with diluent. Pipette out 2 mL of resultant solution in 100 mL of volumetric flask and dilute it up to the mark with diluent.

Preparation of test solution: Weigh accurately 20 tablets of Paracetamol. Determine average weight and crush tablets to fine powder. Weigh accurately and transfer tablets powder equivalent to 500mg of Paracetamol into 100 mL volumetric flask. Add 70 mL of diluent, sonicate it for 10 minutes, cool to room temperature and make up to volume with diluent. Mix well and centrifuge a portion of solution at 5000 rpm for 10 minutes, then pipette out and transfer 5ml centrifugate into a 50ml volumetric flask, make up to volume with diluent.

Preparation of Placebo solution: Weigh accurately and transfer placebo equivalent to 500mg of Paracetamol into 100 mL volumetric flask. Add 70 mL of diluent, sonicate it for 10 minutes, cool to room temperature and make up to volume with diluent. Mix well and centrifuge a portion of solution at 5000 rpm for 10 minutes, then pipette out and transfer 5ml centrifugate into a 50ml volumetric flask, make up to volume with diluent.

Chromatographic conditions:

Column	:	Inertsil ODS-3V, 250 x 4.6mm, 5µm or equivalents
Column temperature	:	35°C
Flow rate	:	1.0 mL/min
Detection	:	225 nm
Injection volume	:	20 µL
Run time	:	90 min

Procedure: Inject 20 µL portion of the blank (one injection), Placebo solution(One injection), standard preparation (six injections) and test preparation (one injection) into the chromatographic system, record the chromatograms and measure the responses for major peak.

Note: Disregard peaks due to placebo and blank.

System suitability:

- Theoretical plates should not be less than 2000.
- Tailing factor from standard chromatogram should not be more than 2.0.
- The RSD of Paracetamol peak areas from six replicate injections of standard should NMT 5.0 %.

Calculation:

$$\% \text{ impurity} = \frac{A}{B} \times \frac{Ws}{100} \times \frac{5}{50} \times \frac{2}{100} \times \frac{100}{Wt} \times \frac{50}{5} \times \frac{Aw}{L} \times \frac{P}{100} \times \frac{1}{RRF} \times 100$$

A = Peak area of impurity obtained from test solution.
B = Average peak area of Paracetamol in the chromatogram from standard solution.
Ws = Weight of Paracetamol standard taken, in mg for standard preparation
Wt = Weight of tablet powder taken for test preparation in mg.
P = Potency of Paracetamol on as is basis
L = Labeled amount of Paracetamol in mg, per Tablet
Aw = Average Weight in mg.
RRF = Relative response factor of impurity

Total impurities = Sum of all the known impurities and unknown impurities.

3. Specification for related substances:

Let us assume that the specification for related substances for paracetamol tablet is as below.

Table 2: Specification of impurity in %

Name of impurities	Name of impurities	
	Release specification	Shelf-life specification
Impurity A	0.5%	1.0%
Impurity B	0.3%	0.6%
HUI	0.20%	0.20%
Total impurity	NMT 2.0%	NMT 3.0%

Note: HUI- Highest unknown impurity

PREPARATION OF CONCENTRATION MATRIX:

For the Related Substances Test Procedure, parameters such as specificity, precision, detection limit (DL), quantitation limit (QL), linearity, and accuracy all require a well-defined concentration matrix. We will now proceed to prepare the concentration matrix for each of these validation parameters.

The following points are covered as part of the concentration matrix for related substances:

1. General information about product
2. Standard and Test concentration
2.1. Standard concentration
2.2. Test concentration
3. Specification for related substances
4. Concentration mapping for validation parameters
4.1. Specificity/Seletivity
4.2. System suitability
4.3. Precision
4.4. Response/Linearity
4.5. Accuracy

1. General information about the product:

At the beginning of concentration matrix, provide general information such as the product name, label claim, placebo weight, etc.

Fig. 1: Excel sheet screenshot for general information about the product

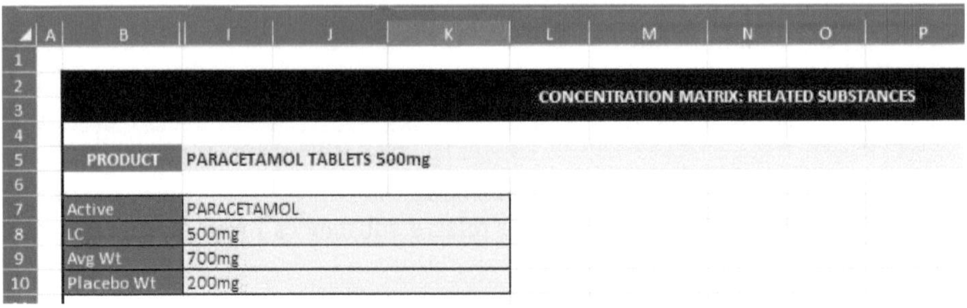

CONCENTRATION MATRIX: RELATED SUBSTANCES

PRODUCT	PARACETAMOL TABLETS 500mg
Active	PARACETAMOL
LC	500mg
Avg Wt	700mg
Placebo Wt	200mg

2. Standard and Test Concentration:

It is also a good idea to map the concentration of standard and test solution preparation. This will help to prepare linearity, accuracy and specificity related solutions.

2.1 Standard Concentration:

- Weigh 50 mg of paracetamol and dilute to 100 mL → Standard stock solution
- Take 5 mL of this standard stock and dilute to 50 mL → Intermediate standard solution
- Take 2 mL of this Intermediate standard solution and dilute to 100 mL → Standard solution

Calculate the resulting concentration of standard stock in ppm using the formula below

$$\text{Standard stock conc (ppm)} = \frac{\text{Standard Weight (mg)}}{\text{Dilution Volume (mL)}} \times 1000$$

$$\text{Conc of standard stock (ppm)} = \frac{50}{100} \times 1000 = 500 \text{ ppm}$$

Note: The potency of the API standard is generally close to 100%, and for simplification, it has been excluded from the initial concentration matrix calculations. However, please remember that while calculating actual results after performing validation experiments, the standard potency must be considered wherever applicable.

In contrast, impurity standards often have potencies significantly lower than 100%, which is why their potency has been included in the Excel sheet while preparing the concentration matrix. You must also account for the impurity potency during result calculations, wherever it applies.

Standard weight: 50 mg *(Refer cell C15 from Fig. 2)*
Standard stock dilution: 100 mL *(Refer cell C16 from Fig. 2)*

Similarly, calculate the concentration of intermediate standard solution and standard solution

$$\text{Resulting conc (ppm)} = \frac{\text{Standard Weight (mg)}}{\text{Dilution Volume (mL)}} \times \frac{\text{Pipetted Volume (mL)}}{\text{Dilution Volume (mL)}} \times 1000$$

Conc. of int. standard solution (ppm)= ---------------- x ------------------ x 1000 =

Conc. of standard solution (ppm)= ---------------- x ----------------- x ----------------- x 1000 =

Note: While calculating the concentration of the intermediate standard solution and standard solution, make sure to use the weight taken and the dilution details of the standard stock solution. This should be followed by any subsequent dilutions, such as 5 mL to 50 mL and 2 mL to 100 mL, as applicable.

Table 3: Tabulate the concentration of standard stock, intermediate and standard solution in below table

Step	Weight/ Volume	Description	Resulting Concentration (ppm)
1	50 mg / 100 mL	Standard stock solution	----------------------------------
2	5 mL / 50 mL	Intermediate standard solution	----------------------------------
3	2 mL / 100 mL	Standard solution	----------------------------------

Fig. 2: excel sheet screenshot to calculate standard concentration.

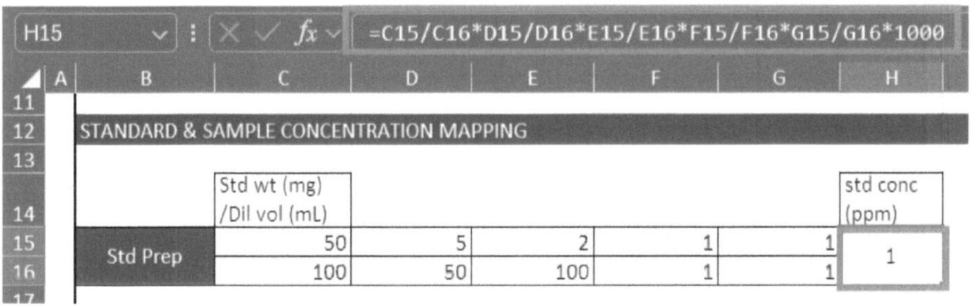

2.2 Test Concentration:

- Weigh and crush 20 paracetamol tablets and weigh powder equivalent to 500 mg of paracetamol and dilute to 100 mL→ Test stock solution
- Take 5 mL of test stock solution and dilute to 50 mL → Test solution

Calculate the resulting concentration of paracetamol in test stock in ppm using the formula below

$$\text{Resulting conc (ppm)} = \frac{\text{Weight (mg)}}{\text{Dilution Volume (mL)}} \times 1000$$

$$\text{Conc of paracetamol in test stock in ppm} = \frac{500}{100} \times 1000 = 5000 \text{ ppm}$$

Weight of Paracetamol in test sample: 500 mg *(Refer cell C19 from Fig. 3)*
Dilution of test stock: 100 mL *(Refer cell C20 from Fig. 3)*

Similarly calculate the concentration of paracetamol in test solution

$$\text{Paracetamol conc in test sol. (ppm)} = \frac{\text{Weight (mg)}}{\text{Dilution Volume (mL)}} \times \frac{\text{Pipetted Volume (mL)}}{\text{Dilution Volume (mL)}} \times 1000$$

$$\text{Paracetamol conc in test sol. (ppm)} = \text{-----------} \times \text{-----------} \times 1000 =$$

Note: While calculating the concentration of the test solution, make sure to use the weight of paracetamol present in test sample (and not the weight of drug product). This should be followed by any subsequent dilutions, such as 5 mL to 50 mL as applicable.

Table 4: Tabulate the concentration of test stock and test solution in the table below

Step	API weight / Volume	Description	Resulting Concentration (ppm)
1	500 mg / 100 mL	Test stock solution	----------------
2	5 mL / 50 mL	Test solution	----------------

Fig. 3: Please check excel sheet screenshot to calculate test concentration.

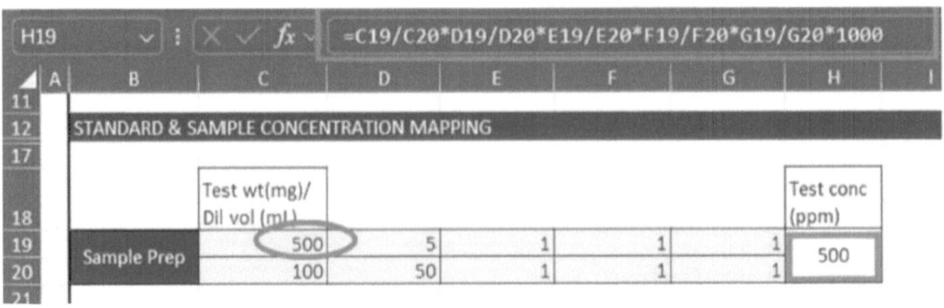

Let us assume that the specification for related substances for paracetamol tablet is as below.

Table 5: Specification of impurity in %

Name of impurities	Specification in %	
	Release specification	Shelf-life specification
Impurity A	0.5%	1.0%
Impurity B	0.3%	0.6%
HUI	0.20%	0.20%
Total impurity	NMT 2.0%	NMT 3.0%

Note: HUI- Highest unknown impurity

Since we will be using ppm as the unit for all solutions (such as standard and test solution), it is necessary to convert the impurity specification from % to ppm.

Let's go ahead and perform this conversion.

$$\textit{Impurity specification in ppm} = \frac{\textit{(Impurity limit in \%) x (Test conc. in ppm)}}{100}$$

Let us calculate impurity A, impurity B, and HUI specification in ppm

$$\textit{Impurity A specification in ppm at release specification} = \frac{0.5\ \%\ x\ 500\ ppm}{100} = 2.5\ ppm$$

Where:
- Impurity A release specification in % = 0.5% *(Refer cell D28, Fig. 4)*
- Test concentration in ppm = 500 ppm *(Refer cell H19, Fig. 3)*

Now, you can calculate the Impurity B and HUI specification in ppm

Tabulate the impurity A, impurity B, and HUI specification both in % and in ppm below

Table 6: Impurity specification both in % and in ppm

Name of impurities	Specification in %		Specification in ppm	
	Release specification	Shelf-life specification	Release specification	Shelf-life specification
Impurity A	0.5%	1.0%	2.5 ppm	---------- ppm
Impurity B	0.3%	0.6%	---------- ppm	---------- ppm
HUI	0.20%	0.20%	---------- ppm	---------- ppm

Fig. 4: Excel sheet screenshot to calculate specifications of impurities in ppm.

F28 =D28*$H$19

SPECIFICATION

Test Name	Impurity Name	Limit in (%)		Limit in (ppm)	
		Release	Stability	Release Spec	Stability
RS	Impurity A	0.5%	1.0%	2.5	5.0
	Impurity B	0.3%	0.6%	1.5	3.0
	HUI	0.20%	0.20%	1.0	1.0
				0.0	0.0
				0.0	0.0
				0.0	0.0
				0.0	0.0
				0.0	0.0
				0.0	0.0
				0.0	0.0
				0.0	0

Impurity Name	B. No/Lot No	Expiry date	Potency
Impurity A	JSDHF6665	20/08/2026	100
Impurity B	FJFJK365	20-SEP-2027	100
HUI	WS/012	15-JAN-2026	100
0			
0			
0			
0			
0			
0			
0			
0			

To convert the impurity specification from percentage to ppm, the proposed formula is: (Impurity % × Test Concentration in ppm) / 100. In the above figure, the impurity concentration in ppm is shown as 'Impurity % × Test Concentration (ppm)'. You might wonder why the division by 100 is not shown explicitly. That's because the impurity value is already expressed in percentage (e.g. Impurity A: 0.5%), and this is factored into the calculation, so dividing by 100 is not required.

Additional rows have been intentionally included to record details of any extra impurities present in the product. The figure also captures important information about the impurities, such as batch number, expiry date, and potency. Since the unknown impurity and HUI (Highest Unknown Impurity) are calculated against the API standard, the relevant details of the API standard are also provided.

4. CONCENTRATION MAPPING FOR VALIDATION PARAMETERS:

Let's now start mapping the concentration required for each validation parameter

4.1. Specificity/Selectivity:

Specificity/Selectivity is all about checking whether the method can clearly identify the target analyte, even when other substances like excipients, impurities, or diluent are present. We are going to prepare standard solution, test solution, blank/diluent, placebo solution, individual impurity identification solution, and impurity spiked test solution for specificity/selectivity of related substances by HPLC. Forced degradation solutions preparation are not considered here, we will discuss it in a separate chapter. The below solutions are prepared specifically

a. Standard solution

b. Test solution

c. Blank/diluent

d. Placebo solution

e. Individual known impurity solutions

f. Impurity spiked test solution

Table 7: Specification solution preparation

Solution Name	Solution Name	Weight in mg	Dilution 1	Dilution 2	Conc. ppm (w.r.t sample)
Standard Solution	Follow the test procedure	------------	100 mL	5 mL → 50 mL Dilution 3 2 mL → 100 mL	------------
Test Solution	Follow the test procedure. Weight equivalent to 500 mg paracetamol shall be considered	------------	100 mL	5 mL → 50 mL	------------
Blank/ diluent	Follow the test preparation procedure by omitting sample	------------	100 mL	5 mL → 50 mL	------------
Placebo solution	Follow the test preparation procedure by replacing sample by placebo. To determine the placebo content in the test solution, it is important to note that 500 mg of paracetamol contains 200 mg of placebo. Therefore, for a test solution using 500 mg of paracetamol, the placebo content will be (200/500)×500=200 mg of placebo.	------------	100 mL	5 mL → 50 mL	------------
Impurity A Identification Solution	Prepare impurity A identification solution at its release specification level, which is 0.5 % or 2.5 ppm	100 mL	100 mL (Imp A stock Sol)	5mL → 200mL	2.5 ppm
Impurity B Identification Solution	Prepare impurity B identification solution at its release specification level, which is ___ % or ___ ppm	------------	------------ (Imp B stock Sol)	___mL → ___mL	______ ppm
Impurity spiked test solution	Test solution shall be spiked with or added with impurity A and impurity B at their respective release specifications.	Weight of a sample eq. 500 mg of paracetamol + _____ mL of impurity A stock + ____mL of impurity B stock	100 mL	5mL → 50mL	Paracetamol is _____ ppm Impurity A is _____ ppm Impurity B is _____ ppm

Follow the test preparation procedures outlined in the STP while preparing for the spiked test, and placebo solutions. However, you can adjust the weight and dilution of the impurity to achieve the desired concentration. Another important point is the dilution process. Ensure that impurity is soluble in the diluent used (especially while making impurity stock solution). If Impurity is not soluble in the test diluent, you may use another diluent in which the impurity is soluble when preparing the stock solution. However, the final solution, which will be analyzed, should preferably be prepared in the diluent used for the test solution.

Note: The test solution and impurity-spiked test solution can alternatively be prepared using the API and placebo, in case the test sample is unsuitable or unavailable. In such cases, use placebo and API as per the product composition. In the current case, use 200 mg of placebo and 500 mg of Paracetamol API to prepare the test solution. Similarly, for the impurity-spiked test solution, use 200 mg of placebo, 500 mg of Paracetamol API, and the respective impurity stock solutions.

a. Standard Solution: Follow the STP

b. Test solution: Follow the STP

c. Diluent: Follow the test solution preparation by omitting test sample.

d. Placebo solution preparation: Follow the test solution preparation by replacing test sample by placebo.

Fig. 5: Excel sheet screenshot for placebo solution preparation.

C54 | =F30

1. SPECIFICITY

	Placebo Wt (mg) /Dil vol (mL)				
Placebo Preparation	200	5	1	1	1
	100	50	1	1	1

e. Individual impurity solution preparation: For preparation of individual impurity solutions, below two steps are involved:

i. Preparation of the Impurity Identification Stock Solution, and
ii. Preparation of the Impurity Identification Solution

Please refer to Fig. 6 covering these two key steps.

Fig. 6: Excel sheet screenshot for individual impurity solution preparation

B48 | Individual Impurity Solution Preparation

Individual Impurity Solution Preparation

Impurity Identification Stock Solution							Impurity Identification Solution prepration									
Impurity Name	Release Spec conc (ppm)	Wt (mg)	Dil to (mL)	Pipetted (mL)	Dil to (mL)	Imp Stock Conc (ppm)	Imp Stock Vol (ml)	Dil to (mL)	Pipetted (mL)	Dil to (mL)	Pipetted (mL)	Dil to (mL)	Pipetted (mL)	Dil to (mL)	Resulted Imp Conc (ppm)
Impurity A	2.50	10	100	1	1	100.00	5.00	200	1	1	1	1	1	1	2.50
Impurity B	1.50	10	100	1	1	100.00	3.00	200	1	1	1	1	1	1	1.50
HUI	1.00					#DIV/0!	#DIV/0!								#DIV/0!
0	0.00					#DIV/0!	#DIV/0!								#DIV/0!
0	0.00					#DIV/0!	#DIV/0!								#DIV/0!
0	0.00					#DIV/0!	#DIV/0!								#DIV/0!
0	0.00					#DIV/0!	#DIV/0!								#DIV/0!
0	0.00					#DIV/0!	#DIV/0!								#DIV/0!
0	0.00					#DIV/0!	#DIV/0!								#DIV/0!
0	0.00					#DIV/0!	#DIV/0!								#DIV/0!

The screenshot above may not be very clear to read, so I will explain it step by step below.

i. Preparation of Impurity identification Stock Solution:

The screenshot below (Fig. 7) guides the preparation of individual impurity stock solutions. These stock solutions are primarily used for the preparation of impurity identification solutions during specificity testing. Additionally, the same stocks can be used to prepare solutions for validation parameters such as precision, linearity, and accuracy if applicable.

Since impurity quantity is often limited in many labs, it's important for analysts to plan their usage wisely. A practical approach is to prepare a common impurity stock solution, which can then be used to prepare different validation solutions as needed.

These stock solutions should be prepared in a suitable diluent in which impurity remains stable. Typically, organic solvents like acetonitrile or methanol are found to be appropriate choices.

Typically, 10–20 mg of an impurity is used to prepare the stock solution, depending on the required concentration. The stock solution is always at a much higher concentration compared to the actual impurity levels needed in validation solutions (such as those for specificity, linearity, etc.).

Once prepared, these stock solutions should be stored under refrigerated or cool conditions to prevent degradation (or as proposed by impurity manufacturer). It is important that analysts label each solution with all essential details, including the impurity name, date of preparation, concentration, and the name of the person who prepared it.

Now, let's understand how to prepare the impurity identification solution. In the current example, the impurity stock solution has been prepared at a concentration of 100 ppm for both Impurity A and Impurity B.

$$\text{Stock sol. conc (ppm)} = \frac{\text{Weight (mg)}}{\text{Dilution Volume (mL)}} \times \frac{\text{Purity}}{100} \times 1000$$

Let us calculate the concentration of Impurity A identification stock solution

$$\text{Impurity A identification stock sol. conc (ppm)} = \frac{10 \text{ mg}}{100 \text{ mL}} \times \frac{100\ \%}{100} \times 1000 = 100 \text{ ppm}$$

Where:

- Weight of impurity A = 10 mg (Refer cell D52 from Fig. 7)
- Impurity A dilution = 100 mL (Refer cell E52 from Fig. 7)
- Impurity A Purity = 100% (Refer cell L28 from Fig. 4)

Similarly calculate the concentration of impurity B identification stock solution

Impurity B identification stock sol. conc (ppm) = ----------- x ----------- x 1000 = --------- ppm

Fig. 7: Excel sheet screenshot for impurity identification stock solution preparation.

H52 | =D52/E52*F52/G52*L28/100*1000

	A	B	C	D	E	F	G	H
47								
48		Individual Impurity Solution Preparation						
49								
50		Impurity Identification Stock Solution						
51		Impurity Name	Release Spec conc (ppm)	Wt (mg)	Dil to (mL)	Pipetted (mL)	Dil to (mL)	Imp Stock Conc (ppm)
52		Impurity A	2.50	10	100	1	1	100.00
53		Impurity B	1.50	10	100	1	1	100.00
54		HUI	1.00					#DIV/0!
55		0	0.00					#DIV/0!
56		0	0.00					#DIV/0!
57		0	0.00					#DIV/0!
58		0	0.00					#DIV/0!
59		0	0.00					#DIV/0!
60		0	0.00					#DIV/0!
61		0	0.00					#DIV/0!

ii.Preparation of Individual Impurity Identification Solution:

This section of the Excel sheet outlines the process for preparing individual impurity solutions at the desired concentrations. It involves two key steps:

Step 1: Calculation of the required volume of impurity stock solution.

Step 2: Verification of the resulted impurity identification solution concentration

Let's go through each of these steps one by one.

Step 1: Calculation of the required volume of impurity stock solution:

After preparing the impurity stock solution (as described above), the next step is to calculate the required volume of stock to achieve the desired impurity concentration through dilution.

In this example, we've selected a dilution volume of 200 mL for both Impurity A and Impurity B. You are free to choose the dilution volume as per requirement. The target concentrations are:

- **Impurity A:** 2.50 ppm (release specification conc.)
- **Impurity B:** 1.50 ppm (release specification conc.)

To calculate the required volume of impurity stock solution for each impurity, use the following formula:

$$\textit{Required volume of impurity stock (mL)} = \frac{\textit{Expected conc (ppm) x Dilution volume (mL)}}{\textit{Impurity stock conc (ppm)}}$$

Let us calculate the required volume of impurity A stock to get its concentration in ppm at release specification

$$\textit{Required volume of impurity A stock (mL) to get its release spec conc} = \frac{2.50 \textit{ ppm x } 200 \textit{ mL}}{100 \textit{ ppm}} = 5 \textit{ mL}$$

Where:
- Expected conc. of impurity A as per release spec. = 2.50 ppm *(Refer cell C52, Fig. 7)*
- Dilution volume (mL) = 200 mL *(Refer cell J52, Fig. 8)*
- Impurity A stock conc. (ppm) = 100 ppm *(Refer cell H52, Fig. 7)*

Fig. 8: Excel sheet screenshot for impurity stock solution volume calculation

I52 | fx | =C52*J52/H52

Individual Impurity Solution Preparation

	Impurity Identification Solution prepration								
	I	J	K	L	M	N	O	P	Q
51	Imp Stock Vol (ml)	Dil to (mL)	Pipetted (mL)	Dil to (mL)	Pipetted (mL)	Dil to (mL)	Pipetted (mL)	Dil to (mL)	Resulted Imp Conc (ppm)
52	5.00	200	1	1	1	1	1	1	2.50
53	3.00	200	1	1	1	1	1	1	1.50
54	#DIV/0!								#DIV/0!
55	#DIV/0!								#DIV/0!
56	#DIV/0!								#DIV/0!
57	#DIV/0!								#DIV/0!
58	#DIV/0!								#DIV/0!
59	#DIV/0!								#DIV/0!
60	#DIV/0!								#DIV/0!
61	#DIV/0!								#DIV/0!

Step 2: Verification of the resulted impurity identification solution concentration:

It is the final check- verifying the prepared impurity solution concentration.
So far, we have prepared the impurity stock solution and calculated the volume of stock needed to achieve the desired impurity concentration in its identification solution.

Now, it's time to verify the final concentration of the impurity solution using actual values including the stock concentration, the volume taken from the stock, and the total dilution volume.

We'll use the following formula to confirm the concentration of the resulted identification solution.

$$\text{Conc of resulted solution (ppm)} = \text{Conc of stock (ppm)} \times \frac{\text{Vol. of stock (mL)}}{\text{Dilution vol.(mL)}} \times \frac{\text{Pipetted vol (mL)}}{\text{Dilution vol (mL)}}$$

Let us calculate the resulted concentration of impurity A identification solution

$$\text{Conc of resulted solution (ppm) of imp A} = 100 \text{ ppm} \times \frac{5 \text{ mL}}{200 \text{ mL}} = 2.5 \text{ ppm}$$

Where:
- Impurity A stock concentration = 100 ppm *(Refer cell H52 from Fig. 7)*
- Impurity A stock volume = 5 mL *(Refer cell I52 from Fig. 8)*
- Dilution volume = 200 mL *(Refer cell J52 from Fig. 8)*

- Target concentration = 2.50 ppm *(as per release specification, refer cell C52, Fig. 7)*

Conclusion:

The resulted concentration of Impurity A (refer cell Q52, Fig. 8) matches the expected or target concentration in ppm (refer cell C52, Fig. 7). Therefore, the selected Impurity A stock solution and the proposed dilution are appropriate and accurate.

Similarly, you can calculate the resulted concentration for impurity B

- Stock concentration = ... ppm
- Volume taken from the stock = ... mL
- Final dilution volume = ... mL
- Target concentration = ... ppm

Conc of resulted solution (ppm) of imp B = ... ppm x $\frac{\text{......... mL}}{\text{............ mL}}$ *= .... ppm*

Conclusion:

Fig. 9: Excel sheet screenshot for resulted impurity concentration calculation

Q52 | =H52*I52/J52*K52/L52*M52/N52*O52/P52

Individual Impurity Solution Preparation

Impurity Identification Solution prepration								
Imp Stock Vol (ml)	Dil to (mL)	Pipetted (mL)	Dil to (mL)	Pipetted (mL)	Dil to (mL)	Pipetted (mL)	Dil to (mL)	Resulted Imp Conc (ppm)
5.00	200	1	1	1	1	1	1	2.50
3.00	200	1	1	1	1	1	1	1.50
#DIV/0!								#DIV/0!
#DIV/0!								#DIV/0!
#DIV/0!								#DIV/0!
#DIV/0!								#DIV/0!
#DIV/0!								#DIV/0!
#DIV/0!								#DIV/0!
#DIV/0!								#DIV/0!
#DIV/0!								#DIV/0!

By calculating the resulting impurity concentration, we've confirmed whether the selected stock solution and dilution give us the expected result. This serves as a critical checkpoint, as accurate concentration is essential during method validation. It might seem like an extra step, but it's better to double-check than to risk preparing incorrect solutions.

f.Impurity spiked test solution for specificity:

In specificity (or selectivity) testing, known impurities must be spiked into the test solution to demonstrate that they do not interfere with each other or with the API. In this example, the impurities will be spiked at their release specification concentrations.

In the screenshot below (Fig. 10) two key activities are covered

i. Preparation of the Impurity Identification Stock Solution for Specificity
ii. Preparation of the Impurity Spiked Sample Solution for Specificity

Fig. 10: Excel sheet screenshot for spiked sample solution preparation.

Spiked Sample Preparation

IMPURITY STOCK SOLUTION PREPARATION							SPIKED SAMPLE PREPARATION							
Impurity Name	Release Spec conc (ppm)	Impurity Wt (mg)	Dil to (ml)	Pipetted (ml)	Dil to (ml)	Imp Stock Conc (ppm)	Sample Wt (mg)	Imp Stock Vol (ml)	Dil to (mL)	Pipetted (mL)	Dil to (mL)	Pipetted (mL)	Dil to (mL)	Resuletd Imp Conc (ppm)
Impurity A	2.5	10	100	1	1	100	700mg	25	100	5	50	1	1	2.5
Impurity B	1.5	10	100	1	1	100		15						1.5
HUI	1.0					#DIV/0!		#DIV/0!						#DIV/0!
0	0.0					#DIV/0!		#DIV/0!						#DIV/0!
0	0.0					#DIV/0!		#DIV/0!						#DIV/0!
0	0.0					#DIV/0!		#DIV/0!						#DIV/0!
0	0.0					#DIV/0!		#DIV/0!						#DIV/0!
0	0.0					#DIV/0!		#DIV/0!						#DIV/0!
0	0.0					#DIV/0!		#DIV/0!						#DIV/0!
0	0.0					#DIV/0!		#DIV/0!						#DIV/0!

The screenshot above may not be very clear to read, so I will explain it step by step below.

i. Preparation of the impurity stock solution for specificity

We have already discussed impurity stock preparation earlier, so we will not discuss it again here. Please refer to the "Individual impurity solution preparation" (fig. 6) for the preparation of impurity stock solution. The same impurity stock solutions are used for preparation of impurity spiked test solutions. Below Fig. 11 provides information on impurity stock solutions which will be further used for preparation of 'impurity spiked test solution' at their release specification.

Fig. 11: Excel sheet screenshot for impurity stock preparation to be used for spiked test preparation.

Spiked Sample Preparation

IMPURITY STOCK SOLUTION PREPARATION						
Impurity Name	Release Spec conc (ppm)	Impurity Wt (mg)	Dil to (mL)	Pipetted (mL)	Dil to (mL)	Imp Stock Conc (ppm)
Impurity A	2.5	10	100	1	1	100
Impurity B	1.5	10	100	1	1	100
HUI	1.0					#DIV/0!
0	0.0					#DIV/0!
0	0.0					#DIV/0!
0	0.0					#DIV/0!
0	0.0					#DIV/0!
0	0.0					#DIV/0!
0	0.0					#DIV/0!
0	0.0					#DIV/0!

ii. Preparation of impurity spiked test solution for specificity:

This section of the Excel sheet outlines the process for preparing impurity spiked test solutions at the desired concentrations (at the impurity release specification).

It involves two key steps:

Step 1: Calculation of the required impurity stock solution volume

Step 2: Verification of the resulted spiked impurity concentration in test solution

Let's go through each of these steps one by one.

Step 1: Calculation of the required impurity stock solution volume

After preparing the impurity stock solution (as described above), the next step is to calculate the required volume of stock to achieve the spiked test solution with desired impurity concentration through dilution. Please note, we must follow the test solution preparation procedure while preparing impurity spiked test solution.

Test preparation:

- Weigh and crush 20 paracetamol tablets and weigh powder equivalent to 500 mg of paracetamol and dilute to 100 mL→ Test stock solution
- Take 5 mL of test stock solution and dilute to 50 mL → Test solution

The target concentrations are:

- **Impurity A:** 2.50 ppm (release specification conc.)
- **Impurity B:** 1.50 ppm (release specification conc.)

To calculate the required volume of impurity stock solution for each impurity, use the following formula:

$$\text{Vol. of impurity stock (mL)} = \text{Expected impurity conc (ppm)} \times \frac{\text{Diluted vol (mL)}}{\text{Impurity stock conc (ppm)}} \times \frac{\text{Dilution vol (mL)}}{\text{Pipetted vol (mL)}}$$

$$\text{Vol. of impurity A stock (mL)} = 2.50\text{ppm} \times \frac{100\ \text{mL}}{100\ \text{ppm}} \times \frac{50\ \text{mL}}{5\ \text{mL}} = 25\ \text{mL}$$

Where:

- Expected concentration of impurity A (release spec conc.) = 2.5ppm (cell C68 from Fig. 11)
- Impurity A stock concentration (ppm) = 100 ppm *(cell H68 from Fig. 11).*
- Dilution volume of the impurity A stock solution = 100 mL *(cell L68 from Fig. 12)*
- Pipetted volume of the resultant solution = 5 mL *(cell M68 from Fig. 12)*
- Further dilution of the pipetted solution = 50 mL *(cell N68 from Fig. 12)*

Similarly, you can calculate the volume of impurity B stock solution to achieve desired concentration (1.5ppm) as below

$$\text{Vol. of impurity B stock (mL)} = \text{-------} \times \frac{\ldots\ldots\ldots\ \text{mL}}{\ldots\ldots\ldots\ \text{ppm}} \times \frac{\ldots\ldots\ldots\ \text{mL}}{\ldots\ldots\ldots\ \text{mL}} = \ldots\ldots\ldots\ldots\ \text{mL}$$

Fig. 12: Excel sheet screenshot for impurity stock volume calculation

K68 =C68*$P$68/$O$68*$N$68/$M$68*$L$68*1/H68

Spiked Sample Preparation

SPIKED SAMPLE PREPARATION							
Sample Wt (mg)	Imp Stock Vol (ml)	Dil to (mL)	Pipetted (mL)	Dil to (mL)	Pipetted (mL)	Dil to (mL)	Resuletd Imp Conc (ppm)
	25						2.5
	15						1.5
	#DIV/0!						#DIV/0!
	#DIV/0!						#DIV/0!
700mg	#DIV/0!	100	5	50	1	1	#DIV/0!
	#DIV/0!						#DIV/0!
	#DIV/0!						#DIV/0!
	#DIV/0!						#DIV/0!
	#DIV/0!						#DIV/0!
	#DIV/0!						#DIV/0!

Note: If the test sample already contains some amount of impurity, then the volume of impurity stock solution to be added must be adjusted accordingly. This adjustment ensures that the final impurity concentration in the spiked test solution matches the desired target. For more clarity on how to perform this adjustment, please refer to the Repeatability Study section, where the method for calculating the appropriate stock volume is explained in detail.

Step 2: Verification of the resulted impurity concentration in spiked test solution for specificity:

It is the final check- verifying the prepared impurity solution concentration in the spiked test solution.

So far, we have prepared the impurity stock solution and calculated the volume of stock needed to achieve the desired concentration in a spiked test solution.

Now, it's time to verify the final concentration of the impurity solution using actual values including the stock concentration, the volume taken from the stock, and the total dilution volume.

We'll use the following formula to confirm the result:

$$\text{Conc of resulted solution (ppm)} = \text{Conc of stock (ppm)} \times \frac{\text{Vol. of stock (mL)}}{\text{Dilution vol.(mL)}} \times \frac{\text{Pipetted vol (mL)}}{\text{Dilution vol (mL)}}$$

Let's take Impurity A as an example:
- Impurity A stock concentration = 100 ppm *(cell H68 from Fig. 11)*
- Volume taken from the stock = 25 mL *(cell K68 from Fig. 13)*
- Test stock dilution volume = 100 mL *(cell L68 from Fig. 13)*
- Test stock pipetted volume = 5 mL *(cell M68 from Fig. 13)*
- Further test solution dilution volume = 50 mL *(cell N68 from fig. 13)*

$$\text{Conc of resulted solution (ppm) of imp A} = 100\ \text{ppm} \times \frac{25\ \text{mL}}{100\ \text{mL}} \times \frac{5\ \text{mL}}{50\ \text{mL}} = 2.5\ \text{ppm}$$

Target concentration for impurity A = 2.50 ppm (cell C68 from Fig. 11)

Conclusion:

The resulted concentration of Impurity A matches the expected value. Therefore, the selected Impurity A stock solution and the proposed dilution are appropriate and accurate.

Similarly, you can calculate the resulted concentration for impurity B
- Stock concentration = ______________ppm
- Volume taken from the stock = ____________mL
- Test stock dilution volume = _________mL
- Test stock pipetted volume = ______________mL
- Further test solution dilution volume =_______________mL
- Target concentration for impurity B = ____________ ppm

Conc of resulted solution (ppm) of imp B = ………… ppm x (……… mL / ………… mL) x (………… mL / ……… mL) = ……….. ppm

Conclusion:

Fig. 13: Excel sheet screenshot for resulted impurity concentration calculation

Q68 | fx | =H68*K68/$L$68*$M$68/$N$68*$O$68/$P$68

Spiked Sample Preparation

Row	SPIKED SAMPLE PREPARATION							
67	Sample Wt (mg)	Imp Stock Vol (ml)	Dil to (mL)	Pipetted (mL)	Dil to (mL)	Pipetted (mL)	Dil to (mL)	Resuletd Imp Conc (ppm)
68		25						2.5
69		15						1.5
70		#DIV/0!						#DIV/0!
71		#DIV/0!						#DIV/0!
72	700mg	#DIV/0!	100	5	50	1	1	#DIV/0!
73		#DIV/0!						#DIV/0!
74		#DIV/0!						#DIV/0!
75		#DIV/0!						#DIV/0!
76		#DIV/0!						#DIV/0!
77		#DIV/0!						#DIV/0!

By calculating the resulting impurity concentration, we've confirmed whether the selected stock solution and dilution give us the expected result.

4.2. System Suitability

Prepare the standard solution or system suitability solutions as per STP

Fig. 14: Excel sheet screenshot for system suitability solution preparation

2. SYSTEM SUITABILITY

Just Prepare stdandard solution as above

4.3. Precision:

Precision can be considered at three levels: repeatability, intermediate precision and reproducibility. For all three levels you can use the same concentration matrix as concentration of standard, test, or method of preparation remains one and the same.

Repeatability should be assessed using a minimum of 9 determinations covering the reportable range for the procedure (e.g., 3 concentrations/3 replicates each) or a minimum of 6 determinations at 100% of the test concentration.
We are going to prepare the concentration matrix for the solutions below

4.3.1 Preparation of repeatability solutions using finished product

4.3.2 Preparation of repeatability solutions using (API + Placebo)

4.3.3. Preparation of repeatability solution for unknown impurity

Below table provides the concentration matrix for preparation of test at 100% of the test concentration.

Table 8: Concentration matrix for preparation of repeatability test at 100% of the test concentration

Solution Name	Solution Name	Weight in mg	Dilution 1	Dilution 1	Conc. (ppm)
Unspiked Test Solution	Follow the test procedure. Weight equivalent to 500 mg paracetamol shall be considered	............mg	100 mL	5 mL → 50 mL	............ppm
Impurity A Stock Solution	Prepare impurity A stock solution at 200 ppm concentration	20mg	100 mL	Not applicable	200 ppm
Impurity B Stock Solution	Prepare impurity B stock solution at 200 ppm concentration	............mg	............mL	Not applicable	............ppm
Impurity spiked test solution	Test solution shall be spiked with or added with impurity A and impurity B at their respective release specifications.	Weight of a sample eq. 500 mg of paracetamol + ______ mL of impurity A stock + ______mL of impurity B stock	100 mL	5 mL → 50 mL	Paracetamol is ______ppm Impurity A is ______ppm Impurity B is ______ ppm
API stock solution	Prepare API stock solution at 5000ppm concentration	50 mg	10 mL	Not applicable	............ppm
Unknown impurity precision solution	Follow the test procedure. Weight of the placebo (200 mg), eq. to 500 mg paracetamol.	Weight of a placebo eq. 500 mg of paracetamol + ______ mL of API stock	100 mL	5 mL → 50 mL	............ppm

Please follow the accuracy section to understand the concentration matrix for precision with 9 determinations covering the reportable range for the procedure (e.g., 3 concentrations/3 replicates each)

4.3.1 Preparation of repeatability solutions using finished product:

The repeatability using finished product can be studied by spiking the test solution with impurity to achieve the impurity at about their respective release specification concentration. In this example, the impurities are spiked at their release specification levels, which are typically lower than the concentrations specified for stability specification. Lower concentrations tend to show higher variability, so if the method proves to be precise at the release specification level, it provides confidence that it will remain precise at the higher concentration used for the stability specification.

To understand the spiking need, one must calculate the concentration of the impurity present in as such test sample or unspiked test sample.

Fig. 15: Excel sheet screenshot for precision covering preparation of repeatability solution at 100%.

3. REPEATABILITY

a. Repeatability using Finished Product: Prepare sample solutions for 6 times

	IMPURITY STOCK SOLUTION PREPARATION									SPIKED SAMPLE PREPARATION								
89	Impurity Name	Release Spec Conc (ppm)	Impurity Wt (mg)	Dil to (mL)	Pipetted (mL)	Dil to (mL)	Imp Stock Conc (ppm)	Imp in unspiked sample	Imp in unspiked sample (ppm)	Imp. To be spiked (ppm)	Sample wt (mg)	Imp Stock Vol (mL)	Dil to (mL)	Pipetted (mL)	Dil to (mL)	Pipetted (mL)	Dil to (mL)	Resulted Imp Conc (Spiked+Unspiked) (ppm)
90	Impurity A	2.5	20	100	1	1	200	0.10%	0.5	2.0	700mg	10.00	100	5	50	1	1	2.5
91	Impurity B	1.5	20	100	1	1	200	0.10%	0.5	1.0		5.00						1.5
92	MUI	1.0					#DIV/0!		0	1.0		#DIV/0!						#DIV/0!
93	0	0.0					#DIV/0!		0	0.0		#DIV/0!						#DIV/0!
94	0	0.0					#DIV/0!		0	0.0		#DIV/0!						#DIV/0!
95	0	0.0					#DIV/0!		0	0.0		#DIV/0!						#DIV/0!
96	0	0.0					#DIV/0!		0	0.0		#DIV/0!						#DIV/0!
97	0	0.0					#DIV/0!		0	0.0		#DIV/0!						#DIV/0!
98	0	0.0					#DIV/0!		0	0.0		#DIV/0!						#DIV/0!
99	0	0.0					#DIV/0!		0	0.0		#DIV/0!						#DIV/0!

The screenshot above may not be very clear to read, so I will explain it step by step below.

i. Preparation of the impurity stock solution: Individual impurity stock solutions are prepared for spiking in test solution. In the given example impurity A and impurity B stock solution is prepared at 200 ppm concentration.

- Impurity A stock solution concentration: 200 ppm (cell H90 from Fig. 16)
- Impurity B stock solution concentration: 200 ppm (cell H91 from Fig. 16)

Fig. 16: Excel sheet screenshot for impurity stock preparation to be used for spiked test preparation

D56

	B	C	D	E	F	G	H
83							
84	3. REPEATABILITY						
85							
86	a. Repeatability using Finished Product: Preapre sample solutions for 6 times						
87							
88	IMPURITY STOCK SOLUTION PREPARATION						
89	Impurity Name	Release Spec conc (ppm)	Impurity Wt (mg)	Dil to (mL)	Pipetted (mL)	Dil to (mL)	Imp Stock Conc (ppm)
90	Impurity A	2.5	20	100	1	1	200
91	Impurity B	1.5	20	100	1	1	200
92	HUI	1.0					#DIV/0!
93	0	0.0					#DIV/0!
94	0	0.0					#DIV/0!
95	0	0.0					#DIV/0!
96	0	0.0					#DIV/0!
97	0	0.0					#DIV/0!
98	0	0.0					#DIV/0!
99	0	0.0					#DIV/0!

ii. Preparation of impurity spiked test solution for repeatability:

This section of the Excel sheet outlines the process for preparing impurity spiked test solutions at the desired concentrations (at the impurity release specification). It involves three key steps:

Step 1: Calculation of the impurity concentration (in ppm) present in unspiked test sample

Step 2: Calculation of the impurity to be spiked for preparation of impurity spiked repeatability solution

Step 3: Calculation of impurity stock volume to be spiked in repeatability test solution

Step 4: Verification of the resulted spiked impurity concentration in repeatability test solution

Let's go through each of these steps one by one.

Step1: Calculation of the impurity concentration (in ppm) present in unspiked test sample

Before deciding how much impurity stock solution to spike into the test sample, it is essential to first determine the amount of impurity already present in the unspiked (or as such) sample.

In most testing procedures, impurities are typically reported in percentage (%). However, in the concentration matrix, impurity levels are expressed in ppm. Therefore, the first step is to convert the impurity concentration present in the unspiked test sample from % to ppm using the following formula:

$$\text{Impurity conc in unspiked test (in ppm)} = \frac{\text{Conc. of impurity in unspiked test (\%)} \times \text{Conc. of API in test (ppm)}}{100}$$

This calculation provides the impurity level in the unspiked sample (in ppm), which is essential for determining the appropriate spiking volume.

Let's now calculate the concentration of Impurity A present in the unspiked test sample, expressed in ppm. Assume that the level of Impurity A in the unspiked sample is 0.10%, and the paracetamol concentration in the test sample is 500 ppm (please refer to the sample preparation procedure for details on test concentration).

Using the previously mentioned formula, we can now convert the impurity concentration from % to ppm.

$$\text{Impurity A conc in unspiked test (in ppm)} = \frac{0.10\% \times 500 \text{ ppm}}{100} = 0.5 \text{ ppm}$$

- Conc. of impurity A in unspiked test (%): 0.10% *(cell I90 from Fig. 17)*
- Conc. of API in test (ppm): 500 ppm *(cell H19 from Fig. 3)*

Similarly calculate the impurity B conc. in unspiked test as below

$$\text{Impurity B conc in unspiked test (in ppm)} = \frac{x}{100} = \ldots\ldots\ldots\ldots\ldots \text{ ppm}$$

Fig. 17: Excel sheet screenshot for impurity concentration (in ppm) present in unspiked test.

J90 | =I90*$H$19

3. REPEATABILITY

a. Repeatability using Finished Product: Preapre sample solutions for 6 times

	IMPURITY	SPIKED SAMPLE PREPARATION										
89	Impurity Name	Imp in unspiked sample	Imp in unspiked sample (ppm)	Imp. To be spiked (ppm)	Sample wt (mg)	Imp Stock Vol (ml)	Dil to (mL)	Pipetted (mL)	Dil to (mL)	Pipetted (mL)	Dil to (mL)	Resulted Imp Conc (Spiked+Unspiked) (ppm)
90	Impurity A	0.10%	0.5	2.0		10.00						2.5
91	Impurity B	0.10%	0.5	1.0		5.00						1.5
92	HUI		0	1.0		#DIV/0!						#DIV/0!
93	0		0	0.0		#DIV/0!						#DIV/0!
94	0		0	0.0	700mg	#DIV/0!	100	5	50	1	1	#DIV/0!
95	0		0	0.0		#DIV/0!						#DIV/0!
96	0		0	0.0		#DIV/0!						#DIV/0!
97	0		0	0.0		#DIV/0!						#DIV/0!
98	0		0	0.0		#DIV/0!						#DIV/0!
99	0		0	0.0		#DIV/0!						#DIV/0!

Step 2: Calculation of the impurity to be spiked for preparation of impurity spiked repeatability solution:

To calculate the amount of impurity to be added (spiked) into the test sample, use the following formula:

A = B – C

Where:

- A = Impurity to be spiked in sample
- B= Expected impurity concentration in spiked sample
- C = Existing impurity concentration in unspiked sample

Let us calculate the required impurity A stock solution volume for preparation of impurity spiked repeatability solution.

Impurity A to be spiked in sample = 2.5 ppm – 0.5 ppm = 2.0 ppm

Where:

- B = Expected impurity concentration in spiked sample = 2.5 *ppm (cell C90 from Fig. 16)*
- C = Existing impurity A concentration in unspiked sample = 0.5 ppm *(cell J90 from Fig. 17)*

Similarly, calculate the required impurity B stock solution volume for preparation of impurity spiked repeatability solution.

Impurity B to be spiked in sample = …………… ppm – …………… ppm = …………… ppm

Fig. 18: Excel sheet screenshot for impurity to be spiked for preparation of impurity spiked repeatability solution.

K90 =C90-J90

3. REPEATABILITY

a. Repeatability using Finished Product: Preapre sample solutions for 6 times

IMPURITY STOCK SOLUTION PREPARATION									
Impurity Name	Release Spec conc (ppm)	Impurity Wt (mg)	Dil to (mL)	Pipetted (mL)	Dil to (mL)	Imp Stock Conc (ppm)	Imp in unspiked sample	Imp in unspiked sample (ppm)	Imp. To be spiked (ppm)
Impurity A	2.5	20	100	1	1	200	0.10%	0.5	2.0
Impurity B	1.5	20	100	1	1	200	0.10%	0.5	1.0
HUI	1.0					#DIV/0!		0	1.0
0	0.0					#DIV/0!		0	0.0
0	0.0					#DIV/0!		0	0.0
0	0.0					#DIV/0!		0	0.0
0	0.0					#DIV/0!		0	0.0
0	0.0					#DIV/0!		0	0.0
0	0.0					#DIV/0!		0	0.0
0	0.0					#DIV/0!		0	0.0

Step 3: Calculation of impurity stock volume to be spiked in repeatability test solution:

Up to this point, we have prepared the impurity stock solution, determined the existing level of a specific impurity in the test sample, and calculated the additional amount of impurity that needs to be spiked. In this step, we will calculate the exact volume of the impurity stock solution to be added to the test solution to achieve the target impurity concentration corresponding to the release specification.

Use the below formula to calculate the impurity stock volume to be spiked in repeatability test solution

$$\text{Impurity stock vol (mL)} = \frac{\text{Impurity to be spiked in test (ppm)}}{\text{Impurity stock conc (ppm)}} \times \text{Test stock dilution (mL)} \times \frac{\text{Diluted to vol (mL)}}{\text{Pipetted vol (mL)}}$$

Let us calculate the volume of impurity A stock to be spiked in repeatability test solution

$$\text{Volume of Impurity A stock (mL)} = \frac{2.0\ ppm}{200\ ppm} \times 100\ mL \times \frac{50\ mL}{5\ mL} = 10.0\ mL$$

Where:

- Impurity A to be spiked in test (ppm) = 2.0 ppm (cell K90 from Fig. 18)
- Impurity A stock conc (ppm) = 200 ppm (cell H90 from Fig. 16)
- Test stock dilution (mL) = 100 mL (cell N90 from Fig. 19)
- Test further Diluted to volume (mL) = 50 mL (cell P90 from Fig. 19)
- Pipetted volume of test stock (mL) = 5 mL (cell O90 from Fig. 19)

It means, if 10 mL of an Impurity A stock solution (having 200ppm concentration) is added to a test solution that already contains 0.5 ppm of impurity A, and the total volume is made up to 100 mL, and further when the 5 mL of the resulted solution is diluted to 50 mL, then the final concentration of impurity A in the solution will be 2.5 ppm. This matches the target concentration for impurity A in the repeatability spiked test solution.

In the next step, we will verify if this concentration has been achieved. Before moving ahead, you can try calculating the volume of impurity B stock solution required to reach its target concentration in the repeatability test solution *(refer cell C90, Fog. 18).*

Similarly calculate the volume of impurity B stock

$$\text{Volume of Impurity B stock (mL)} = \frac{\ldots\ldots\ldots\ldots\ ppm}{\ldots\ldots\ldots\ldots\ ppm} \times \ldots\ldots\ldots\ldots\ mL \times \frac{\ldots\ldots\ldots\ldots\ mL}{\ldots\ldots\ldots\ldots\ mL} = \ldots\ldots\ldots\ mL$$

Fig. 19: Excel sheet screenshot for impurity stock volume to be spiked for preparation of impurity spiked repeatability solution

M90 =K90*$N$90*$R$90/$Q$90*$P$90/$O$90*1/H90

3. REPEATABILITY

a. Repeatability using Finished Product: Preapre sample solutions for 6 times

	SPIKED SAMPLE PREPARATION							
89	Sample wt (mg)	Imp Stock Vol (ml)	Dil to (mL)	Pipetted (mL)	Dil to (mL)	Pipetted (mL)	Dil to (mL)	Resulted Imp Conc (Spiked+Unspiked) (ppm)
90	700mg	10.00	100	5	50	1	1	2.5
91		5.00						1.5
92		#DIV/0!						#DIV/0!
93		#DIV/0!						#DIV/0!
94		#DIV/0!						#DIV/0!
95		#DIV/0!						#DIV/0!
96		#DIV/0!						#DIV/0!
97		#DIV/0!						#DIV/0!
98		#DIV/0!						#DIV/0!
99		#DIV/0!						#DIV/0!

Step 4: Verification of the resulted spiked impurity concentration in repeatability test solution:

It is the final check- verifying the prepared impurity spiked solution concentration in the spiked test solution.

We'll use the following formula to confirm the result:

$$\text{Conc of resulted solution (ppm)} = A \times \frac{B}{C} \times \frac{D}{E} + F$$

Where:

- A = Impurity stock concentration (ppm)
- B = Volume of the impurity stock (mL)
- C = Test stock dilution volume (mL)
- D = Test stock pipetted volume (mL)
- E = Further test solution dilution volume (mL)
- F = Amount of impurity present in unspiked sample (ppm)

Let us calculate resulted concentration of impurity A in spiked sample

$$\text{Conc of resulted solution (ppm) of imp A} = \left[200\ \text{ppm} \times \frac{10\ \text{mL}}{100\ \text{mL}} \times \frac{5\ \text{mL}}{50\ \text{mL}}\right] + 0.5\ \text{ppm} = 2.5\ \text{ppm}$$

Where:

- A= Impurity A stock concentration = 200 ppm *(cell H90 from Fig. 16)*
- B= Volume taken from the stock = 10 mL *(cell M90 from Fig. 20)*
- C= Test stock dilution volume = 100 mL *(cell N90 from Fig. 20)*
- D= Test stock pipetted volume = 5 mL *(cell O90 from Fig. 20)*
- E= Further test solution dilution volume = 50 mL *(cell P90 from fig. 20)*
- F= Amount of impurity present in unspiked sample = 0.5 ppm *(cell J90 from Fig. 18)*

Target concentration for impurity A = 2.50 ppm *(cell C90 from Fig. 18)*

Conclusion:

The resulted concentration of Impurity A matches the expected value. Therefore, the selected Impurity A stock solution and the proposed dilution are appropriate and accurate.

Similarly, you can calculate the resulted concentration for impurity B

- A= Impurity B stock concentration = ____________________
- B= Volume taken from the stock = ____________________
- C= Test stock dilution volume = ____________________
- D= Test stock pipetted volume = ____________________
- E= Further test solution dilution volume = ____________________
- F= Amount of impurity present in unspiked sample = ____________________
- Target concentration for impurity B = ____________________

Conc of resulted solution (ppm) of imp B =

Conclusion:

Fig. 20: Excel sheet screenshot for resulted impurity concentration calculation

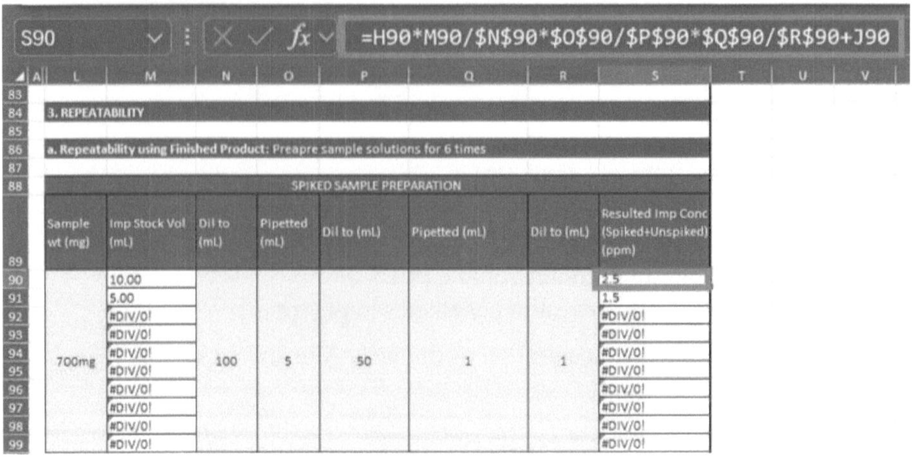

S90 =H90*M90/$N$90*$O$90/$P$90*$Q$90/$R$90+J90

3. REPEATABILITY

a. Repeatability using Finished Product: Preapre sample solutions for 6 times

SPIKED SAMPLE PREPARATION							
Sample wt (mg)	Imp Stock Vol (mL)	Dil to (mL)	Pipetted (mL)	Dil to (mL)	Pipetted (mL)	Dil to (mL)	Resulted Imp Conc (Spiked+Unspiked) (ppm)
700mg	10.00	100	5	50	1	1	2.5
	5.00						1.5
	#DIV/0!						#DIV/0!
	#DIV/0!						#DIV/0!
	#DIV/0!						#DIV/0!
	#DIV/0!						#DIV/0!
	#DIV/0!						#DIV/0!
	#DIV/0!						#DIV/0!
	#DIV/0!						#DIV/0!
	#DIV/0!						#DIV/0!

4.3.2 Preparation of repeatability solutions using (API + Placebo):

If the test sample is unavailable or unsuitable, you can use a combination of placebo and API based on the product's composition. The first step involves accurately weighing the required quantities of placebo and API to prepare the sample. From there, the procedure follows the same steps as described earlier for "Repeatability Using Finished Product."

Fig. 21: Excel sheet screenshot for repeatability using API + Placebo

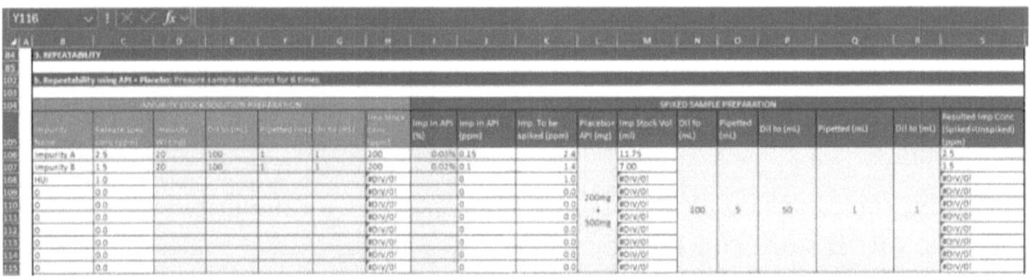

3. REPEATABILITY

b. Repeatability using API + Placebo: Preapre sample solutions for 6 times

IMPURITY STOCK SOLUTION PREPARATION							SPIKED SAMPLE PREPARATION										
Impurity Name	Release spec conc (ppm)	Impurity Wt (mg)	Dil to (mL)	Pipetted (mL)	Dil to (mL)	Imp Stock Conc (ppm)	Imp in API (%)	Imp in API (ppm)	Imp. To be spiked (ppm)	Placebo+API (mg)	Imp Stock Vol (ml)	Dil to (mL)	Pipetted (mL)	Dil to (mL)	Pipetted (mL)	Dil to (mL)	Resulted Imp Conc (Spiked+Unspiked) (ppm)
Impurity A	2.5	20	100	1	1	200	0.03%	0.15	2.4	200mg + 500mg	11.75	100	5	50	1	1	2.5
Impurity B	1.5	20	100	1	1	200	0.02%	0.1	1.4		7.00						1.5
HUI	1.0					#DIV/0!		0	1.0		#DIV/0!						#DIV/0!
0	0.0					#DIV/0!		0	0.0		#DIV/0!						#DIV/0!
0	0.0					#DIV/0!		0	0.0		#DIV/0!						#DIV/0!
0	0.0					#DIV/0!		0	0.0		#DIV/0!						#DIV/0!
0	0.0					#DIV/0!		0	0.0		#DIV/0!						#DIV/0!
0	0.0					#DIV/0!		0	0.0		#DIV/0!						#DIV/0!
0	0.0					#DIV/0!		0	0.0		#DIV/0!						#DIV/0!
0	0.0					#DIV/0!		0	0.0		#DIV/0!						#DIV/0!

The screenshot above may not be very clear to read, so I will explain it step by step below.

i. Preparation of the Impurity Stock Solution: Individual impurity stock solutions are prepared for spiking in test solution. In the given example impurity A and impurity B stock solution is prepared at 200 ppm concentration.

- Impurity A stock solution concentration: 200 ppm *(cell H106 from Fig. 22)*
- Impurity B stock solution concentration: 200 ppm *(cell H107 from Fig. 22)*

Fig. 22: Excel sheet screenshot for impurity stock preparation to be used for (API + Placebo) spiked test preparation.

	A	B	C	D	E	F	G	H
84		3. REPEATABILITY						
85								
102		b. Repeatability using API + Placebo: Preapre sample solutions for 6 times						
103								
104		IMPURITY STOCK SOLUTION PREPARATION						
105		Impurity Name	Release Spec conc (ppm)	Impurity Wt (mg)	Dil to (mL)	Pipetted (mL)	Dil to (mL)	Imp Stock Conc (ppm)
106		Impurity A	2.5	20	100	1	1	200
107		Impurity B	1.5	20	100	1	1	200
108		HUI	1.0					#DIV/0!
109		0	0.0					#DIV/0!
110		0	0.0					#DIV/0!
111		0	0.0					#DIV/0!
112		0	0.0					#DIV/0!
113		0	0.0					#DIV/0!
114		0	0.0					#DIV/0!
115		0	0.0					#DIV/0!

ii. Preparation of Impurity Spiked (API + Placebo) Solution for Repeatability:

This section of the Excel sheet outlines the process for preparing impurity spiked 'API + Placebo' solutions at the desired concentrations (at the impurity release specification). It involves three key steps:

Step 1: Calculation of the impurity conc. (in ppm) present in unspiked test sample (API + Placebo)

Step 2: Calculation of the impurity to be spiked for preparation of impurity spiked (API + Placebo) repeatability solution

Step 3: Calculation of impurity stock volume to be spiked in (API + Placebo) repeatability solution

Step 4: Verification of the resulted spiked impurity concentration in (API + Placebo) repeatability solution

Follow above procedure as we followed during "Repeatability Using Finished Product."

Fig. 23: Excel sheet screenshot for impurity spiked preparations using (API + Placebo) for repeatability

	A	I	J	K	L	M	N	O	P	Q	R	S
83												
84		3. REPEATABILITY										
85												
102		b. Repeatability using API + Placebo: Preapre sample solutions for 6 times										
103												
104		SPIKED SAMPLE PREPARATION										
105		Imp in API (%)	Imp in API (ppm)	Imp. To be spiked (ppm)	Placebo+ API (mg)	Imp Stock Vol (ml)	Dil to (mL)	Pipetted (mL)	Dil to (mL)	Pipetted (mL)	Dil to (mL)	Resulted Imp Conc (Spiked+Unspiked) (ppm)
106		0.03%	0.15	2.4	200mg + 500mg	11.75	100	5	50	1	1	2.5
107		0.02%	0.1	1.4		7.00						1.5
108			0	1.0		#DIV/0!						#DIV/0!
109			0	0.0		#DIV/0!						#DIV/0!
110			0	0.0		#DIV/0!						#DIV/0!
111			0	0.0		#DIV/0!						#DIV/0!
112			0	0.0		#DIV/0!						#DIV/0!
113			0	0.0		#DIV/0!						#DIV/0!
114			0	0.0		#DIV/0!						#DIV/0!
115			0	0.0		#DIV/0!						#DIV/0!

In this case, the impurity levels present in the API are considered as the baseline impurity levels in the unspiked sample (impurity A at 0.03% and impurity B at 0.02%). (Refer cell I106 and I107 from fig 23). These values are then converted to ppm impurity A corresponds to 2.4 ppm and impurity B to 1.4 ppm. (Refer cell K106, and K107 from fig 23).

Next, the volumes of impurity stock solutions required to achieve the target concentrations in the 'API + Placebo' mixture are calculated. A test sample is prepared by weighing 200 mg of placebo and 500 mg of API (Paracetamol). To this, 11.75 mL of impurity A stock and 7.00 mL of impurity B stock are added. (Refer cell M106, and M107 from fig 23).

As a result, the final concentrations achieved in the (API + Placebo) sample are 2.5 ppm for impurity A and 1.5 ppm for impurity B. (Refer cell S106 and S107 from fig 23). These values match the expected target concentrations, confirming the accuracy of the spiking procedure.

4.3.3. Preparation of repeatability solutions for unknown impurity:

The unknown impurity refers to any unidentified impurity present in a given sample. Since it is unknown, a specific reference standard for it is not available. Therefore, the API itself is used as a surrogate standard for the unknown impurity, assuming that the impurity is structurally related to the API. Repeatability for unknown impurity is evaluated by preparing an API solution at the concentration specified for the highest unknown impurity (HUI) limit.

Fig. 24: Excel sheet screenshot for 'preparation for unknown impurity repeatability solutions'

3. REPEATABILITY

c. Preparation for HUI repeatability solutions

	API STOCK SOLUTION PREPARATION							SPIKED SAMPLE PREPARATION							
	API Name	Release Spec conc (ppm)	API Wt (mg)	Dil to (mL)	Pipetted (mL)	Dil to (mL)	API Stock Conc (ppm)	Placebo Wt (mg)	API Stock Vol (ml)	Dil to (mL)	Pipetted (mL)	Dil to (mL)	Pipetted (mL)	Dil to (mL)	Resulted Imp Conc (Spiked) (ppm)
123	Paracetamol	1.0	50	100	1	1	500	200mg	2.00	100	5	50	1	1	1.0
124							#DIV/0!		#DIV/0!						#DIV/0!
125							#DIV/0!		#DIV/0!						#DIV/0!
126							#DIV/0!		#DIV/0!						#DIV/0!
127							#DIV/0!		#DIV/0!						#DIV/0!
128							#DIV/0!		#DIV/0!						#DIV/0!
129							#DIV/0!		#DIV/0!						#DIV/0!
130							#DIV/0!		#DIV/0!						#DIV/0!
131							#DIV/0!		#DIV/0!						#DIV/0!
132							#DIV/0!		#DIV/0!						#DIV/0!

The screenshot above may not be very clear to read, so I will explain it step by step below.

The specification for the Highest Unknown Impurity (HUI) is 0.20% in percentage terms, which corresponds to 1.0 ppm with respect to 500 ppm API concentration. Therefore, in the repeatability study for unknown impurity, the target concentration of the API should be 1.0 ppm. To achieve this, the placebo (as present in the actual test sample) is weighed and combined with an appropriate quantity of API to prepare a solution with the desired concentration.

Before preparing the unknown impurity/HUI repeatability solution, a suitable API stock solution should be prepared. As shown in Fig. 25, a 500 ppm API stock solution is used for this purpose (cell H123 from Fig. 25).

Fig. 25: Please check excel sheet screenshot for 'preparation of API stock solution'

H123 | fx | =D123/E123*F123/G123*1000

3. REPEATABILITY

c. Preparation for HUI repeatability solutions

	API STOCK SOLUTION PREPARATION						
122	API Name	Release Spec conc (ppm)	API Wt (mg)	Dil to (mL)	Pipetted (mL)	Dil to (mL)	API Stock Conc (ppm)
123	Paracetamol	1.0	50	100	1	1	500
124							#DIV/0!
125							#DIV/0!
126							#DIV/0!
127							#DIV/0!
128							#DIV/0!
129							#DIV/0!
130							#DIV/0!
131							#DIV/0!
132							#DIV/0!

The required volume of the 500 ppm API stock solution is calculated as illustrated in Fig. 26. Based on the calculation, 2 mL of the API stock solution (cell K123 from Fig. 26) and 200 mg of placebo are needed. These quantities are processed according to the test sample preparation procedure.

As a confirmatory step, the resulted concentration of API in the prepared solution is calculated and found to be 1.0 ppm (cell Q123 from Fig. 26), which aligns with the expected concentration for the HUI repeatability study.

Fig. 26: Excel sheet screenshot for 'resulted impurity conc in spiked sample'

K123 — fx =C123*$P$123/$O$123*$N$123/$M$123*$L$123/H123

3. REPEATABILITY

c. Preparation for HUI repeatability solutions

Row	SPIKED SAMPLE PREPARATION							
122	Placebo Wt. (mg)	API Stock Vol (ml)	Dil to (mL)	Pipetted (mL)	Dil to (mL)	Pipetted (mL)	Dil to (mL)	Resulted Imp Conc (Spiked) (ppm)
123		2.00						1.0
124		#DIV/0!						#DIV/0!
125		#DIV/0!						#DIV/0!
126		#DIV/0!						#DIV/0!
127	200mg	#DIV/0!	100	5	50	1	1	#DIV/0!
128		#DIV/0!						#DIV/0!
129		#DIV/0!						#DIV/0!
130		#DIV/0!						#DIV/0!
131		#DIV/0!						#DIV/0!
132		#DIV/0!						#DIV/0!

4.2 Response/linearity:

In the current example, the linearity study is conducted from the LOQ, 50% level up to 150%, ensuring that it covers both release and shelf-life specifications. It must be performed for each known impurity as well as for unknown impurities. Since a reference standard for unknown impurities is not available, the API is used as a surrogate.

To systematically design the linearity concentration matrix, follow these key steps:

Step 1: Preparation of linearity stock solutions

Step 2: Calculation of lowest and highest linearity level concentration

Step 3: Calculation of expected concentration across various linearity levels

Step 4: Preparation of linearity solutions

Step 5: Verification of resulted solution at various linearity levels

Begin by preparing a linearity stock solution at a concentration higher than the highest level required. Ideally, prepare a combined stock containing both the known impurity and API. This approach minimizes pipetting steps and simplifies the preparation of multiple linearity levels.

Once the stock solution is ready, prepare individual linearity samples through dilution using calculated volumes.

The final and crucial step is to verify the resulted concentration of each prepared solution to ensure they meet the expected linearity levels.

Step 1: Preparation of linearity stock solutions:

Please refer to Fig. 27 for preparation of linearity stock solution for known and unknown impurity. The API is used for preparation of linearity stock for unknown impurity (cell B141 from Fig 27).

Conc. of linearity stock can be calculated by the below formula

$$\text{Conc of linearity stock (ppm)} = \frac{\text{Impurity wt. (mg)}}{\text{Dilution vol (mL)}} \times \frac{\text{Purity in \%}}{100} \times 1000$$

Let us calculate the conc. of impurity A linearity stock by using the above formula

$$\text{Conc of impurity A linearity stock (ppm)} = \frac{12.5\ mg}{100\ mL} \times \frac{100\ \%}{100} \times 1000 = 1.25\ ppm$$

Impurity A weight for stock preparation: 125 mg *(cell E139 from Fig. 27)*
Impurity A stock dilution volume: 100 mL *(cell F139 from Fig. 27)*
Impurity A purity = 100 % *(cell L28 from Fig. 4)*

Similarly calculate the conc. of linearity stock for Impurity B and unknown impurity

$$\text{Conc of impurity B linearity stock (ppm)} = \frac{\dots\dots\dots\ mg}{\text{---------}\ mL} \times \text{----------------} \times 1000 = \dots\dots\dots\dots ppm$$

$$\text{Conc of unknown impurity stock (ppm)} = \frac{\dots\dots\dots\ mg}{\text{----------}\ mL} \times \text{--------------} \times 1000 = \dots\dots\dots\dots\ ppm$$

Fig. 27: Excel sheet screenshot for 'preparation of linearity stock'

K139 =E139/F139*G139/H139*I139/J139*L28/100*1000

4. RESPONSE/LINEARITY

	Linearity Stock Preparations									
138	Impurity Name	Release Spec conc (ppm)	Stability Spec conc (ppm)	Std. Wt (mg)	Dil to (mL)	Pipetted (mL)	Dil to (mL)	Pipetted (mL)	Dil to (mL)	Conc (ppm)
139	Impurity A	2.5	5.0	12.5	100	1	1	1	1	125
140	Impurity B	1.5	3.0	7.5	100	1	1	1	1	75
141	Unk. Imp	1.0	1.0	5	100	1	1	1	1	50
142	0	0.0	0.0							#DIV/0!
143	0	0.0	0.0							#DIV/0!
144	0	0.0	0.0							#DIV/0!
145	0	0.0	0.0							#DIV/0!
146	0	0.0	0.0							#DIV/0!
147	0	0.0	0.0							#DIV/0!
148	0	0.0	0.0							#DIV/0!
149	0	0.0	0.0							#DIV/0!

Step 2: Calculation of lowest and highest linearity level concentration:

The linearity in case of related substances must cover reporting level or QL/LOQ

(Quantitation Limit) to minimum 120% of stability specification concentration (refer, ICH Q2(R2). However, in the current example, we will cover linearity level from LOQ, 50% to 150% level.

The first step is to calculate the concentration of a specific impurity at specified linearity level.

$$\textit{Impurity conc at specified level (ppm)} = \frac{\textit{Impurity conc in ppm at the specified level x linearity level}}{100}$$

Let us now calculate the Impurity A conc in ppm at lowest level- 50% and highest level- 150%. Please note that the actual lowest level is LOQ in this case, but as we don't have LOQ value in hand, we have considered 50% as the measurable lowest level.

$$\textit{Impurity A conc. in ppm at 50\% of release spec} = \frac{2.5 \textit{ ppm x } 50}{100} = 1.25 \textit{ ppm}$$

Impurity A conc. in ppm at release spec: 2.5 ppm *(refer cell C139, Fig. 27)*
Lowest level for which conc is to be measured: 50% *(refer cell N139, Fig. 28)*
Similarly, calculate the lowest and highest concentration for other impurities and tabulate below

Table 9: Lowest and highest concentration of impurities for linearity

Name of impurities	**Lowest level**	**Highest level**	**Lowest level conc w.r.t release spec**	**Highest level conc w.r.t shelf-life spec**
Impurity A	50%	150%	1.25 ppm	---------- ppm
Impurity B	50%	150%	---------- ppm	---------- ppm
HUI	50%	150%	---------- ppm	---------- ppm

Fig. 28: Excel sheet screenshot for 'calculation of lowest and highest-level conc.'

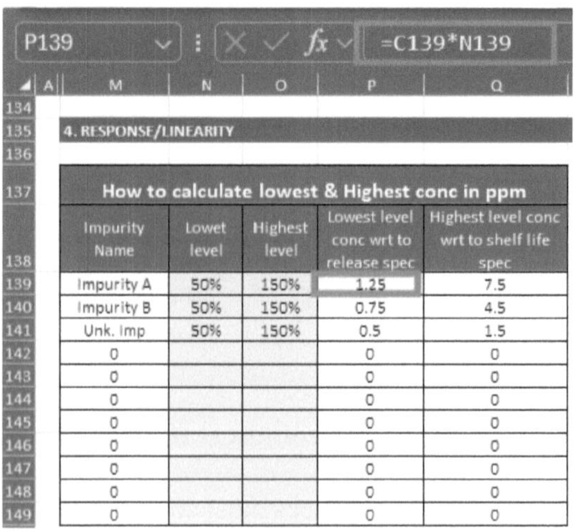

P139 =C139*N139

4. RESPONSE/LINEARITY

How to calculate lowest & Highest conc in ppm

Impurity Name	Lowet level	Highest level	Lowest level conc wrt to release spec	Highest level conc wrt to shelf life spec
Impurity A	50%	150%	1.25	7.5
Impurity B	50%	150%	0.75	4.5
Unk. Imp	50%	150%	0.5	1.5
0			0	0
0			0	0
0			0	0
0			0	0
0			0	0
0			0	0
0			0	0
0			0	0

Step 3: Calculation of expected concentration across various linearity levels:

Once the lowest and highest concentrations for each impurity are identified across the linearity range, the next step is to select a minimum of five concentration levels, including the LOQ.

In this example, we have chosen to study seven linearity levels. Since the exact LOQ value will be determined during the method validation, the concentration for the LOQ level is currently left blank.

If you refer to Figure 29, you'll notice that the linearity levels are not listed as 50% to 150% instead, they range from 50% to 300%. At first glance, this might seem like a typo, but it's not.
Here's why:

The percentage linearity levels are calculated based on the release specification concentration. For instance, if the release specification for Impurity A is 2.5 ppm, then 150% of this would be 3.75 ppm.

However, in this case, we aim to cover 150% of the shelf-life specification (5 ppm), which might be 7.5 ppm. When you compare this 7.5 ppm against the release specification (2.5 ppm), it actually corresponds to 300% of the release spec.

So, the 300% level you see in the table or figure is not an error it's simply a reflection of how the linearity levels are scaled based on the release specification as the reference point.

So, while it may appear unusual, this method ensures you're evaluating the method across the entire range from LOQ all the way to the highest specification limit, covering both release and shelf-life requirements.
Let us now calculate the expected impurity concentration at various linearity levels.

$$\text{Expected impurity conc. (ppm)} = \frac{\text{Linearity level in (\%) x conc. at release specification in (ppm)}}{100}$$

Let us calculate the expected concentration for impurity A at 50% linearity level

$$\text{Expected impurity A conc. (ppm) at 50\% level} = \frac{50\ \%\ x\ 2.5\ ppm}{100} = 1.25\ ppm$$

Linearity level in (%) for impurity A = 50 % *(Refer cell B155 from Fig. 29)*
Impurity A conc. at release specification = 2.5 ppm *(Refer cell C139 from Fig. 27)*

Similarly, calculate the concentration for impurity A, impurity B, and unknown impurity at other levels and tabulate below.

Table 10: Expected impurity concentration across various linearity levels.

	Expected impurity conc. in ppm		
Linearity Level	Impurity A	Impurity B	Unknown impurity
LOQ			
50%	1.25 ppm		
75%			
100%			
125%			
150%			
300%			

Fig. 29: Excel sheet screenshot for 'calculation of expected impurity conc. across linearity levels'

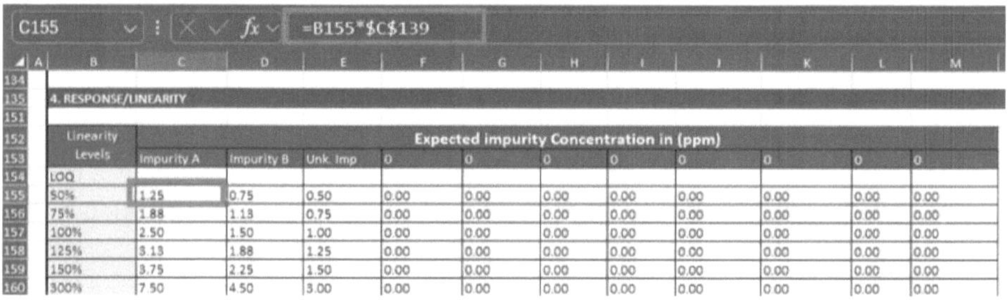
C155 =B155*$C$139

4. RESPONSE/LINEARITY

Linearity Levels	Expected impurity Concentration in (ppm)										
	Impurity A	Impurity B	Unk. Imp	0	0	0	0	0	0	0	0
LOQ											
50%	1.25	0.75	0.50	0.00	0.00	0.00	0.00	0.00	0.00	0.00	0.00
75%	1.88	1.13	0.75	0.00	0.00	0.00	0.00	0.00	0.00	0.00	0.00
100%	2.50	1.50	1.00	0.00	0.00	0.00	0.00	0.00	0.00	0.00	0.00
125%	3.13	1.88	1.25	0.00	0.00	0.00	0.00	0.00	0.00	0.00	0.00
150%	3.75	2.25	1.50	0.00	0.00	0.00	0.00	0.00	0.00	0.00	0.00
300%	7.50	4.50	3.00	0.00	0.00	0.00	0.00	0.00	0.00	0.00	0.00

Step 4: Preparation of linearity solutions:

Once we have identified the expected linearity concentrations, the next step is to prepare the linearity solutions. These can be prepared using the linearity stock solutions as outlined in Fig. 27. The concentrations of the linearity stock solutions are as follows: 125 ppm for Impurity A, 75 ppm for Impurity B, and 50 ppm for the unknown impurity. (Refer cell K139, K140, K141, Fig. 27).

As discussed earlier, the API will serve as a surrogate for the unknown impurity. Therefore, a 50 ppm API stock solution will be sufficient for preparing the unknown impurity linearity levels.

Use the formula below to prepare the linearity solutions at the desired concentrations.

$$\textit{Volume of linearity stock (mL)} = \frac{A}{B} \times C \times \frac{D}{E}$$

- A = Expected impurity concentration in ppm
- B = Concentration of Impurity stock in ppm
- C = Dilution volume of impurity stock solution in mL
- D = Further dilution in mL
- E = Pipetted volume in mL

Let us calculate the volume of impurity A stock required for preparation of linearity level 50%

$$\text{Volume of Impurity A linearity stock (mL) for 50\% level} = \frac{A}{B} \times C \times \frac{D}{E}$$

A= Expected impurity concentration in ppm = 1.25 ppm *(Refer cell C155, Fig. 29)*
B= Concentration of Impurity stock in ppm = 125 ppm *(Refer cell K139, Fig. 27)*
C = Dilution volume of impurity stock solution in mL = 100 mL (Refer cell N167, Fig. 30)
D= Further dilution in mL = 50 mL *(Refer cell P167, Fig. 30)*
E= Pipetted volume in mL = 10 mL *(Refer cell O167, Fig. 30)*

$$\text{Volume of Impurity A linearity stock (mL) for 50\% level} = \frac{1.25\ ppm}{125\ ppm} \times 100\ mL \times \frac{50\ mL}{10\ mL} = 5\ mL$$

Similarly calculate the volume of impurity A linearity stock, impurity B linearity stock, unknown impurity linearity stock for the rest of the linearity levels and tabulate below

Table 11: Impurity stock volume to be taken across various linearity levels.

	Impurity stock volume to be taken in mL		
Linearity Level	Impurity A linearity stock	Impurity B linearity stock	Unknown impurity linearity stock
LOQ			
50%	5 mL		
75%			
100%			
125%			
150%			
300%			

Fig. 30: Excel sheet screenshot for 'preparation of linearity solutions'

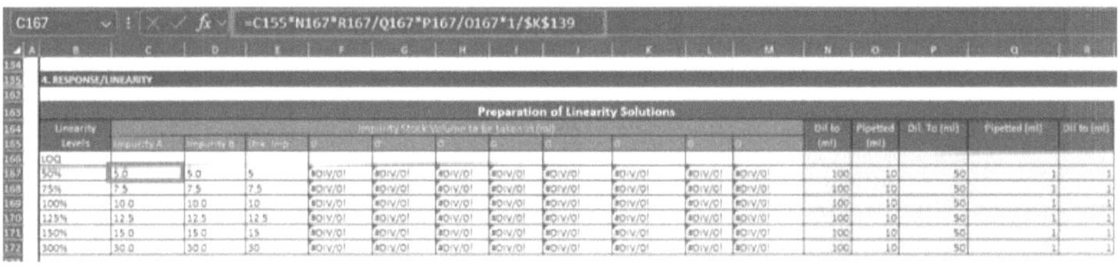

Step 5: Verification of concentration of resulted solution at various linearity levels:

The final step is to confirm whether the expected linearity concentrations are achieved using the prepared stock solutions and their respective dilutions. The resulting impurity concentration can be calculated using the formula below.

$$\text{Resulted conc (ppm)} = A \times \frac{B}{C} \times \frac{D}{E}$$

Where:

- A= Concentration of Impurity stock in ppm
- B = Volume of Impurity A linearity stock (mL)
- C = Dilution volume of impurity stock solution in mL
- D = Pipetted volume in mL
- E = Further dilution in mL

Let us calculate the resulted conc. of impurity A at linearity level 50%

$$\text{Resulted conc (ppm) of Impurity A at 50\% linearity} = 125 \text{ ppm} \times \frac{5 \text{ mL}}{100 \text{ mL}} \times \frac{10 \text{ mL}}{50 \text{ mL}} = 1.25 \text{ ppm}$$

A= Concentration of Impurity stock in ppm = 125 ppm *(Cell K139, Fig. 27)*
B = Volume of Impurity A linearity stock (mL) = 5 mL *(Cell C167, Fig. 30)*
C = Dilution volume of impurity stock solution in mL = 100 mL *(Cell N167, Fig. 30)*
D= Pipetted volume in mL = 10 mL *(Cell O167, Fig. 30)*
E= Further dilution in mL = 50 mL *(Cell P167, Fig. 30)*

Conclusion:

The resulting concentration of Impurity A at the 50% level *(Refer Cell C177, Fig. 31)* matches the expected value of 1.25 ppm *(Refer Cell C155, Fig. 29)*.
Similarly, calculate the resulted concentration for impurity A, impurity B, and unknown impurity and tabulate below
Table 12: Impurity stock volume to be taken across various linearity levels.

	Resulted concentration of impurity in ppm		
Linearity Level	Impurity A conc	Impurity B conc	Unknown impurity conc
LOQ			
50%	1.25 ppm		
75%			
100%			
125%			
150%			
300%			

Fig. 31: Excel sheet screenshot for 'calculation of resulted impurity conc. across linearity levels'

C177 =$K$139*C167/N167*O167/P167*Q167/R167

4. RESPONSE/LINEARITY

Linearity Levels	Resulted Concentration of Impurities in ppm										
	Impurity A	Impurity B	Unk. Imp	0	0	0	0	0	0	0	0
LOQ											
50%	1.25	0.75	0.50	#DIV/0!	#DIV/0!	#DIV/0!	#DIV/0!	#DIV/0!	#DIV/0!	#DIV/0!	#DIV/0!
75%	1.88	1.13	0.75	#DIV/0!	#DIV/0!	#DIV/0!	#DIV/0!	#DIV/0!	#DIV/0!	#DIV/0!	#DIV/0!
100%	2.50	1.50	1.00	#DIV/0!	#DIV/0!	#DIV/0!	#DIV/0!	#DIV/0!	#DIV/0!	#DIV/0!	#DIV/0!
125%	3.13	1.88	1.25	#DIV/0!	#DIV/0!	#DIV/0!	#DIV/0!	#DIV/0!	#DIV/0!	#DIV/0!	#DIV/0!
150%	3.75	2.25	1.50	#DIV/0!	#DIV/0!	#DIV/0!	#DIV/0!	#DIV/0!	#DIV/0!	#DIV/0!	#DIV/0!
300%	7.50	4.50	3.00	#DIV/0!	#DIV/0!	#DIV/0!	#DIV/0!	#DIV/0!	#DIV/0!	#DIV/0!	#DIV/0!

4.3 Accuracy:

We are going to prepare concentration matrix for below accuracy solutions

4.3.1 Accuracy using drug product/test sample

4.3.2 Accuracy using (API + Placebo)

4.3.2 Accuracy for unknown impurity

4.3.1 Accuracy using drug product/test sample

To systematically design the accuracy concentration matrix using drug product, follow these key steps:

Step 1: Preparation of accuracy stock solutions

Step 2: Calculation of lowest and highest accuracy level concentration

Step 3: Calculation of expected concentration across various accuracy levels

Step 4: Preparation of accuracy solutions by using test sample

Step 5: Verification of concentration of resulted solution at various accuracy levels

Let us discuss each step in detail

Step 1: Preparation of accuracy stock solutions:

Please refer Fig. 32 for preparation of accuracy stock solution for known and unknown impurity.

Conc. of accuracy stock can be calculated by the formula below

$$\text{Conc of accuracy stock (ppm)} = \frac{\text{Impurity wt. (mg)}}{\text{Dilution vol (mL)}} \times \frac{\text{Purity (\%)}}{100} \times 1000$$

Concentration of impurity A accuracy stock = 250 ppm *(Refer cell K189, Fig. 32)*

Concentration of impurity B accuracy stock = 150 ppm *(Refer cell K190,, Fig. 32)*

Fig. 32: Excel sheet screenshot for 'preparation of accuracy stock'

5. ACCURACY

Accuracy Stock Preparations

	Impurity Name	Release Spec conc (ppm)	Shelf life Spec conc (ppm)	Wt (mg)	Dil to (mL)	Pipetted (mL)	Dil to (mL)	Pipetted (mL)	Dil to (mL)	Conc (ppm)
189	Impurity A	2.5	5.0	12.5	50	1	1	1	1	250
190	Impurity B	1.5	3.0	7.5	50	1	1	1	1	150
191	Unk. Imp	1.0	1.0							#DIV/0!
192	0	0.0	0.0							#DIV/0!
193	0	0.0	0.0							#DIV/0!
194	0	0.0	0.0							#DIV/0!
195	0	0.0	0.0							#DIV/0!
196	0	0.0	0.0							#DIV/0!
197	0	0.0	0.0							#DIV/0!
198	0	0.0	0.0							#DIV/0!
199	0	0.0	0.0							#DIV/0!

Step 2: Calculation of lowest and highest accuracy level concentration

The accuracy in case of related substances, must cover reporting level or QL/LOQ (Quantitation Limit) to minimum 120% of stability specification concentration (ICH Q2(R2). However, in the current example, we will cover linearity level from LOQ, 50% to 150% level. The first step is to calculate the concentration of a specific impurity at its release spec and shelf-life specification in ppm.

$$\textit{Impurity conc at specified level (ppm)} = \frac{\textit{Impurity conc in ppm at the specified level x linearity level}}{100}$$

Let us calculate Impurity A conc. in ppm at 50% of release specification by using above formula

$$\textit{Impurity A conc. in ppm at 50\% of release spec} = \frac{2.5 \textit{ ppm x } 50}{100} = 1.25 \textit{ ppm}$$

Where:

- Impurity A conc. in ppm at release spec = 2.5 ppm *(Refer cell C189, Fig. 32)*
- Linearity level for which conc is to be measured = 50% Refer *(cell N189, Fig. 33)*

Calculate the lowest and highest concentration for other impurities and tabulate below

Table 13: Lowest and highest concentration of impurities for accuracy

Name of impurities	Lowest level	Highest level	Lowest level conc w.r.t release spec	Highest level conc w.r.t shelf-life spec
Impurity A	50%	150%		
Impurity B	50%	150%		

Fig. 33: Excel sheet screenshot for 'calculation of lowest and highest conc. in ppm'

P189 | fx =C189*N189

	M	N	O	P	Q
185	5. ACCURACY				
186					
187	How to calculate lowest & Highest conc in ppm				
188	Impurity Name	Lowet level	Highest level	Lowest level conc wrt to release spec	Highest level conc wrt to shelf life spec
189	Impurity A	50%	150%	1.25	7.5
190	Impurity B	50%	150%	0.75	4.5
191	Unk. Imp			0	0
192	0			0	0
193	0			0	0
194	0			0	0
195	0			0	0
196	0			0	0
197	0			0	0
198	0			0	0
199	0			0	0

Step 3: Calculation of expected concentration across various accuracy levels

Once the lowest and highest concentrations for each impurity are identified across the accuracy levels, the next step is to select a minimum of 3 concentration levels, including the LOQ.

In this example, we have chosen to study 7 accuracy levels. Since the exact LOQ value will be determined during the method validation, the concentration for the LOQ level is currently left blank.

If you refer to Figure 34, you'll notice that the linearity levels are not listed as 50% to 150% instead, they range from 50% to 300%. (Please refer to the linearity section for the discussion)

Let us now calculate the expected impurity concentration at various accuracy levels.

$$\textit{Expected impurity conc. (ppm)} = \frac{\textit{Accuracy level in (\%) x conc. at release specification in (ppm)}}{100}$$

Let us calculate the expected concentration for impurity A at 50% accuracy level

$$\textit{Expected impurity A conc. (ppm) at 50\% level} = \frac{50\ \%\ x\ 2.5\ ppm}{100} = 1.25\ ppm$$

Where:

- Accuracy level in (%) for impurity A = 50% *(Refer cell B205, Fig. 34)*
- Impurity A conc. at release specification = 2.5 ppm *(Refer cell C189, Fig 32)*

Similarly, calculate the concentration for impurity A, impurity B, and unknown impurity at other levels and tabulate below.

Table 14: Expected impurity concentration across various accuracy levels.

	Expected impurity conc. in ppm		
Linearity Level	Impurity A	Impurity B	Unknown impurity
LOQ			
50%	1.25 ppm		
75%			
100%			
125%			
150%			
300%			

Fig. 34: Excel sheet screenshot for 'calculation of expected impurity conc. across accuracy levels'

C205 | =B205*$C$189

5. ACCURACY

Accuracy Levels	Expected impurity Concentration in (ppm) across accuracy levels									
	Impurity A	Impurity B	Unk. Imp	0	0	0	0	0	0	0
LOQ										
50%	1.25	0.75	0.50	0.00	0.00	0.00	0.00	0.00	0.00	0.00
75%	1.88	1.13	0.75	0.00	0.00	0.00	0.00	0.00	0.00	0.00
100%	2.50	1.50	1.00	0.00	0.00	0.00	0.00	0.00	0.00	0.00
125%	3.13	1.88	1.25	0.00	0.00	0.00	0.00	0.00	0.00	0.00
150%	3.75	2.25	1.50	0.00	0.00	0.00	0.00	0.00	0.00	0.00
300%	7.50	4.50	3.00	0.00	0.00	0.00	0.00	0.00	0.00	0.00

Step 4: Accuracy using drug product/test sample:

Accuracy using the finished product can be evaluated by spiking the test solution with impurities at specific accuracy levels. In this example, impurities are spiked at their release specification levels 50%, 75%, 100%, 125%, 150%, and 300% along with the LOQ level. The required amount of impurity is added using the accuracy stock solution to achieve the target spiking concentration. Please ensure that all accuracy solutions are prepared by strictly following the 'test sample preparation' as defined in standard test procedure, using the exact quantity of test sample as defined.

Use the formula below to prepare the accuracy solutions at the desired concentrations by spiking accuracy stock solutions (for accuracy stock preparation- refer step 1).

$$\textit{Volume of accuracy stock (mL)} = \frac{A}{B} \times C \times \frac{D}{E}$$

Where;

- A = Expected impurity spiking concentration in ppm
- B = Concentration of Impurity stock in ppm
- C = Dilution volume of impurity stock solution in mL (It is nothing but the test stock preparation)
- D = Further dilution in mL
- E = Pipetted volume in mL

Let us calculate the volume of impurity A stock required for preparation of accuracy level 50%

$$\textit{Volume of Impurity A accuracy stock (mL) for 50\% level} = \frac{A}{B} \times C \times \frac{D}{E}$$

A = Expected impurity spiking concentration in ppm = 1.25 ppm *(Refer cell C205, Fig. 34)*
B = Concentration of Impurity stock in ppm = 250 ppm *(Refer cell K189, Fig. 32)*
C = Dilution volume of impurity stock solution in mL = 100 mL *(Refer cell N217, Fig. 35)*
D = Further dilution in mL = 50 mL *(Refer cell P217, Fig. 35)*
E = Pipetted volume in mL = 5 mL *(Refer cell O217, Fig. 35)*

$$\textit{Volume of Impurity A accuracy stock (mL) for 50\% level} = \frac{1.25}{250} \times 100 \times \frac{50}{5} = 5\ mL$$

Similarly, calculate the volume of impurity A accuracy stock, and impurity B accuracy stock for the rest of the accuracy levels and tabulate below

Table 15: Impurity stock volume to be taken across various accuracy levels.

Accuracy Level	Expected impurity conc. in ppm	
	Impurity A accuracy stock	Impurity B accuracy stock
LOQ		
50%	5 mL	
75%		
100%		
125%		
150%		
300%		

Fig. 35: Excel sheet screenshot for 'volume of impurity stock to be spiked across accuracy levels'

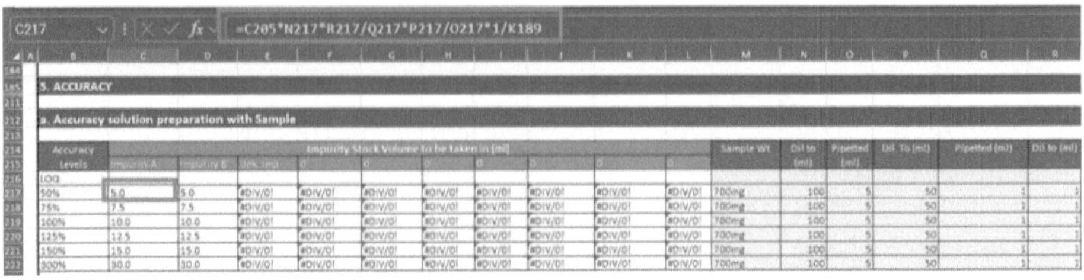

Accuracy Levels	Impurity Stock Volume to be taken in (ml)											Sample Wt	Dil to (ml)	Pipetted (ml)	Dil To (ml)	Pipetted (ml)	Dil to (ml)
	Impurity A	Impurity B	Unk. imp	0	0	0	0	0	0	0						
LOQ																
50%	5.0	5.0	#DIV/0!	#DIV/0!	#DIV/0!	#DIV/0!	#DIV/0!	#DIV/0!	#DIV/0!	#DIV/0!	700mg	100	5	50	1	1
75%	7.5	7.5	#DIV/0!	#DIV/0!	#DIV/0!	#DIV/0!	#DIV/0!	#DIV/0!	#DIV/0!	#DIV/0!	700mg	100	5	50	1	1
100%	10.0	10.0	#DIV/0!	#DIV/0!	#DIV/0!	#DIV/0!	#DIV/0!	#DIV/0!	#DIV/0!	#DIV/0!	700mg	100	5	50	1	1
125%	12.5	12.5	#DIV/0!	#DIV/0!	#DIV/0!	#DIV/0!	#DIV/0!	#DIV/0!	#DIV/0!	#DIV/0!	700mg	100	5	50	1	1
150%	15.0	15.0	#DIV/0!	#DIV/0!	#DIV/0!	#DIV/0!	#DIV/0!	#DIV/0!	#DIV/0!	#DIV/0!	700mg	100	5	50	1	1
300%	30.0	30.0	#DIV/0!	#DIV/0!	#DIV/0!	#DIV/0!	#DIV/0!	#DIV/0!	#DIV/0!	#DIV/0!	700mg	100	5	50	1	1

Step 5: Verification of concentration of resulted solution at various accuracy levels

The final step is to confirm whether the expected accuracy concentrations are achieved using the prepared stock solutions and their respective dilutions. The resulting impurity concentration can be calculated using the formula below.

$$\text{Resulted conc (ppm)} = A \times \frac{B}{C} \times \frac{D}{E}$$

Where:

- A = Concentration of Impurity stock in ppm
- B = Volume of Impurity A accuracy stock (mL)
- C = Dilution volume of impurity stock solution in mL (It is nothing but the test stock preparation)
- D = Pipetted volume in mL
- E = Further dilution in mL

Let us calculate the resulted conc. of impurity A at accuracy level 50%

$$\text{Resulted conc (ppm) of Impurity A at 50\% accuracy level} = 250 \times \frac{5}{100} \times \frac{5}{50} = 1.25 \text{ ppm}$$

A= Concentration of Impurity A stock in ppm = 250 ppm *(Refer cell K189, Fig. 32)*

B = Volume of Impurity A accuracy stock (mL) = 5 mL *(Refer cell C217, Fig. 35)*

C = Dilution volume of impurity A stock solution in mL = 100 mL *(Refer cell N217, Fig. 35)*

D= Pipetted volume in mL = 5 mL *(Refer cell O217, Fig. 35)*

E= Further dilution in mL = 50 mL *(Refer cell P217, Fig. 35)*

Conclusion:

The resulting concentration of Impurity A at the 50% level (refer Cell C227, Fig. 36) matches the expected value of 1.25 ppm (refer Cell C205, Fig. 34).

Similarly, calculate the resulted concentration for impurity A, and impurity B and tabulate below.

Table 16: Impurity stock volume to be taken across various accuracy levels.

Accuracy Level	Resulted concentration of impurity in ppm	
	Impurity A conc	Impurity B conc
LOQ		
50%	1.25 ppm	
75%		
100%		
125%		
150%		
300%		

Fig. 36: Excel sheet screenshot for 'calculation of resulted impurity conc. across accuracy levels'

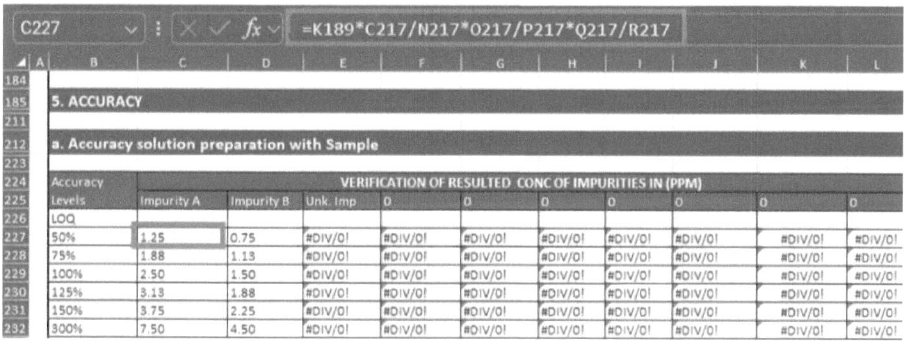
C227 =K189*C217/N217*O217/P217*Q217/R217

5. ACCURACY

a. Accuracy solution preparation with Sample

Accuracy Levels	VERIFICATION OF RESULTED CONC OF IMPURITIES IN (PPM)									
	Impurity A	Impurity B	Unk. Imp	0	0	0	0	0	0	0
LOQ										
50%	1.25	0.75	#DIV/0!	#DIV/0!	#DIV/0!	#DIV/0!	#DIV/0!	#DIV/0!	#DIV/0!	#DIV/0!
75%	1.88	1.13	#DIV/0!	#DIV/0!	#DIV/0!	#DIV/0!	#DIV/0!	#DIV/0!	#DIV/0!	#DIV/0!
100%	2.50	1.50	#DIV/0!	#DIV/0!	#DIV/0!	#DIV/0!	#DIV/0!	#DIV/0!	#DIV/0!	#DIV/0!
125%	3.13	1.88	#DIV/0!	#DIV/0!	#DIV/0!	#DIV/0!	#DIV/0!	#DIV/0!	#DIV/0!	#DIV/0!
150%	3.75	2.25	#DIV/0!	#DIV/0!	#DIV/0!	#DIV/0!	#DIV/0!	#DIV/0!	#DIV/0!	#DIV/0!
300%	7.50	4.50	#DIV/0!	#DIV/0!	#DIV/0!	#DIV/0!	#DIV/0!	#DIV/0!	#DIV/0!	#DIV/0!

4.3.2 Accuracy using (API + Placebo):

If the test sample is unavailable or unsuitable, you can use a combination of placebo and API based on the product's composition. The first step involves accurately weighing the required quantities of placebo and API to prepare the sample. From there, the procedure follows the same steps as described earlier for "Repeatability Using Finished Product."

To systematically design the accuracy concentration matrix using (API + Placebo), follow these key steps:

Step 1: Preparation of accuracy stock solutions

Step 2: Calculation of lowest and highest accuracy level concentration

Step 3: Calculation of expected concentration across various accuracy levels

Step 4: Preparation of accuracy solutions by using (API + Placebo)

Step 5: Verification of concentration of resulted solution at various accuracy levels

"Please note that Step 1, Step 2, and Step 3 will not be repeated here, as they are already included in the Excel sheet under section 4.3.1 (Accuracy using drug product/test sample).

Step 4: Preparation of accuracy solutions by using (API + Placebo)

Accuracy using (API + Placebo) can be evaluated by spiking the (API + Placebo) solution with impurities at specific accuracy levels. In this example, impurities are spiked at their release specification levels 50%, 75%, 100%, 125%, 150%, and 300% along with the LOQ level.

Note: Further, please follow the procedure as given under Step 4 from the "Accuracy using drug product/test sample" (4.3.1)

Use the formula below to prepare the accuracy solutions at the desired concentrations by spiking accuracy stock solutions *(refer step 1).*

$$\text{Volume of accuracy stock (mL)} = \frac{A}{B} \times C \times \frac{D}{E}$$

Where:
- A = Expected impurity spiking concentration in ppm
- B = Concentration of Impurity stock in ppm
- C = Dilution volume of impurity stock solution in mL
- D = Further dilution in mL
- E = Pipetted volume in mL

Let us calculate the volume of impurity A stock required for preparation of accuracy level 50%

$$\text{Volume of Impurity A accuracy stock (mL) for 50\% level} = \frac{A}{B} \times C \times \frac{D}{E}$$

A= Expected impurity spiking concentration in ppm = 1.25 ppm *(Refer cell C205, Fig. 34)*
B= Concentration of Impurity stock in ppm = 250 ppm *(Refer cell K189, Fig. 32)*
C = Dilution volume of impurity stock solution in mL = 100 mL *(Refer cell O241, Fig. 37)*
D= Further dilution in mL = 50 mL *(Refer cell Q241, Fig. 37)*
E= Pipetted volume in mL = 5 mL *(Refer cell P241, Fig. 37)*

$$\text{Volume of Impurity A accuracy stock (mL) for 50\% level} = \frac{1.25}{250} \times 100 \times \frac{50}{5} = 5 \text{ mL}$$

Calculate the volume of impurity A accuracy stock, and impurity B accuracy stock for the rest of the accuracy levels and tabulate below

Table 17: Impurity stock volume to be taken across various accuracy levels using 'API + Placebo'.

Accuracy Level	**Impurity stock volume to be taken in mL**	
	Impurity A accuracy stock	Impurity B accuracy stock
LOQ		
50%		
75%		
100%		
125%		
150%		
300%		

Fig. 37: Excel sheet screenshot for accuracy using API + Placebo

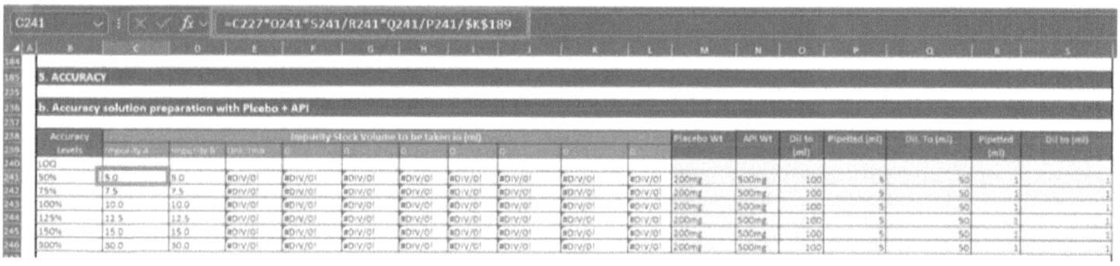

In this case, the impurity levels present in the API are considered as the impurity levels in the unspiked sample. The volumes of impurity stock solutions required to achieve the target concentrations in the 'API + Placebo' mixture is calculated. A test sample is prepared by weighing 200 mg of placebo and 500 mg of API (Paracetamol).

Step 5: Verification of concentration of resulted solution at various accuracy levels using API+ Placebo

The final step is to confirm whether the expected accuracy concentrations are achieved using the prepared stock solutions and their respective dilutions. The resulting impurity concentration can be calculated using the formula below.

$$Resulted\ conc\ (ppm) = A \times \frac{B}{C} \times \frac{D}{E}$$

Where:

- A = Concentration of Impurity stock in ppm
- B = Volume of Impurity A accuracy stock (mL)
- C = Dilution volume of impurity stock solution in mL
- D = Pipetted volume in mL
- E = Further dilution in mL

Let us calculate the resulted conc. of impurity A at accuracy level 50%

$$\text{Resulted conc (ppm) of Impurity A at 50\% accuracy level} = 250 \times \frac{5}{100} \times \frac{5}{50} = 1.25 \text{ ppm}$$

A= Concentration of Impurity stock in ppm = 250 ppm *(Refer cell K189, Fig. 32)*
B = Volume of Impurity Accuracy stock (mL) = 5 mL *(Refer cell C241, Fig. 37)*
C = Dilution volume of impurity stock solution in mL = 100 mL *(Refer cell O241, Fig. 37)*
D= Pipetted volume in mL = 5 mL *(Refer cell P241, Fig. 37)*
E= Further dilution in mL = 50 mL *(Refer cell Q241, Fig. 37)*

Conclusion:

The resulting concentration of Impurity A at the 50% level (refer cell C251, Fig. 38) matches the expected value of 1.25 ppm (refer cell C205, Fig. 34).
Similarly, calculate the resulted concentration for impurity A, and impurity B and tabulate below

Table 18: Impurity stock volume to be taken across various accuracy levels using 'API + Placebo'.

Accuracy Level	Resulted concentration of impurity in ppm	
	Impurity A conc	Impurity B conc
LOQ		
50%	1.25 ppm	
75%		
100%		
125%		
150%		
300%		

Fig. 38: Excel sheet screenshot for 'calculation of resulted impurity conc. across accuracy levels' with Placebo + API

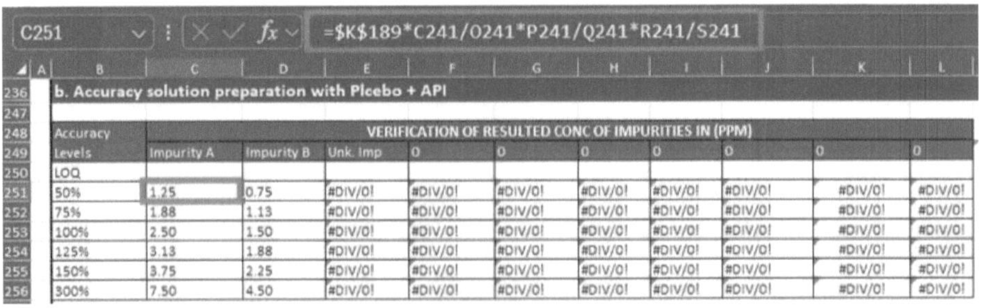

C251 =$K$189*C241/O241*P241/Q241*R241/S241

b. Accuracy solution preparation with Plcebo + API

Accuracy Levels	VERIFICATION OF RESULTED CONC OF IMPURITIES IN (PPM)									
	Impurity A	Impurity B	Unk. Imp	0	0	0	0	0	0	0
LOQ										
50%	1.25	0.75	#DIV/0!	#DIV/0!	#DIV/0!	#DIV/0!	#DIV/0!	#DIV/0!	#DIV/0!	#DIV/0!
75%	1.88	1.13	#DIV/0!	#DIV/0!	#DIV/0!	#DIV/0!	#DIV/0!	#DIV/0!	#DIV/0!	#DIV/0!
100%	2.50	1.50	#DIV/0!	#DIV/0!	#DIV/0!	#DIV/0!	#DIV/0!	#DIV/0!	#DIV/0!	#DIV/0!
125%	3.13	1.88	#DIV/0!	#DIV/0!	#DIV/0!	#DIV/0!	#DIV/0!	#DIV/0!	#DIV/0!	#DIV/0!
150%	3.75	2.25	#DIV/0!	#DIV/0!	#DIV/0!	#DIV/0!	#DIV/0!	#DIV/0!	#DIV/0!	#DIV/0!
300%	7.50	4.50	#DIV/0!	#DIV/0!	#DIV/0!	#DIV/0!	#DIV/0!	#DIV/0!	#DIV/0!	#DIV/0!

4.3.2 Accuracy for unknown impurity:

The unknown impurity refers to any unidentified impurity present in a given sample. Since it is unknown, a specific reference standard for it is not available. Therefore, the API itself is used as a surrogate standard for the unknown impurity, assuming that the impurity is structurally related to the API. Accuracy for unknown impurity is evaluated by preparing an API solution at the concentration specified for the highest unknown impurity (HUI) limit.

To systematically design the accuracy concentration matrix for unknown impurity, follow these key steps:

Step 1: Preparation of accuracy stock solutions for unknown impurity

Step 2: Calculation of lowest and highest accuracy level concentration

Step 3: Calculation of expected concentration across various accuracy levels

Step 4: Preparation of accuracy solutions by using API and Placebo

Step 5: Verification of concentration of resulted solution at various accuracy levels

Step1: Preparation of accuracy stock solutions for unknown impurity:
Please refer to Fig. 39 for preparation of an 'accuracy stock solution' for unknown impurity.
Conc. of accuracy stock can be calculated by the formula below

$$\text{Conc of accuracy stock (ppm)} = \frac{\text{API Standard weight (mg)}}{\text{Dilution vol (mL)}} \times \frac{\text{Purity (\%)}}{100} \times 1000$$

The concentration of 'accuracy stock for unknown impurity' = 500 ppm *(Refer cell K264, Fig. 39)*

Fig. 39: Excel sheet screenshot for 'preparation of accuracy stock for unknown impurity'

	B	C	D	E	F	G	H	I	J	K
184										
185	5. ACCURACY									
259										
260	c. Preparation of API accuracy solution for unknown impurity									
261										
262	Accuracy Stock Preparations									
263	API Name	Release Spec conc (ppm)	Shelf life Spec conc (ppm)	Wt (mg)	Dil to (mL)	Pipetted (mL)	Dil to (mL)	Pipetted (mL)	Dil to (mL)	Conc (ppm)
264	Paracetamol	1.0	1.0	25	50	1	1	1	1	500
265		0.0	0.0							#DIV/0!
266		0.0	0.0							#DIV/0!
267		0.0	0.0							#DIV/0!
268		0.0	0.0							#DIV/0!
269		0.0	0.0							#DIV/0!
270		0.0	0.0							#DIV/0!
271		0.0	0.0							#DIV/0!
272		0.0	0.0							#DIV/0!
273		0.0	0.0							#DIV/0!

Step 2: Calculation of lowest and highest accuracy level concentration for unknown impurity
The accuracy in case of related substances, must cover reporting level or LOQ/QL (Quantitation Limit) to minimum 120% of stability specification concentration. However, in the current example, we will cover linearity level from LOQ, 50% to 150% level. The first step is to calculate the concentration of a highest unknown impurity at its release specification in ppm.

$$\text{Unknown impurity conc at specified level (ppm)} = \frac{\text{Unkn. impurity conc (ppm) at spec. x accuracy level}}{100}$$

Let us calculate the unknown Impurity conc. in ppm at 50% of release specification by using the above formula

$$\text{Unknown impurity conc. in ppm at 50\% of release spec} = \frac{1.0 \text{ ppm x } 50\ \%}{100} = 0.5 \text{ ppm}$$

Where:

- Unknown impurity conc. in ppm at release spec: 1.0 ppm *(Refer cell C264, Fig. 39)*
- Lowest level for which conc is to be measured: 50% *(Refer cell N264, Fig. 40)*

Calculate the lowest and highest concentration for highest unknown impurity and tabulate below

Table 19: Lowest and highest concentration of unknown impurity for accuracy

Name of impurities	Lowest level	Highest level	Lowest level conc w.r.t release spec	Highest level conc w.r.t shelf-life spec
HUI	50%	150%	0.5 ppm	---------- ppm

Fig. 40: Please check excel sheet screenshot for 'calculation of lowest and highest conc. in ppm'

P264 =C264*N264

	A	M	N	O	P	Q	R	S
184								
185		5. ACCURACY						
259								
260		c. Preparation of API accuracy solution for unknown impurity						
261								
262		How to calculate lowest & Highest conc in ppm						
263		Impurity Name	Lowet level	Highest level	Lowest level conc wrt to release spec	Highest level conc wrt to shelf life spec		
264		Paracetamol	50%	150%	0.5	1.5		
265		0			0	0		
266		0			0	0		
267		0			0	0		
268		0			0	0		
269		0			0	0		
270		0			0	0		
271		0			0	0		
272		0			0	0		
273		0			0	0		

Step 3: Calculation of expected concentration across various accuracy levels for unknown impurity

Once the lowest and highest concentrations for unknown impurity are identified across the accuracy levels, the next step is to select a minimum of 3 concentration levels, including the LOQ.

In this example, we have chosen to study 7 accuracy levels. Since the exact LOQ value will be determined during the method validation, the concentration for the LOQ level is currently left blank.

Let us now calculate the expected unknown impurity concentration at various accuracy levels.

$$\text{Expected unknown impurity conc. (ppm)} = \frac{\text{Accuracy level in (\%) x conc. at release spec. in (ppm)}}{100}$$

Let us calculate the expected concentration for unknown impurity at 50% accuracy level

$$\text{Expected unknown impurity conc. (ppm) at 50\% level} = \frac{50\,\% \times 1.0\ ppm}{100} = 0.5\ ppm$$

Where:
- Accuracy level in (%) for unknown impurity = 50% (Refer cell B279, Fig. 41)
- Unknown impurity conc. at release specification = 1.0 ppm (Refer cell C264, Fig. 39)

Similarly, calculate the concentration for unknown impurity at other accuracy levels and tabulate below.

Table 20: Expected unknown impurity concentration across various accuracy levels.

Accuracy Level	Unknown impurity conc (ppm)
LOQ	
50%	
75%	
100%	
125%	
150%	
300%	

Fig. 41: Excel sheet screenshot for 'calculation of expected unknown impurity conc. across accuracy levels'

C279 =$C$264*B279

5. ACCURACY

c. Preparation of API accuracy solution for unknown impurity

Accuracy Levels	Expected API Concentration in (ppm)									
	Paracetamol	0.0	0	0	0	0	0	0	0	0
LOQ										
50%	0.50	0.00	0.00	0.00	0.00	0.00	0.00	0.00	0.00	0.00
75%	0.75	0.00	0.00	0.00	0.00	0.00	0.00	0.00	0.00	0.00
100%	1.00	0.00	0.00	0.00	0.00	0.00	0.00	0.00	0.00	0.00
125%	1.25	0.00	0.00	0.00	0.00	0.00	0.00	0.00	0.00	0.00
150%	1.50	0.00	0.00	0.00	0.00	0.00	0.00	0.00	0.00	0.00
300%	3.00	0.00	0.00	0.00	0.00	0.00	0.00	0.00	0.00	0.00

Step 4: Preparation of accuracy solutions by using API and Placebo:

To evaluate the accuracy for unknown impurities, placebo (200 mg) is added with API at every accuracy levels. In this example, the API is spiked at concentrations corresponding to the highest unknown impurity release specification covering 50%, 75%, 100%, 125%, 150%, and 300%, along with the LOQ level. The required amount of API is added using the API accuracy stock solution to achieve the target concentration.

Please ensure all accuracy solutions are prepared exactly as per the 'test sample preparation' outlined in the standard test procedure. This includes using the same quantity of placebo as specified for the test sample.

Use the formula below to prepare accuracy solutions at the desired concentrations by appropriately diluting the accuracy stock solution *(prepared under step 1).*

$$\text{Volume of API accuracy stock (mL)} = \frac{A}{B} \times C \times \frac{D}{E}$$

Where:

- A= Expected API spiking concentration in ppm
- B = Concentration of API accuracy stock in ppm
- C = Dilution volume of API accuracy stock solution in mL
- D = Further dilution in mL
- E = Pipetted volume in mL

Let us calculate the volume of API accuracy stock for preparation of accuracy level 50%

$$\text{Volume of API accuracy stock (mL) for 50\% level} = \frac{A}{B} \times C \times \frac{D}{E}$$

A = Expected API spiking concentration in ppm at 50% = 0.50 ppm *(Refer cell C279, Fig. 41)*
B = Concentration of API stock in ppm = 500 ppm *(Refer cell K264, Fig. 39)*
C = Dilution volume of API stock solution in mL = 100 mL *(Refer cell O290, Fig. 42)*
D = Further dilution in mL = 50 mL *(Refer cell Q290, Fig. 42)*

E = Pipetted volume in mL = 5 mL *(Refer cell P290, Fig. 42)*

$$\text{Volume of API accuracy stock (mL) for 50\% level} = \frac{0.50}{500} \times 100 \times \frac{50}{5} = 1.0\ mL$$

Calculate the volume of API accuracy stock for the rest of the accuracy levels and tabulate below

Table 21: Impurity stock volume to be taken across various accuracy levels.

Accuracy Level	API accuracy stock (mL)
LOQ	
50%	1.0 mL
75%	
100%	
125%	
150%	
300%	

Fig. 42: Excel sheet screenshot for accuracy of unknown impurity using API and Placebo

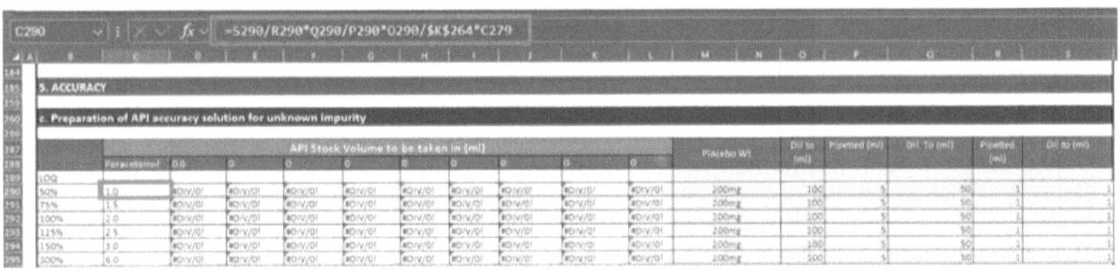

Step 5: Verification of conc. of resulted solution at various accuracy levels for unknown impurity

The final step is to confirm whether the expected accuracy concentrations are achieved using the prepared stock solutions and their respective dilutions. The resulting API concentration (as a surrogate for unknown impurity) can be calculated using the formula below.

$$\text{Resulted conc (ppm)} = A \times \frac{B}{C} \times \frac{D}{E}$$

Where:

- A= Concentration of API accuracy stock in ppm
- B = Volume of API accuracy stock (mL)
- C = Dilution volume of API accuracy stock solution in mL
- D = Pipetted volume in mL
- E = Further dilution in mL

Let us calculate the resulted conc. of API at accuracy level 50%

$$\text{Resulted conc (ppm) of API at 50\% accuracy level} = 500 \times \frac{1}{100} \times \frac{5}{50} = 0.5\ ppm$$

Where:
- A = Concentration of API accuracy stock in ppm = 500 ppm *(Refer cell K264, Fig. 39)*
- B = Volume of Impurity Accuracy stock (mL) = 1 mL *(Refer cell C290, Fig. 42)*
- C = Dilution volume of API stock solution in mL = 100 mL *(Refer cell O290, Fig. 42)*
- D = Pipetted volume in mL = 5 mL *(Refer cell P290, Fig. 42)*
- E= Further dilution in mL = 50 mL *(Refer cell Q290, Fig. 42)*

Conclusion:

The resulting concentration of API at the 50% level matches (refer cell C300, Fig. 43) the expected value of 0.5 ppm (refer cell C279, Fig. 41).

Similarly, calculate the resulted concentration for API at other levels and tabulate below

Table 22: Impurity stock volume to be taken across various accuracy levels for unknown impurity.

Accuracy Level	Resulted conc. of API (in ppm)
LOQ	
50%	0.5 ppm
75%	
100%	
125%	
150%	
300%	

Fig. 43: Excel sheet screenshot for 'calculation of resulted impurity conc. across accuracy levels' for unknown impurity using API and Placebo

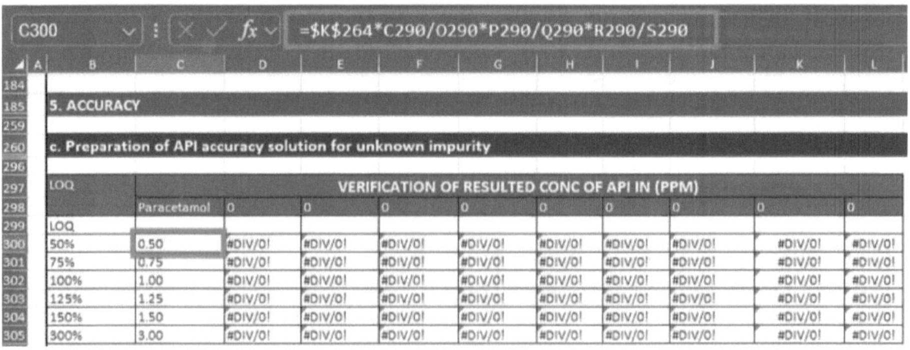

LOQ	VERIFICATION OF RESULTED CONC OF API IN (PPM)									
	Paracetamol	0	0	0	0	0	0	0	0	0
LOQ										
50%	0.50	#DIV/0!	#DIV/0!	#DIV/0!	#DIV/0!	#DIV/0!	#DIV/0!	#DIV/0!	#DIV/0!	#DIV/0!
75%	0.75	#DIV/0!	#DIV/0!	#DIV/0!	#DIV/0!	#DIV/0!	#DIV/0!	#DIV/0!	#DIV/0!	#DIV/0!
100%	1.00	#DIV/0!	#DIV/0!	#DIV/0!	#DIV/0!	#DIV/0!	#DIV/0!	#DIV/0!	#DIV/0!	#DIV/0!
125%	1.25	#DIV/0!	#DIV/0!	#DIV/0!	#DIV/0!	#DIV/0!	#DIV/0!	#DIV/0!	#DIV/0!	#DIV/0!
150%	1.50	#DIV/0!	#DIV/0!	#DIV/0!	#DIV/0!	#DIV/0!	#DIV/0!	#DIV/0!	#DIV/0!	#DIV/0!
300%	3.00	#DIV/0!	#DIV/0!	#DIV/0!	#DIV/0!	#DIV/0!	#DIV/0!	#DIV/0!	#DIV/0!	#DIV/0!

Conclusion:

In this example, we learned how to create a concentration matrix for related substances method validation using paracetamol tablets. The same approach can be applied to other dosage forms like oral liquids, injectables, and semi-solids.

This method is also suitable for drug substances. However, since placebo is not applicable in drug substances, it should be excluded during the preparation of validation solutions.

CHAPTER: 06

CONCENTRATION MATRIX FOR DISSOLUTION BY HPLC

★ Objective

This chapter is designed as a workbook, where you will fill in the blanks, calculate concentrations, and build your own validation concentration matrix for dissolution.

To help you understand and calculate concentrations of standard and sample solutions, I am going to take a practical case study where we are going to prepare a concentration matrix for dissolution of Paracetamol in paracetamol tablets 500 mg by HPLC.

For preparing concentration matrix, you need the key information below.

1. Product composition
2. Standard Test Procedure (STP)
3. Specification

1. Product Composition:

The excipients used in paracetamol tablets are maize starch, potassium sorbate, purified talc, hydroxypropyl methylcellulose.

Table 1: Composition of a drug product

Name	Conc. Of Telmisartan
Paracetamol	500 mg
Maize starch	100 mg
Potassium sorbate	20 mg
hydroxypropyl methylcellulose	50 mg
Purified talc	30 mg
Total Weight	700 mg

2. Standard Test Procedure (STP) for Dissolution of Paracetamol in Paracetamol Tablets 500 mg by HPLC:

Chemicals / Reagents:

Potassium dihydrogen phosphate : AR Grade
Triethylamine : HPLC Grade
Acetonitrile : HPLC Grade
Orthophosphoric acid : HPLC Grade
Sodium hydroxide : AR Grade
Water : Milli Q

Preparation of Buffer:

Accurately weigh and transfer 2.7 g of potassium dihydrogen phosphate and 2 mL of triethylamine in 1000 ml of water, dissolve and adjust the pH to 2.50 ± 0.05 with Orthophosphoric acid.

Mobile phase preparation:

Mix buffer and acetonitrile in the ratio 70: 30 v/v, sonicate and degas for 10 min.

Diluent:

Prepare a mixture of water and acetonitrile in the ratio 50:50 v/v.

Preparation Dissolution media:

Accurately weigh and dissolve 6.8 g of potassium dihydrogen orthophosphate and 9.0g of sodium hydroxide in 1000ml of water. Adjust the pH to 6.80 ± 0.05 with the help of sodium hydroxide or orthophosphoric acid.

Preparation of Standard stock solution:

Accurately weigh and transfer 56 mg of Paracetamol working standard into 100 mL volumetric flask, add 70 mL of diluents, sonicate to dissolve and dilute it up to the mark with diluent.

Preparation of Standard solution:

Pipette out 5 mL of standard stock solution in 50 mL volumetric flask and dilute to volume with dissolution media.

Chromatographic conditions:

Column	:	Nucleosil 100-5 CN , 250 x 4.6 mm, 5μ or equivalent
Column temperature	:	25°C
Detection	:	225 nm
Flow rate	:	1.0 mL/min
Injection volume	:	10μL
Run time	:	15 min
Needle wash	:	Water: Methanol (50:50 v/v)

Dissolution Parameters:

Medium	:	pH 6.8 phosphate buffer
Quantity	:	900 mL
Apparatus	:	USP II (Paddle)
RPM	:	50 RPM
Temperature	:	37 ± 0.5 °C
Time	:	30min

Sample preparation:

Transfer one unit into each of 6 dissolution bowl containing 900ml of the dissolution medium, pre-equilibrated to 37 ± 0.5 °C. Start the dissolution apparatus and withdraw 10ml of the sample after 30 minutes. Centrifuge the sample and further dilute 5ml of the centrifuged sample to 50ml with dissolution medium.

Procedure:

Inject 10 µL portion of the dissolution media as blank (one injection), standard preparation (five injections) and test preparation (one injection) into the chromatograph, record the chromatograms and measure the responses for major peak.

System suitability:

(a) Tailing factor from standard chromatogram should not be more than 2.0.

(b) Theoretical plates should not be less than 2000.

(c) The relative standard deviation for five replicate injections of standard preparation should not be more than 2.0 %

Calculation:

$$\text{Quantity of Paracetamol dissolved as \% of labeled amount} = \frac{A}{B} \times \frac{Ws}{100} \times \frac{5}{50} \times \frac{900}{1} \times \frac{50}{5} \times \frac{1}{L} \times \frac{P}{100} \times 100$$

A = Peak area of Paracetamol from test preparation.

B = Average peak area of Paracetamol from standard preparation.

Ws = Weight of Paracetamol standard taken, in mg for standard preparation.

P = Potency of Paracetamol on as is basis

L = Labeled amount of Paracetamol, in mg, per tablets.

3. Specification:

Let us assume that the specification for dissolution of paracetamol tablet is as below.

- Not Less Than 80% in 30 minutes

PREPARATION OF CONCENTRATION MATRIX:

For dissolution test procedure specificity, precision, linearity, and accuracy needs a concentration matrix. So, now we are going to prepare concentration matrix for each parameter.

The following points are covered as part of the concentration matrix for related substances:

1. General information about product
2. Standard and Test concentration

2.1. Standard concentration

2.2. Test concentration

3. Concentration mapping for validation parameters

3.1. Specificity/Selectivity

3.2. System suitability

3.3. Precision

3.4. Response/Linearity

3.5. Accuracy

1. General information about the product:

At the beginning of concentration matrix, provide general information such as the product name, label claim, placebo weight, etc.

Fig. 1: Excel sheet screenshot for product details.

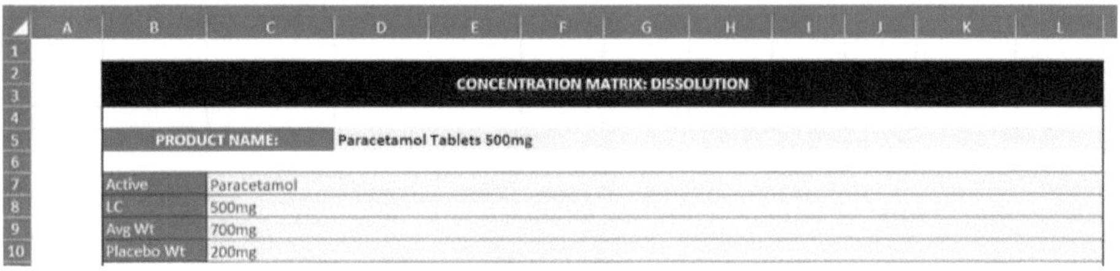

2. Standard and Test Concentration:

It is also a good idea to map the concentration of standard and test solution preparation. This will help to prepare linearity, accuracy and specificity related solutions.

2.1 Standard Concentration

- Weigh 56 mg of paracetamol and dilute to 100 mL → Standard stock solution
- Take 5 mL of this standard stock and dilute to 50 mL → Standard solution

$$\textit{Resulting standard conc (ppm)} = \frac{\textit{Weight (mg)}}{\textit{Dilution Volume (mL)}} \times \frac{\textit{Pipetted Volume (mL)}}{\textit{Dilution Volume (mL)}} \times 1000$$

Where:

- Standard weight: 56 mg *(Refer cell C29, Fig. 2)*
- Standard stock dilution: 100 mL *(Refer cell C30, Fig. 2)*
- Pipetted standard volume (mL): 5 mL *(Refer cell D29, Fig. 2)*
- Further standard dilution volume (mL): 50 mL *(Refer cell D30, Fig. 2)*

Table 2: Standard solution preparation steps

Step	Weight/Volume	Description	Resulting Concentration (ppm)
1	56 mg / 100 mL	Standard stock solution	------------------------
2	5 mL / 50 mL	Standard solution	------------------------

Note: The potency of the API standard is generally close to 100%, and for simplification, it has been excluded from the initial concentration matrix calculations. However, please remember that while calculating actual results after performing validation experiments, the standard potency must be considered wherever applicable.

2.2 Test Concentration:

- One tablet in 900 mL dissolution medium → Test stock solution
- Take 5 mL of test stock solution and dilute to 50 mL → Test solution

The weight of paracetamol per tablet is 500 mg (LC)

$$\textit{Resulting test conc (ppm)} = \frac{\textit{LC (mg)}}{\textit{Dissolution medium (mL)}} \times \frac{\textit{Pipetted Volume (mL)}}{\textit{Dilution Volume (mL)}} \times 1000$$

Where:

- LC of paracetamol (mg) = 500 mg *(Refer cell C33, Fig. 2)*
- Dissolution medium (mL) =9000 mL *(Refer cell C34, Fig. 2)*

- Volume pipetted from test stock: 5 mL *(Refer cell D33, Fig. 2)*
- Final dilution volume for test solution: 50 mL *(Refer cell D34, Fig. 2)*

Table 3: Test solution preparation steps

Step	API weight / Volume	Description	Resulting Concentration (ppm)
1	500 mg / 900 mL	Test stock solution	------------------------
2	5 mL / 50 mL	Test solution	------------------------

Fig. 2: Excel sheet screenshot for standard and sample concentration.

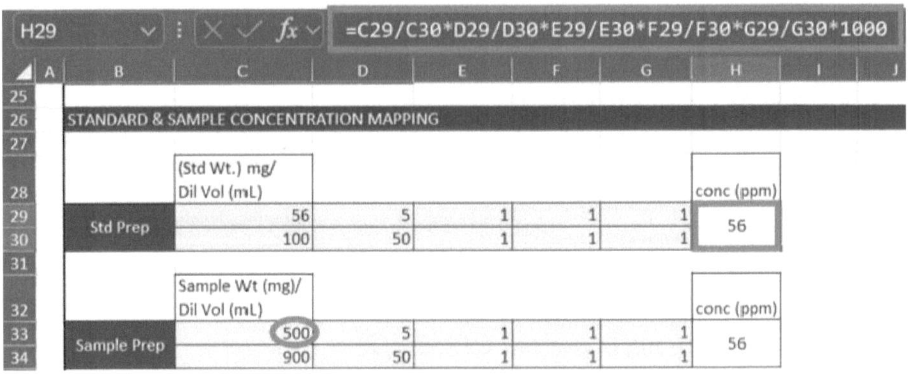

Please note, here 500 mg is not the sample weight, but it is the weight of paracetamol present in a tablet.

3. CONCENTRATION MAPPING FOR VALIDATION PARAMETERS

3.1. Specificity/Selectivity:

Specificity/Selectivity is all about checking whether the method can clearly identify the target analyte, even when other substances like excipients, dissolution medium, or diluent is present. We are going to prepare a standard solution, test solution, placebo solution, blank, for specificity/selectivity of dissolution by HPLC.

a. Standard solution

b. Test solution

c. Blank/diluent

d. Placebo solution

Table 4: Specificity/Selectivity solutions preparation

Solution Name	Discussion	Weight in mg	Dilution 1	Dilution 2	Conc. (ppm)
Standard Solution	Follow the test procedure	----------	100 mL	5mL → 50mL	----------
Test Solution	Follow the test procedure.		900 mL	5mL → 50mL	----------
Blank/ diluent	Follow the test preparation procedure by omitting sample				
Placebo solution	Follow the test preparation procedure by replacing sample by placebo. To determine the placebo content in the test solution, it is important to note that 500 mg of paracetamol contains 200 mg of placebo. Therefore, 200mg of the placebo shall be used	----------	900 mL	5mL → 50mL	

While preparing the standard, test, blank, and placebo solutions, you must follow the standard and test preparation procedures outlined in the STP.

Note: The test solution can alternatively be prepared using the API and placebo, in case the test sample is unsuitable or unavailable. In the above case, use 200 mg of placebo and 500 mg of Paracetamol API to prepare the test solution with 'Placebo + API' approach.

Fig. 3: Excel sheet screenshot for specificity (placebo preparation).

	A	B	C	D	E	F	G	H
39		1. SPECIFICITY						
40								
41			Placebo Wt (mg)					
42		Placebo	200mg	5	1	1	1	
43		Preparation	900	50	1	1	1	

3.2. System Suitability

Prepare the standard solution or system suitability solutions as per STP

Fig. 4: Excel sheet screenshot for system suitability.

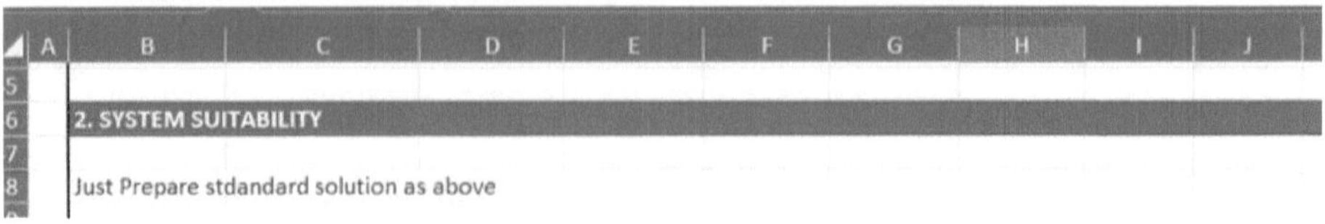

3.3. Precision:

Precision can be considered at three levels: repeatability, intermediate precision and reproducibility. For all three levels you can use the same concentration matrix as concentration of standard, test, or method of preparation remains one and the same.

Repeatability should be assessed using a minimum of 9 determinations covering the reportable range for the procedure (e.g., 3 concentrations/3 replicates each) or a minimum of 6 determinations at 100% of the test concentration. Below table provides the concentration matrix for preparation of test at 100% of the test concentration.

We are going to prepare the concentration matrix for the solutions below

3.3.1 Preparation of repeatability solutions using finished product

3.3.2 Preparation of repeatability solutions using (Placebo +API)

Table 5: Repeatability solution preparation

Solution Name	Discussion	Weight in mg	Dilution 1	Dilution 2	Conc. (ppm)
Test Solution	Follow the test procedure with six units	----------	900 mL	5mL → 50mL	----------
Test solution using Placebo + API	Placebo Weight + Paracetamol Weight	Placebo Wt. ---------- API Wt. ----------	900 mL	5mL → 50mL	----------

Follow the accuracy section to understand the concentration matrix for precision with 9 determinations covering the reportable range for the procedure (e.g., 3 concentrations/3 replicates each)

3.3.1 Preparation of repeatability solutions using finished product:

The repeatability using finished product can be studied by analyzing test solutions as per STP.

3.3.2 Preparation of repeatability solutions using (API + Placebo):

If the test sample is unavailable or unsuitable, you can use a combination of placebo and API based on the product's composition. The first step involves accurately weighing the required quantities of placebo and API to prepare the sample. From there, the procedure follows the same steps as described earlier for "Repeatability Using Finished Product."

Note: In the current example, the amount of placebo is 200 mg and amount of API is 500 mg

Let us understand the paracetamol concentration in repeatability solution using (Placebo + API)

Paracetamol conc. in ppm = (500 mg/900 mL) x (5 mL/50 mL) x 1000 = 56 ppm

Where:

- Placebo wt. (mg) = 200 mg (Refer cell C57, Fig. 5)
- Paracetamol wt. (mg) = 500 mg (Refer cell D57, Fig. 5)
- Dissolution medium volume (mL) = 900 mL (Refer cell C58, Fig. 5)
- Pipetted volume (mL) = 5 mL (Refer cell E57, Fig. 5)
- Further dilution volume (mL) = 50 mL (Refer cell E58, Fig. 5)

Fig. 5: Excel sheet screenshot for precision covering preparation of repeatability solution at 100%.

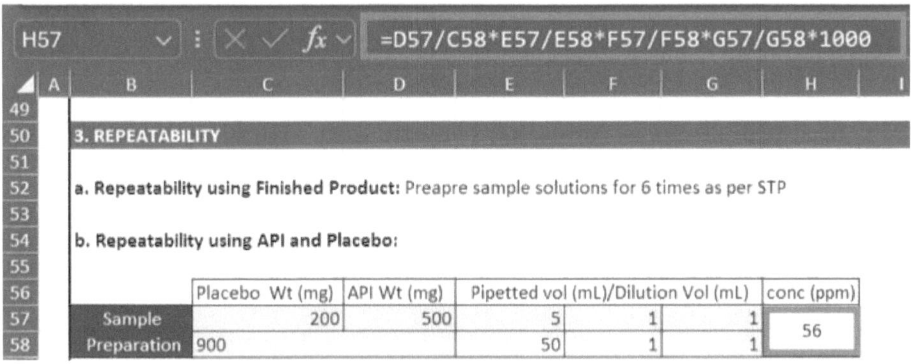

3.4 Response/Linearity:

The response of an analytical procedure is its ability (within a given range) to obtain a signal which is effectively related to the concentration (amount) or activity of analyte in the sample by some known mathematical function. (ICH Q2)

To systematically design the linearity concentration matrix, follow these key steps:

Step 1: Deciding linearity levels

Step 2: Preparation of linearity stock solutions

Step 3: Calculation of expected concentration across various linearity levels

Step 4: Required volume of linearity stock solution for the preparation of linearity solutions

Step 5: Verification of resulted linearity solution at various linearity levels

Let us discuss each step in detail.

Step 1: Deciding linearity levels

From the stock solution, we will be preparing 5 linearity levels as below (25%, 75%, 100%, 125%, and 150%)

Step 2: Preparation of linearity stock solutions

Prepare a stock solution from which further linearity solutions at different levels can be prepared. This approach helps in avoid multiple errors.

The concentration of linearity stock solution can be calculated using below formula

$$\textit{Linearity stock conc. (ppm)} = \frac{\textit{Weight of compound (mg)}}{\textit{Dilution volume (mL)}} \times 1000$$

Let us understand the paracetamol concentration in linearity stock solution
Where:
- Weight of Paracetamol for linearity stock preparation = 56 mg *(Refer cell C64, Fig. 6)*
- Dilution volume (mL)= 100 mL *(Refer cell C65, Fig. 6)*

Table 6: Linearity stock preparation

Solution Name	Discussion	Weight in mg	Dilution 1	Conc. (ppm)
Linearity stock	Paracetamol	56 mg	100 mL	----------------

Fig. 6: Excel sheet screenshot for linearity stock solution preparation

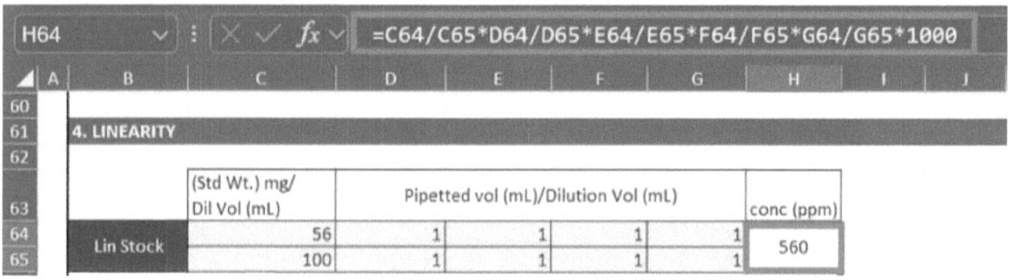

H64 =C64/C65*D64/D65*E64/E65*F64/F65*G64/G65*1000

4. LINEARITY

	(Std Wt.) mg/ Dil Vol (mL)	Pipetted vol (mL)/Dilution Vol (mL)				conc (ppm)
Lin Stock	56	1	1	1	1	560
	100	1	1	1	1	

Step 3: Calculation of expected concentration across various linearity levels

The expected concentration of paracetamol at specified linearity level can be calculated as below
Expected conc. in ppm = [Linearity level (%) x Test conc (ppm)]/100
The expected concentration in ppm at 25% = [25 %x 56 ppm]/100 = 14 ppm
Where:
- Linearity level = 25% *(Refer cell B68, Fig. 7)*
- Test conc. (ppm) = 56 ppm *(Refer cell H33, Fig. 2)*

Fig. 7: Excel sheet screenshot for expected concentration of a paracetamol at various linearity levels

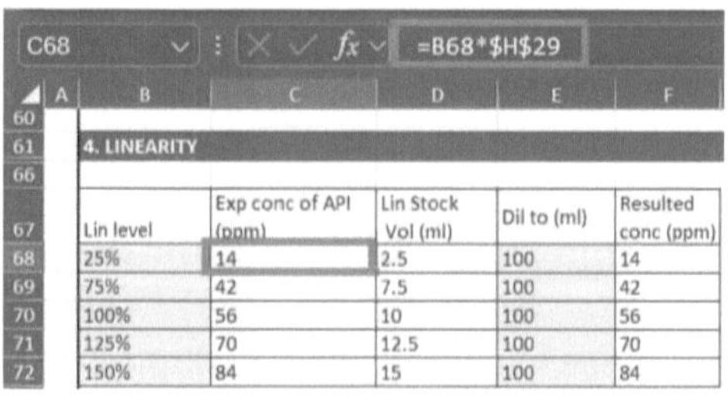

C68 =B68*$H$29

4. LINEARITY

Lin level	Exp conc of API (ppm)	Lin Stock Vol (ml)	Dil to (ml)	Resulted conc (ppm)
25%	14	2.5	100	14
75%	42	7.5	100	42
100%	56	10	100	56
125%	70	12.5	100	70
150%	84	15	100	84

Step 4: Required volume of linearity stock solution for the preparation of linearity solutions

The required volume of linearity stock solution for the preparation of linearity solutions is calculated as below

$$\textit{Required Vol. of Linearity stock solution in (mL)} = \frac{A \times B}{C}$$

Where:

- A = Expected concentration of API at a specified linearity level (in ppm)
- B = Dilution of 'linearity stock' to prepare a specified linearity level solution (in mL)
- C = Conc. of linearity stock solution (in ppm)

Let us calculate the required volume of linearity stock for 25% linearity level by using the above formula

Required volume of Linearity stock solution for 25% level= (14 ppm x 100 mL)/560 ppm = 2.5 mL

Where:

- Expected conc. of paracetamol at 25% linearity level = 14 ppm *(Refer cell C68, Fig. 7)*
- Diluted volume = 100 mL *(Refer cell E68, Fig. 8)*
- Concentration of paracetamol linearity stock solution = 560 ppm *(Refer cel H64, Fig. 6)*

Fig. 8: Excel sheet screenshot for required volume of the linearity stock to achieve expected concentration of a paracetamol at various linearity levels

D68 =C68*E68/$H$64

	A	B	C	D	E	F
60						
61		4. LINEARITY				
66						
67		Lin level	Exp conc of API (ppm)	Lin Stock Vol (ml)	Dil to (ml)	Resulted conc (ppm)
68		25%	14	2.5	100	14
69		75%	42	7.5	100	42
70		100%	56	10	100	56
71		125%	70	12.5	100	70
72		150%	84	15	100	84

Step 5: Verification of resulted linearity solution at various linearity levels

The resulting concentration of API at specified linearity level can be calculated as below

$$\textit{Resulted conc. in ppm} = \frac{\textit{Conc. of linearity stock (ppm) x Linearity stock volume (mL)}}{\textit{Dilution Volume (mL)}}$$

Let us calculate the resulted conc. in ppm for paracetamol at 25% linearity level by using the above formula

The Resulted conc. of paracetamol in ppm at 25% level = 560 ppm x 2.5 mL/100 mL = 14 ppm

Where:

- Conc. of linearity stock (in ppm) = 560 ppm (Refer cell H64, Fig. 6)
- Linearity stock volume (mL) = 2.5 mL (Refer cell D68, Fig. 9)
- Dilution Volume (mL) = 100 mL (Refer cell E68, Fig. 9)

Conclusion:

The resulting solution, prepared using the above details, achieves the expected concentration of paracetamol at the 25% linearity level (see cell F68, Fig. 9).

Fig. 9: Excel sheet screenshot for resulted concentration of paracetamol at various linearity levels

F68 fx =$H$64*D68/E68

	A	B	C	D	E	F
60						
61		4. LINEARITY				
66						
67		Lin level	Exp conc of API (ppm)	Lin Stock Vol (ml)	Dil to (ml)	Resulted conc (ppm)
68		25%	14	2.5	100	14
69		75%	42	7.5	100	42
70		100%	56	10	100	56
71		125%	70	12.5	100	70
72		150%	84	15	100	84

Based on the above information, calculate the expected concentrations, the required volume of linearity stock, and the resulting concentrations for the remaining linearity levels. Enter the values in the table below.

Table 7: Linearity solution preparation

Linearity Level	Expected conc. of paracetamol in ppm	Linearity stock Vol (ml)	Dil to (ml)	Resulted conc. (ppm)
25%	14 ppm	2.5 mL	100 mL	14 ppm
75%				
100%				
125%				
150%				

3.5. Accuracy:

The accuracy of an analytical procedure expresses the closeness of agreement between the value which is accepted either as a conventional true value or an accepted reference value and the value found. This is sometimes termed trueness. We are going to prepare concentration matrix for below accuracy solutions

3.5.1 Accuracy using (API + Placebo)

To systematically design the accuracy concentration matrix using (API+Placebo), follow these key steps:

Step 1: Deciding accuracy levels

Step 2: Calculation of expected initial concentration across various accuracy stock solutions

Step 3: Calculation of expected final concentration across various accuracy levels

Step 4: Calculating the required weight of API at various accuracy levels

Step 5: Preparation of accuracy solutions

Step 6: Verification of concentration of resulted solution at various accuracy levels

Step 1: Deciding accuracy levels

We can prepare 5 accuracy levels such as 25%, 75%, 100%, 125%, and 150%

Step 2: Calculation of expected initial concentration across various accuracy stock solutions

The expected initial concentration of paracetamol at specified accuracy level can be calculated as below

$$\text{Expected initial conc. in ppm} = \frac{\text{Accuracy level}}{100} \times \frac{\text{API Wt. in dissolution bowl as per test preparation}}{\text{Dissolution medium volume (mL)}} \times 1000$$

$$\text{Expected initial conc. of paracetamol (ppm) at 25\% accuracy} = \frac{25\ \%}{100\ mL} \times \frac{500\ mg}{900\ mL} \times 1000 = 139\ ppm$$

Where:

- Accuracy level= 25 % *(Refer cell B79, Fig. 10)*
- API Wt. in dissolution bowl as per test preparation = 500 mg *(Refer cell C33, Fig. 2)*
- Dissolution medium volume (mL) = 900 mL *(Refer cell C34, Fig. 2)*

Fig. 10: Excel sheet screenshot for the expected initial conc. of paracetamol at various accuracy levels

C79 =B79*$C$33/$C$34*1000

5. ACCURACY

Placebo Wt	200mg									
Acc. level	Exp Initial Conc of API (ppm)	Exp Final Conc (ppm)	API Wt.(mg)	Dil to (V1)	Pipetted (ml)	Dil to (ml)	Pipetted (ml)	Dil to (ml)	Resulted Initial Conc (ppm)	Resulted Final Conc (ppm)
25%	139	14	125	900	5	50	1	1	139	14
75%	417	42	375	900	5	50	1	1	417	42
100%	556	56	500	900	5	50	1	1	556	56
125%	694	69	625	900	5	50	1	1	694	69
150%	833	83	750	900	5	50	1	1	833	83

Step 3: Calculation of expected final concentration across various accuracy levels

The expected final accuracy concentration of API at specified accuracy level can be calculated as below

Expected conc. in ppm = [Accuracy level (%) x Test conc (ppm)]/100

Let us calculate the expected concentration of paracetamol at 25% accuracy level

The expected conc. of paracetamol in ppm at 25% accuracy level = (25 x56)/100 = 14 ppm

Where:

- Accuracy level in percentage (%) = 25% *(Refer cell B79, Fig. 11)*
- Test conc. in ppm = 56 ppm *(Refer cell H33, Fig. 2)*

Fig. 11: Excel sheet screenshot for the expected final conc. of paracetamol at various accuracy levels

D79 fx =B79*$H$33

	B	C	D	E	F	G	H	I	J	K	L
75	5. ACCURACY										
77	Placebo Wt	200mg									
78	Acc. level	Exp Initial Conc of API (ppm)	Exp Final Conc (ppm)	API Wt.(mg)	Dil to (V1)	Pipetted (ml)	Dil to (ml)	Pipetted (ml)	Dil to (ml)	Resulted Initial Conc (ppm)	Resulted Final Conc (ppm)
79	25%	139	14	125	900	5	50	1	1	139	14
80	75%	417	42	375	900	5	50	1	1	417	42
81	100%	556	56	500	900	5	50	1	1	556	56
82	125%	694	69	625	900	5	50	1	1	694	69
83	150%	833	83	750	900	5	50	1	1	833	83

Step 4: Calculating the required weight of API at various accuracy levels

The required weight of API for various accuracy levels is calculated by using the formula below

Required weight of API in mg = [Accuracy level (%) x Weight of API in test preparation]/100

Let us calculate the required API weight for 25% accuracy level.

Required weight of API in mg at 25% accuracy level = [25 x 500 mg]/100 = 125 mg

Where:

- Accuracy level in percentage (%) = 25% *(Refer cell B79, Fig. 11)*
- Wt. of API in test preparation = 500 mg *(Refer cell C33, Fig. 2)*

Fig. 11: Excel sheet screenshot for the required wight of the API at various at various accuracy levels

E79 fx =B79*$C$33

	B	C	D	E	F	G	H	I	J	K	L
75	5. ACCURACY										
77	Placebo Wt	200mg									
78	Acc. level	Exp Initial Conc of API (ppm)	Exp Final Conc (ppm)	API Wt.(mg)	Dil to (V1)	Pipetted (ml)	Dil to (ml)	Pipetted (ml)	Dil to (ml)	Resulted Initial Conc (ppm)	Resulted Final Conc (ppm)
79	25%	139	14	125	900	5	50	1	1	139	14
80	75%	417	42	375	900	5	50	1	1	417	42
81	100%	556	56	500	900	5	50	1	1	556	56
82	125%	694	69	625	900	5	50	1	1	694	69
83	150%	833	83	750	900	5	50	1	1	833	83

Step 5: Preparation of accuracy solutions

The accuracy solutions at various accuracy levels can be prepared by using the API (as calculated in step 3), and the amount of placebo present in test sample. The amount of placebo must be kept the same across all accuracy levels. The 200 mg of the placebo is present in test sample (Refer "Placebo solution" preparation as per Table 4 (specificity) to know the placebo present in test sample). Follow the sample preparation procedure as per STP by using calculated amount of API required at specified accuracy level and 200 mg of placebo. Wight of placebo is given in C77, Fig. 11. The further accuracy solution is prepared as per test preparation procedure.

Fig. 11 (cell E79, E80, E81, E82, E83) provides the required API weight for various accuracy levels.

Step 6: Verification of initial and final concentration of resulted solution at various accuracy levels

The resulted initial concentration of paracetamol at specified accuracy level can be calculated as below

$$\text{Resulted initial conc. in ppm} = \frac{\text{Weight of API in mg}}{\text{Dissolution medium Volume (mL)}} \times 1000$$

The Resulted initial conc. for paracetamol in ppm at 25% = [125 mg/900 mL] x 1000 = 139 ppm

Where:

- Weight of API at 25% Accuracy level = 125 mg *(Refer cell E79, Fig. 12)*
- Dissolution medium volume = 900 mL *(Refer cell F79, Fig. 12)*

Fig. 12: Excel sheet screenshot for the resulted initial conc. of paracetamol at various accuracy levels

K79 | =E79/F79*1000

	A	B	C	D	E	F	G	H	I	J	K	L
74												
75		5. ACCURACY										
76												
77		Placebo Wt	200mg									
78		Acc. level	Exp Initial Conc of API (ppm)	Exp Final Conc (ppm)	API Wt.(mg)	Dil to (V1)	Pipetted (ml)	Dil to (ml)	Pipetted (ml)	Dil to (ml)	Resulted Initial Conc (ppm)	Resulted Final Conc (ppm)
79		25%	139	14	125	900	5	50	1	1	139	14
80		75%	417	42	375	900	5	50	1	1	417	42
81		100%	556	56	500	900	5	50	1	1	556	56
82		125%	694	69	625	900	5	50	1	1	694	69
83		150%	833	83	750	900	5	50	1	1	833	83

Conclusion:

The resulted initial concentration of paracetamol at 25% accuracy level meets the expected concentration at the same level (refer cell C79, Fig. 12)

Verification of final concentration of resulted solution at various accuracy levels can be calculated as below:

$$\text{Resulted final conc. in ppm} = \frac{\text{Weight of API in mg}}{\text{Dissolution medium Volume (mL)}} \times \frac{\text{Pipetted vol (mL)}}{\text{Dilution vol (mL)}} \times 1000$$

The Resulted final conc. for paracetamol (ppm) at 25% = (125 mg/900 mL) x (5 mL/50 mL) x 1000
= 14 ppm

Where:

- Weight of API at 25% Accuracy level = 125 mg *(Refer cell E79, Fig. 13)*
- Dissolution medium volume = 900 mL *(Refer cell F79, Fig. 13)*
- Pipetted volume (mL) = 5 mL *(Refer cell G79, Fig. 13)*
- Further dilution volume (mL) = 50 mL *(Refer cell H79, Fig. 13)*

Conclusion:

The resulted final concentration of paracetamol at 25% accuracy level meets the expected concentration at the same level (refer cell D79, Fig. 13)

Fig. 13: Excel sheet screenshot for the resulted final conc. of paracetamol at various accuracy levels

L79 | fx =E79/F79*G79/H79*I79/J79*1000

5. ACCURACY

Placebo Wt	200mg									
Acc. level	Exp Initial Conc of API (ppm)	Exp Final Conc (ppm)	API Wt.(mg)	Dil to (V1)	Pipetted (ml)	Dil to (ml)	Pipetted (ml)	Dil to (ml)	Resulted Initial Conc (ppm)	Resulted Final Conc (ppm)
25%	139	14	125	900	5	50	1	1	139	14
75%	417	42	375	900	5	50	1	1	417	42
100%	556	56	500	900	5	50	1	1	556	56
125%	694	69	625	900	5	50	1	1	694	69
150%	833	83	750	900	5	50	1	1	833	83

Using the information provided above, complete the table below by entering the appropriate values. This will help ensure that the calculations and preparations are aligned with the required concentrations and procedures

Table 8: Accuracy solution preparation

Acc. level	Exp Initial Conc. of API (ppm)	Exp Final Conc. (ppm)	API Wt. (mg)	Dissolution medium vol. (mL)	Pipetted (ml)	Dil. to (ml)	Resulted Initial Conc. (ppm)	Resulted Final Conc. (ppm)
25%	139 ppm	14 ppm	125 mg	900 mL	5 mL	50 mL	139 ppm	14 ppm
75%								
100%								
125%								
150%								

CHAPTER: 07

CONCENTRATION MATRIX FOR RESIDUAL SOLVENTS BY GC

★ Objective

This chapter is designed as a workbook, where you will fill in the blanks, calculate concentrations, and build your own validation concentration matrix.

To help you understand and calculate concentrations of standard and sample solutions, I am going to take a practical case study where we are going to prepare a concentration matrix for residual solvents of paracetamol tablets 500 mg by GC.

For preparing concentration matrix, you need the key information below.

1. Product composition
2. Standard Test Procedure (STP)
3. Specification

1. Product Composition:

The excipients used in paracetamol tablets are maize starch, potassium sorbate, purified talc, hydroxypropyl methylcellulose.

Table 1: Composition of a drug product

Name	Conc. Of Telmisartan
Paracetamol	500 mg
Maize starch	100 mg
Potassium sorbate	20 mg
hydroxypropyl methylcellulose	50 mg
Purified talc	30 mg
Total Weight	700 mg

2. Standard Test Procedure (STP) for Residual Solvents of Paracetamol Tablets 500 mg by GC:

Chemicals / Reagents:

Benzyl alcohol : HPLC / GC Grade
Ethanol : HPLC / GC Grade
Methanol : HPLC/GC Grade
Dichloromethane : HPLC/GC Grade

Diluent: Benzyl alcohol

Standard stock solution:

Transfer accurately about 500 mg ethanol, 300 mg of methanol, and 60 mg of methylene dichloride (MDC) into a 100 mL volumetric flask containing about 60 mL of diluent, dilute to volume with diluent and mix well.

Standard solution:

Pipette 10 mL of standard stock solution into a 100 mL volumetric flask and dilute to volume with diluent and mix well. Transfer exactly 5.0 mL of the standard solution into six head space vials each and seal immediately with septum using crimper.

Test solution:

Accurately weigh about 500 mg of crushed tablet powder into a head space vial, add exactly 5 mL of diluent and seal immediately with septum using crimper.

Preparation of blank:

Pipette 5 mL of diluent into a head space vial and seal immediately with septum using crimper.

Chromatographic system:

Model : Agilent 7890A
Column : DB-624, 30m x 0.53mm, film thickness 3.0 µm or equivalent.
Detector : Flame Ionization Detector
Carrier gas : Nitrogen
Carrier flow (Column pressure) : 1.5 psi
Make up gas (Nitrogen) : 25 mL/minute
Hydrogen flow : 40 mL/minute
Air flow : 400 mL/minute
Split ratio : 15:01
Run Time : 33.3 minutes
Column oven temperature : 35°C
Program : Initially maintain temperature at 35°C and hold for 10.0 minutes, increase to 60°C at ramp 3°C/minute, then increase to 235 °C at ramp 35 °C/minute, hold for 10.0 minutes.
Injector temperature : 160°C
Detector temperature : 240°C
Head space parameters :
Instrument : Agilent G1888
Oven temperature : 85°C
Loop temperature : 95°C
Transfer line temperature : 120°C
GC-Cycle time : 50.00 minutes
Vial shaking : High
Vial equilibration time : 20.00 minutes
Pressurization time : 1.00 minutes
Pressurization Equilibration time : 0.50 minutes

Loop Fill time : 3.00 minutes
Loop Equilibration time : 1.00 minutes
Sampler injection time : 2.00 minutes
Sequence purge valve : 3.00 minutes
Septum purge flow : 3.00 mL/min

Procedure:

Chromatograph the head space of diluent as blank (one injection), Standard solution (six injections) and Test solution (one injection), record the chromatograms and measure the peaks responses.

System suitability:

(1) Tailing factor for ethanol, methanol, an MDC peak in standard solution should not be more than 2.0.

(2) Theoretical plate count for ethanol, methanol, and MDC should not be less than 5000.

(3) The relative standard deviation of peak areas for ethanol, methanol, and MDC of six replicate injections of standard should not be more than 15 %.

Note: Subtract areas of peak(s), if any for blank, appearing at the retention time of ethanol, methanol, MDC, obtained for standard preparation and test preparation.

Calculations:

$$\text{Residual solvent in ppm} = \frac{(At\text{-}\rho x)}{(As\text{-}\rho x)} \times \frac{Ws}{100} \times \frac{10}{100} \times \frac{5}{Wt} \times \frac{P}{100} \times 10^6$$

At = Peak area of solvent for Test preparation

As = Average peak area of solvent for Standard preparation

ρx = Area of peak, if any appearing at the retention time of solvent from blank.

Ws = Weight of solvent taken in mg for standard stock solution.

Wt = Weight of crushed tablet powder taken in mg, for test preparation.

P = Purity of respective solvent in percentage (%)

3. Specification:

Let us assume that the specification for residual solvents in paracetamol tablet is as below.

- Ethanol: NMT 5000 ppm
- Methanol: NMT 3000 ppm
- MDC: NMT 600 ppm

PREPARATION OF CONCENTRATION MATRIX:

For the Residual solvent test procedure, parameters such as specificity, precision, detection limit (DL), quantitation limit (QL), linearity, and accuracy all require a well-defined concentration matrix. We will now proceed to prepare the concentration matrix for each of these validation parameters.

The following points are covered as part of the concentration matrix for residual solvents:

1. General information about product
2. Standard and Test concentration
2.1. Standard concentration
2.2. Test concentration
3. Specification for related substances
4. Concentration mapping for validation parameters
4.1. Specificity/Selectivity
4.2. System suitability
4.3. Precision
4.4. Response/Linearity
4.5. Accuracy

1. General information about the product:

At the beginning of concentration matrix, provide general information such as the product name, label claim, placebo weight, etc.

Fig. 1: Excel sheet screenshot for general information about the product.

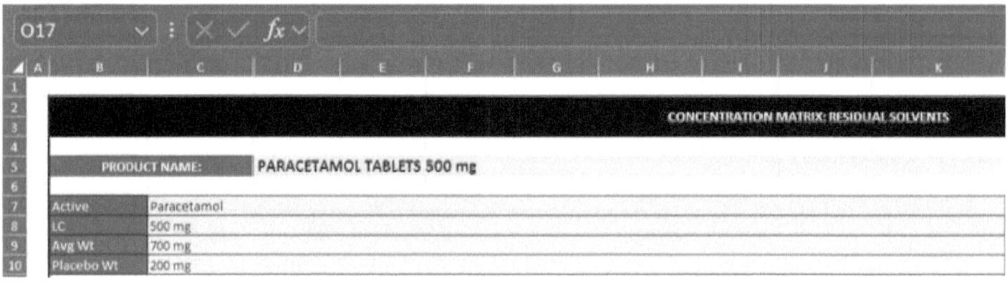

2. Standard and Test Concentration:

It is also a good idea to map the concentration of standard and test solution preparation. This will help to prepare linearity, accuracy and specificity related solutions.

2.1 Standard Concentration:

- Weigh 500 mg, 300 mg, and 60 mg of ethanol, methanol, and methylene dichloride (MDC) and dilute to 100 mL → Standard stock solution

- Take 10 mL of this standard stock and dilute it to 100 mL → Standard solution

Calculate the resulting concentration of residual solvent in ppm with respect to sample using the formula below

$$\text{Resulting conc (ppm)} = \frac{\text{Weight (mg)}}{\text{Dilution Volume (mL)}} \times \frac{\text{Pipetted Vol. (mL)}}{\text{Dilution Vol. (mL)}} \times \frac{\text{Sample Dilution (mL)}}{\text{Sample wt (mg)}} \times 10^6$$

$$\text{Conc of ethanol standard (ppm)} = \frac{500}{100} \times \frac{10}{100} \times \frac{5}{500} \times 10^6 = 5000\ \text{ppm}$$

Where:

- Ethanol standard weight (mg) = 500 mg *(Refer cell C15 from Fig. 2)*

- Ethanol standard stock dilution (mL) = 100 mL *(Refer cell C16 from Fig. 2)*
- Ethanol standard stock pipetted volume (mL) = 10 mL *(Refer cell D15 from Fig. 2)*
- Ethanol standard stock diluted to (mL) = 100 mL *(Refer cell D16 from Fig. 2)*
- Sample dilution (mL) = 5 mL *(Refer cell G15 from Fig. 2)*
- Sample weight (mg) = 500 mg *(Refer cell G16 from Fig. 2)*

Similarly, calculate the concentration of methanol, and MDC standard solutions as below.

Conc. of methanol standard (ppm) = ------------------- x ------------------- x --------------- x 10^6 =

Conc. of MDC standard (ppm) = ------------------- x ------------------- x --------------- x 10^6 =

Note: The purity of the residual solvent standard is typically close to 100%, and hence, it is not considered while defining the standard concentration during the preparation of the concentration matrix. However, if you are using a residual solvent standard with significantly lower purity, you must apply a purity correction factor (purity/100) while calculating the concentration.

Additionally, even though purity is not factored in during concentration mapping for simplicity, it must be taken into account while calculating the final results after the validation study.

✦ Understanding how to prepare residual solvent standard concentration (in ppm) with respect to sample concentration:

Before we get into calculations, let's first understand the basic concept of ppm (parts per million):

- 1 ppm = 1 part in 1,000,000 parts
  - For example:
    - 1 µg of ethanol in 1,000,000 µg of product = 1 ppm
    - 1 µg of ethanol in 1000 mg of product = 1 ppm
    - 1 µg of ethanol in 1 g of product = 1 ppm

Therefore, 1 ppm = 1 microgram per gram (1 µg/g) of sample.

Example: 5000 ppm ethanol in the Sample

5000 ppm means:

- 5000 µg ethanol per 1000 mg of sample
- 2500 µg ethanol per 500 mg of sample (as per current example we are using 500 mg sample)

Thus, 2500 µg or 2.5 mg ethanol in 500 mg sample = 5000 ppm ethanol

Standard Solution Preparation:

500 mg of ethanol dilute to 100 mL → Concentration = 500 mg / 100 mL = 5 mg/mL

Further 10 mL of the above solution is diluted to 100 mL → Final ethanol concentration = 0.5mg/mL

So, this standard solution appears to be 500 ppm in terms of direct dilution. So, this is the direct or absolute concentration of ethanol in that standard solution, with no reference to sample.

Sample Solution Preparation:

500 mg of sample diluted to 5 mL → Sample concentration = 100mg/mL

Converting Standard ppm with Respect to Sample:

Now let's calculate standard ppm with respect to sample concentration using the formula:

$$\text{Ethanol std conc. in ppm (w.r.t sample)} = \frac{\text{ethanol conc. in std (mg/mL)}}{\text{sample conc. (mg/mL)}} \times 10^6$$

$$\text{Ethanol conc. in std (mg/mL)} = \frac{500\ mg}{100\ mL} \times \frac{10\ mL}{100\ mL}$$

$$\text{Sample concentration (mg/mL)} = \frac{500mg}{5\ mL}$$

If we substitute these details in the above equation, we will get below

$$\text{Ethanol std conc. in ppm (wrt sample)} = \frac{\left[\dfrac{500\ mg\ \text{std wt.}}{100\ mL} \times \dfrac{10\ mL}{100\ mL}\right]}{\left[\dfrac{500\ mg\ \text{sample wt.}}{5\ mL\ \text{sample dil.}}\right]} \times 10^6$$

Let us further simplify the above equation

$$\text{Ethanol std conc. in ppm (wrt sample)} = \frac{500\ mg\ \text{std wt.}}{100\ mL} \times \frac{10\ mL}{100\ mL} \times \frac{5\ mL\ \text{sample dil.}}{500\ mg\ \text{sample wt.}} \times 10^6$$

Table 2: Tabulate the concentration of standard stock, and standard solution in below table

Residual solvent	Weight/ Volume	Further dilution	Sample Dilution (mL)/ Sample wt. (mg)	Resulting Concentration w.r.t sample (ppm)
Ethanol	500mg / 100mL	10mL → 100mL	5 mL/ 500 mg	----------------------
Methanol	300mL / 100mL			----------------------
MDC	60mL / 100mL			----------------------

2.2 Test Concentration:

- Weigh about 500 mg of crushed tablet powder, add 5 mL diluent → Test solution

Calculate the resulting concentration of test in ppm using the formula below

$$\text{Resulting conc (ppm)} = \frac{\text{Weight (mg)}}{\text{Dilution Volume (mL)}} \times 1000$$

$$\textit{Conc of test stock in ppm} = \frac{500}{5} \times 1000 = 100000 \textit{ ppm (absolute concentration)}$$

Weight of test sample (mg) = 500 mg *(Refer cell C29 from Fig. 2)*
Dilution of test sample = 5 mL *(Refer cell C30 from Fig. 2)*

Fig. 2: Excel sheet screenshot to calculate standard and test concentration.

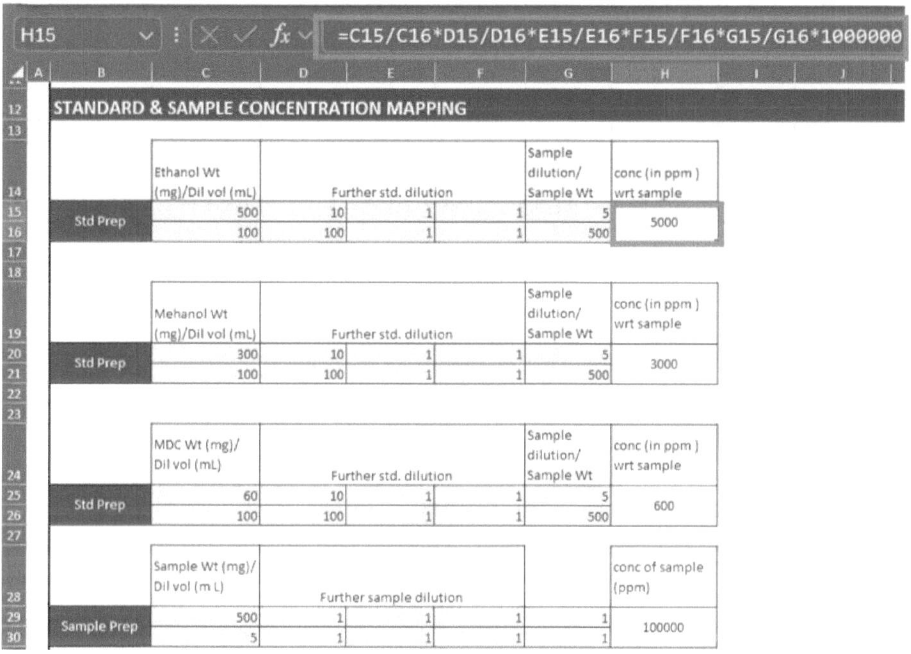

H15 =C15/C16*D15/D16*E15/E16*F15/F16*G15/G16*1000000

STANDARD & SAMPLE CONCENTRATION MAPPING

	Ethanol Wt (mg)/Dil vol (mL)	Further std. dilution			Sample dilution/ Sample Wt	conc (in ppm) wrt sample
Std Prep	500	10	1	1	5	5000
	100	100	1	1	500	

	Mehanol Wt (mg)/Dil vol (mL)	Further std. dilution			Sample dilution/ Sample Wt	conc (in ppm) wrt sample
Std Prep	300	10	1	1	5	3000
	100	100	1	1	500	

	MDC Wt (mg)/ Dil vol (mL)	Further std. dilution			Sample dilution/ Sample Wt	conc (in ppm) wrt sample
Std Prep	60	10	1	1	5	600
	100	100	1	1	500	

	Sample Wt (mg)/ Dil vol (m L)	Further sample dilution				conc of sample (ppm)
Sample Prep	500	1	1	1	1	100000
	5	1	1	1	1	

3. Specification for residual solvents:

Let us assume that the specification for residual solvents for paracetamol tablet is as below.

Table 3: Specification for residual solvents

Name of impurities	Release specification
Ethanol	5000 ppm
Methanol	3000 ppm
MDC	600 ppm

Fig. 3: Excel sheet screenshot for residual solvent specification

SPECIFICATION

Test Name	Res solvent Name	Limit in ppm
RESIDUAL SOLVENT	Ethanol	5000
	Methanol	3000
	MDC	600

4. CONCENTRATION MAPPING FOR VALIDATION PARAMETERS:

Let's now start mapping the concentration required for each validation parameter

4.1. Specificity/Selectivity:

Specificity/Selectivity is all about checking whether the method can clearly identify the target analyte, even when other substances like excipients, impurities, or diluent are present.

We are going to prepare standard solution, test solution, blank/diluent, placebo solution, individual impurity identification solution, and impurity spiked test solution for specificity/selectivity of residual solvent by GC. Forced degradation is generally not required for residual solvent method validation. The below solutions are prepared specifically.

a. Standard solution
b. Test solution
c. Blank/diluent
d. Placebo solution
e. Individual residual solvent indification solutions
f. Residual solvent spiked test solution

Table 4: Specification solution preparation

Solution Name	Solution Name	Weight in mg	Dilution 1	Dilution 2	Conc. ppm (w.r.t sample)
Standard Solution	Follow the test procedure	Ethanol: Methanol: MDC:	100 mL	10mL → 100mL	Ethanol: Methanol: MDC:
Test Solution	Follow the test procedure	----------------	5 mL		
Blank/ diluent	Follow the test preparation procedure by omitting sample				
Placebo solution	Follow the test preparation procedure by replacing sample by placebo. 700 mg of sample contains 200mg placebo, hence 500 mg sample will contain (500 x 200)/700= 143 mg of placebo.	----------------	5 mL		
Ethanol Identification Solution	Prepare ethanol identification solution at its release specification level, which is 5000 ppm	----------------	100 mL	10mL → 100mL	----------------
Methanol Identification Solution	Prepare methanol identification solution at its release specification level, which is 3000 ppm	----------------	100 mL	10mL → 100mL	----------------
MDC Identification solution	Prepare MDC identification solution at its release specification level, which is 600 ppm	----------------	100 mL	10mL → 100mL	----------------
Residual solvent spiked test solution	Test solution shall be prepared in standard solution	----------------	5 mL		

Note: The test solution and residual solvent-spiked test solution can alternatively be prepared using the API and placebo, in case the test sample is unsuitable or unavailable. In the current case, use 143 mg of placebo and 357 mg of Paracetamol API to prepare the test solution. Similarly, for the residual solvent-spiked test solution, use 143 mg of placebo, 357 mg of Paracetamol API, and the standard solution.

a. Standard Solution: Follow the STP

b. Test solution: Follow the STP

c. Diluent: Follow the test solution preparation by omitting test sample.

e. Placebo solution preparation: Follow the test solution preparation by replacing test sample by placebo.

Note: In this case, the API has been excluded from the placebo since all three residual solvents originate from the API itself. However, if the residual solvents are introduced during the drug product manufacturing process, the placebo should contain all excipients and the API—excluding only the residual solvents under analysis.

Fig. 4: Excel sheet screenshot for placebo preparation.

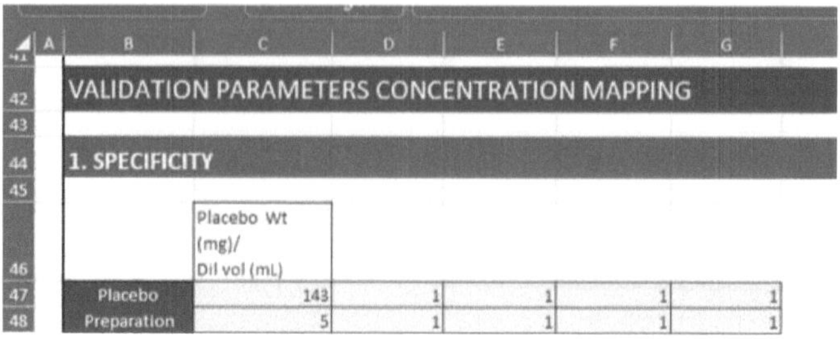

VALIDATION PARAMETERS CONCENTRATION MAPPING

1. SPECIFICITY

	Placebo Wt (mg)/ Dil vol (mL)				
Placebo Preparation	143	1	1	1	1
	5	1	1	1	1

f. Individual residual solvent solution preparation:

Each residual solvent identification solution should be prepared at the specification concentration. If the standard solution is already prepared at the specification level, then the same procedure used for standard solution preparation can be followed for preparing the identification solutions as well. In such cases, individual residual solvent reference standards should be weighed and diluted separately in their respective volumetric flasks. Please refer to the figure below for detailed preparation steps.

Let us calculate the concentration of ethanol identification (ID) solution in ppm (w.r.t sample)

$$\text{Conc. of ethanol ID sol. in ppm (w.r.t sample)} = \frac{500\ mg}{100\ mL} \times \frac{10\ mL}{100\ mL} \times \frac{5\ mL}{500 mg} \times 10^6 = 5000\ ppm$$

Where:

- Weight of ethanol standard wt. (mg) = 500 mg *(Refer cell D54 from Fig. 5)*
- Ethanol stock dilution (ml) = 100 mL *(Refer cell E54 from Fig. 5)*
- Pipetted vol (mL) = 10 mL *(Refer cell F54 from Fig. 5)*
- Further dilution (mL)= 100 mL *(Refer cell G54 from Fig. 5)*
- Sample dilution vol (mL) = 5 mL *(Refer cell H54 from Fig. 5)*
- Sample wt. in (mg)= 500 mg *(Refer cell I54 from Fig. 5)*

Conclusion: The resulted concentration of ethanol matches the expected or target concentration in ppm (w.r.t sample) (refer cell C54, Fig. 5). Therefore, the selected ethanol weight and dilution are appropriate and accurate.

Similarly, you can calculate the Conc. of methanol and MDC ID sol. in ppm (w.r.t sample)

$$\text{Conc. of methanol ID sol. in ppm (w.r.t sample)} = \text{-----------} \times \text{-----------} \times \text{-----------} \times 10^6 =$$

Conc. of MDC ID sol. in ppm (w.r.t sample) = ----------- x ------------ x ----------- x 10^6 =

Fig. 5: Excel sheet screenshot for individual residual solvent solution preparation.

J54 | fx | =D54/E54*F54/G54*H54/I54*1000000

Individual Impurit Slution Preparation

Solvent Identification Solution								
Residual solvent Name	Spec conc (ppm)	Solvent Wt (mg)	Dil to (mL)	Pipetted (mL)	Dil to (mL)	Sample dilution (mL)	Sample Wt (mg)	Conc (ppm) wrt sample
Ethanol	5000	500	100	10	100	5	500	5000
Methanol	3000	300	100	10	100	5	500	3000
MDC	600	60	100	10	100	5	500	600

g. Residual solvent spiked test solution for specificity:

In specificity (or selectivity) testing, residual solvents must be intentionally spiked into the test solution to demonstrate that they do not interfere with each other, the API, or any other components of the sample matrix. In this example, the residual solvents are spiked at their respective release specification concentrations.

A simple and effective way to prepare the residual solvent spiked test solution is by using the same residual solvent stock solution that was prepared during standard preparation. As shown in Figure 6, the stock solutions for ethanol, methanol, and methylene dichloride (MDC) are prepared following the standard procedure. The stock concentrations in mg/mL are calculated in cells H63, H64, and H65 (fig. 6).

The sample weight used is recorded in cell I63, and the volume of residual solvent stock added is noted in cell J63. Specifically, 5 mL of residual solvent stock solution is added to 500 mg of test sample. This results in final concentrations of Ethanol: 5000 ppm, Methanol: 3000 ppm, MDC: 600 ppm (assuming no residual solvent is present in sample) All concentrations are w.r.t sample.

Fig. 6: Excel sheet screenshot for residual solvent spiked sample solution preparation.

K63 | fx | =D63/$E$63*$F$63/$G$63*$J$63/$I$63*1000000

1. SPECIFICITY

Spiked Sample Preparation

RESIDUAL SOLVENTS STOCK SOLUTION PREPARATION							SPIKED SAMPLE PREPARATION		
Residual solvent Name	Spec conc (ppm)	Solvent Wt (mg)	Dil to (mL)	Pipetted (mL)	Dil to (mL)	Solvent Stock Conc (mg/ml)	Sample Wt (mL)	Vol of Stock sol	Resulted conc of solvents (in ppm) wrt sample
Ethanol	5000	500				0.5			5000
Methanol	3000	300	100	10	100	0.3	500	5	3000
MDC	600	60				0.06			600

Verification of the resulted residual solvent concentration in spiked test solution for specificity:

It is the final check- verifying the prepared residual solvent solution concentration in the spiked test solution.

So far, we have prepared the residual solvent stock solution and calculated the volume of stock needed to achieve the desired concentration in a spiked test solution.

Now, it's time to verify the final concentration in ppm w.r.t sample of the residual solvent solution using actual values including the stock concentration, the volume taken from the stock, and the total dilution volume.

$$\text{Conc. of ethanol in ppm (w.r.t sample)} = \frac{500\ mg}{100\ mL} \times \frac{10\ mL}{100\ mL} \times \frac{5\ mL}{500\ mg} \times 10^6 = 5000\ ppm$$

Where:

- Ethanol wt. (mg) = 500 mg *(cell D63 from Fig. 6)*
- Ethanol dilution volume (mL) = 100 mL *(cell E63 from Fig. 6)*
- Ethanol solution pipetted volume (mL) = 10 mL *(cell F63 from Fig. 6)*
- Further dilution (mL) = 100 mL *(cell G63 from Fig. 6)*
- Test wt. (mg) = 500 mg *(cell I63 from fig. 6)*
- Volume of ethanol stock (mL) = 5 mL *(cell J63 from Fig. 6)*

Conclusion:

The resulted concentration of ethanol matches the expected value.

4.2. System Suitability

Prepare the standard solution or system suitability solutions as per STP

Fig. 7: Excel sheet screenshot for system suitability solution preparation

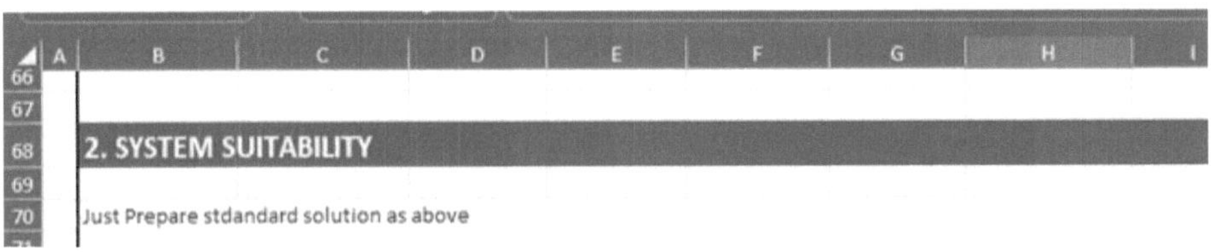

4.3. Precision:

Precision can be considered at three levels: repeatability, intermediate precision and reproducibility. For all three levels you can use the same concentration matrix as concentration of standard, test, or method of preparation remains one and the same.

Repeatability should be assessed using a minimum of 9 determinations covering the reportable range for the procedure (e.g., 3 concentrations/3 replicates each) or a minimum of 6 determinations at 100% of the test concentration.
We are going to prepare the concentration matrix for the solutions below

4.3.1 Preparation of repeatability solutions using finished product

4.3.2 Preparation of repeatability solutions using (API + Placebo)

Below table provides the concentration matrix for preparation of test at 100% of the test concentration.

Table 5: Concentration matrix for preparation of repeatability test at 100% of the test concentration

Solution Name	Discussion	Weight in mg	Dilution 1	Dilution 2	Conc. ppm (w.r.t sample)
Unspiked Test Solution	Follow the test procedure	----------	5 mL		
Repeatab-ility standard solution	Prepare repeatability standard solution containing ethanol, methanol, and MDC at the required concentration. (Refer step 1 under 4.3.1)	Wt. of ethanol: ---------- Wt. of methanol: ---------- Wt. of MDC: ----------	100 mL	10mL → 100mL	Ethanol conc.: ---------- Methanol conc.: ---------- MDC conc.: ----------
Residual solvent spiked test solution	Test solution shall be prep-ared by using repeatability standard solution as a diluent	Weight of sample: ----------	5 mL of repeatabil-ity standard solution		

Please follow the accuracy section to understand the concentration matrix for precision with 9 determinations covering the reportable range for the procedure (e.g., 3 concentrations/3 replicates each)

4.3.1 Preparation of repeatability solutions using finished product:

The repeatability using finished product can be studied by spiking the test solution with residual solvents to achieve the residual solvents at about their respective release specification concentration.

To understand the spiking need, one must calculate the concentration of the residual solvent present in as such test sample or unspiked test sample.

Fig. 8: Excel sheet screenshot for repeatability solution at 100% using finished product

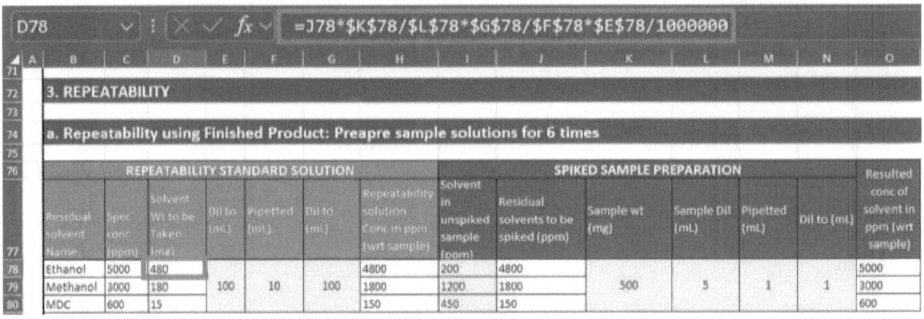

D78 =J78*$K$78/$L$78*$G$78/$F$78*$E$78/1000000

3. REPEATABILITY

a. Repeatability using Finished Product: Preapre sample solutions for 6 times

REPEATABILITY STANDARD SOLUTION							SPIKED SAMPLE PREPARATION						Resulted conc of solvent in ppm (wrt sample)
Residual solvent Name	Spec conc (ppm)	Solvent Wt to be Taken (mg)	Dil to (mL)	Pipetted (mL)	Dil to (mL)	Repeatability solution Conc in ppm (wrt sample)	Solvent in unspiked sample (ppm)	Residual solvents to be spiked (ppm)	Sample wt (mg)	Sample Dil (mL)	Pipetted (mL)	Dil to (mL)	
Ethanol	5000	480				4800	200	4800					5000
Methanol	3000	180	100	10	100	1800	1200	1800	500	5	1	1	3000
MDC	600	15				150	450	150					600

We will prepare the repeatability solution using drug product with the help of the two steps.

Step 1: Residual solvent quantity required for preparation of repeatability standard solution

Step 2: Verification of the resulted spiked residual solvent concentration in repeatability test solution

Let us start from the first…

Step 1: Residual solvent quantity required for preparation of repeatability standard solution

A common repeatability standard solution is prepared containing residual solvents ethanol, methanol, and methylene dichloride (MDC) which will be spiked into the test sample during repeatability testing. In this example, the repeatability stock solution is prepared to contain Ethanol: 4800 ppm, Methanol: 1800 ppm, and MDC: 150 ppm.

Now you may wonder why these specific concentrations?
Here's the rationale:

The test sample already contains certain levels of residual solvents even before spiking. The goal is to spike the repeatability standard solution in such a way that the final concentration of each residual solvent in the spiked sample approaches the expected specification level.

Let's understand the unspiked test sample first. It contains: Ethanol: 200 ppm, Methanol: 1200 ppm, MDC: 450 ppm.

The target concentrations (post-spiking) should be aligned with their respective release specifications: Ethanol: 5000 ppm, Methanol: 3000 ppm, and MDC: 600 ppm

So, the required amount to be spiked should bridge the gap between what's already present and what's expected:
- Ethanol: 5000 – 200 = 4800 ppm
-Methanol: 3000 – 1200 = 1800 ppm
-MDC: 600 – 450 = 150 ppm

Hence, the repeatability stock solution is designed to contain ethanol, methanol, and MDC at 4800 ppm, 1800 ppm, and 150 ppm respectively, so that when spiked into the test solution, the final concentrations match the target levels.

Let us now understand the weight of the residual solvents to be taken for preparing repeatability solutions.

$$\text{Weight of solvent} = A \times \frac{B}{C} \times \frac{D}{E} \times \frac{F}{10^6}$$

Where:
- A = Residual solvent to be spiked in (ppm) w.r.t sample
- B = Sample wt. (mg) as per test procedure
- C = Sample dilution (mL) as per test procedure
- D = Repeatability standard solution final dilution volume (mL)
- E = Pipetted volume of repeatability stock (mL)
- F = Repeatability standard stock volume (mL)

Let us calculate the ethanol weight for preparation of repeatability stock solution

$$\text{Weight of ethanol (mg)} = 4800\ \text{ppm} \times \frac{500\ \text{mg}}{5\ \text{mL}} \times \frac{100\ \text{mL}}{10\ \text{mL}} \times \frac{100\ \text{mL}}{10^6} = 480\ \text{mg}$$

Where:
- A= Residual solvent to be spiked in ppm wrt sample = 4800 ppm *(refer cell J78, Fig 8)*
- B = Sample wt. (mg) = 500 mg *(Refer cell K78, Fig 8)*
- C = Sample dilution (mL) = 5 mL *(Refer cell L78, Fig 8)*
- D = Repeatability std. solution final dilution vol (mL) = 100 mL *(Refer cell G78, Fig 8)*
- E = Pipetted volume of repeatability stock (mL) = 10 mL *(Refer cell F78, Fig 8)*
- F = Repeatability std. stock vol. (mL) = 100 mL *(Refer cell E78, Fig 8)*

Similarly calculate methanol and MDC weight for preparation of repeatability stock solution

Weight of methanol (mg) = ………………… ppm x -------------------- x ---------------------x -------------- =

Weight of MDC (mg) = ………………… ppm x -------------------- x ---------------------x -------------- =

Step 2: Verification of the resulted spiked residual solvent concentration in repeatability test solution

It is the final check- verifying the concentration of residual solvent in the spiked test solution.

We'll use the following formula to confirm the result:

$$\text{Solvent conc (ppm) wrt sample} = \frac{\text{Solvent wt. (mg)}}{\text{Dilution (mL)}} \times \frac{\text{Pipetted vol (mL)}}{\text{Dilution (mL)}} \times \frac{\text{Sample Dil. (mL)}}{\text{Sample wt. (mg)}} \times 10^6 + S_{unspiked}$$

$S_{unspiked}$ = Solvent present in unspiked test in ppm (w.r.t sample)

Let's take ethanol as an example:

$$\text{Ethanol conc (ppm) wrt sample} = \left[\frac{480\ mg}{100\ mL} \times \frac{10\ mL}{100\ mL} \times \frac{5\ mL}{500\ mg} \times 10^{6}\right] + 200\ ppm = 5000\ ppm$$

- Ethanol wt. (mg) = 480 mg *(cell D78 from Fig. 9)*
- Dilution volume (mL) = 100 mL *(cell E78 from Fig. 9)*
- Pipetted volume (mL) = 10 mL *(cell F78 from Fig. 9)*
- Further Dilution (mL) = 100 mL *(cell G78 from Fig. 9)*
- Test solution dilution volume (mL)= 5 mL *(cell L78 from Fig. 9)*
- Test weight (mg) = 500 mg *(cell K78 from Fig. 9)*
- Ethanol present in unspiked sample = 200 ppm *(cell I78, from Fig. 9)*

Conclusion:

The resulted concentration of ethanol matches the expected value. Therefore, the selected ethanol weight and the proposed dilution are appropriate and accurate.

Similarly, you can calculate the resulted concentration for methanol and MDC

Methanol conc (ppm) wrt sample = [--------------- x --------------- x -------------- x 10^6]+ ……………ppm =

MDC conc (ppm) wrt sample = [--------------- x --------------- x -------------- x 10^6]+ ……………ppm =

Conclusion:

Fig. 9: Excel sheet screenshot for calculation of resulted conc of residual solvent using drug product

O78 =D78/$E$78*$F$78/$G$78*$L$78/$K$78*1000000+I78

3. REPEATABILITY

a. Repeatability using Finished Product: Preapre sample solutions for 6 times

REPEATABILITY STANDARD SOLUTION							SPIKED SAMPLE PREPARATION						Resulted conc of solvent in ppm (wrt sample)
Residual solvent Name	Spec conc (ppm)	Solvent Wt to be Taken (mg)	Dil to (mL)	Pipetted (mL)	Dil to (mL)	Repeatability solution Conc in ppm (wrt sample)	Solvent in unspiked sample (ppm)	Residual solvents to be spiked (ppm)	Sample wt (mg)	Sample Dil (mL)	Pipetted (mL)	Dil to (mL)	
Ethanol	5000	480				4800	200	4800					5000
Methanol	3000	180	100	10	100	1800	1200	1800	500	5	1	1	3000
MDC	600	15				150	450	150					600

4.3.2 Preparation of repeatability solutions using (API + Placebo):

If the test sample is unavailable or unsuitable, you can use a combination of placebo and API based on the product's composition. The first step involves accurately weighing the required quantities of placebo and API to prepare the sample. From there, the procedure follows the same steps as described earlier for "Repeatability Using Finished Product."

In the current example, the total weight of the paracetamol tablet is 700 mg, and the label claim specifies 500 mg of paracetamol. Based on this, a 500 mg portion of the sample would contain approximately 357 mg of paracetamol (API) and 143 mg of placebo.

Therefore, each repeatability solution (comprising API and placebo) should be prepared using 357 mg of paracetamol and 143 mg of placebo to accurately reflect the actual formulation.

We will prepare the repeatability solution using 'API + Placebo' with the help of the two steps.

Let's understand the residual solvent content in API. The residual solvent in API will be considered as the residual solvent in 'API + Placebo' (assuming placebo does not contribute to residual solvent). API contains: Ethanol: 500 ppm, Methanol: 200 ppm, MDC: 150 ppm. (Refer cell I86, I87, I88, Fig. 10)

The target concentrations (post-spiking) should be aligned with their respective release specifications: Ethanol: 5000 ppm, Methanol: 3000 ppm, and MDC: 600 ppm

So, the required amount to be spiked should bridge the gap between what's already present and what's expected:
- Ethanol: 5000 – 500 = 4500 ppm
- Methanol: 3000 – 200 = 2800 ppm
- MDC: 600 – 150 = 450 ppm

Hence, the repeatability stock solution is designed to contain ethanol, methanol, and MDC at 4500 ppm, 2800 ppm, and 450 ppm respectively (refer cell H86, H87, H88, Fig. 10), so that when spiked into the test solution, the final concentrations match the target levels. (Refer cell O86, O87, O88, Fig. 10)

Step 1: Residual solvent quantity required for preparation of repeatability standard solution

Follow the "preparation of repeatability solution using drug product"

Fig. 10: Excel sheet screenshot for repeatability solution at 100% using (API + Placebo)

D86 =J86*$K$86/$L$86*$G$86/$F$86*$E$86/1000000

3. REPEATABILITY

b. Repeatability using (API + Placebo): Preapre (API + Placebo) solutions for 6 times

REPEATABILITY STANDARD SOLUTION							SPIKED (API + PLACEBO) PREPARATION						Resulted conc of solvent in ppm (wrt sample)
Residual solvent Name	Spec conc (ppm)	Solvent Wt to be Taken (mg)	Dil to (mL)	Pipetted (mL)	Dil to (mL)	Repeatability solution Conc in ppm (wrt sample)	Solvent in API (ppm)	Residual solvents to be spiked (ppm)	(API + Placebo) wt in mg	Sample Dil (mL)	Pipetted (mL)	Dil to (mL)	
Ethanol	5000	450	100	10	100	4500	500	4500	500	5	1	1	5000
Methanol	3000	280				2800	200	2800					3000
MDC	600	45				450	150	450					600

Step 2: Verification of the resulted spiked residual solvent concentration in repeatability test solution

Follow the "preparation of repeatability solution using drug product"

Fig. 11: Excel sheet screenshot for calculation of resulted conc of residual solvent using (API + Placebo)

O86 =D86/$E$86*$F$86/$G$86*$L$86/$K$86*1000000+I86

3. REPEATABILITY

b. Repeatability using (API + Placebo): Preapre (API + Placebo) solutions for 6 times

REPEATABILITY STANDARD SOLUTION								SPIKED (API + PLACEBO) PREPARATION						
Residual solvent Name	Spec conc (ppm)	Solvent Wt to be Taken (mg)	Dil to (mL)	Pipetted (mL)	Dil to (mL)	Repeatability solution Conc in ppm (wrt sample)	Solvent in API (ppm)	Residual solvents to be spiked (ppm)	(API + Placebo) wt in mg	Sample Dil (mL)	Pipetted (mL)	Dil to (mL)	Resulted conc of solvent in ppm (wrt sample)
Ethanol	5000	450				4500	500	4500					5000
Methanol	3000	280	100	10	100	2800	200	2800	500	5	1	1	3000
MDC	600	45				450	150	450					600

4.2 Response/linearity:

The response of an analytical procedure is its ability (within a given range) to obtain a signal which is effectively related to the concentration (amount) or activity of analyte in the sample by some known mathematical function. (ICH Q2)

The linearity study is conducted from the LOQ, 50% level up to 150% of the release specifications.

To systematically design the linearity concentration matrix, follow these key steps:

Step 1: Preparation of linearity stock solutions

Step 2: Calculation of expected concentration across various linearity levels

Step 3: Preparation of linearity solutions

Step 4: Verification of resulted solution at various linearity levels

Let us start from the step 1…

Step 1: Preparation of linearity stock solutions:

Please refer to Fig. 12 for preparation of linearity stock solution for residual solvents.

Conc. of linearity stock in ppm (w.r.t sample) can be calculated by the formula below

$$\text{Linearity stock conc in ppm wrt sample} = \frac{\text{Solvent wt. (mg)}}{\text{Dilution (mL)}} \times \frac{\text{Sample Dil. (mL)}}{\text{Sample Wt. (mg)}} \times 10^6$$

Let us calculate the conc. of ethanol linearity stock in ppm w.r.t sample by using the above formula

$$\text{Conc of ethanol linearity stock in ppm w.r.t sample} = \frac{500\ mg}{100\ mL} \times \frac{5\ mL}{500\ mg} \times 10^6 = 50000\ ppm$$

Where:

- Ethanol weight for stock preparation: 500 mg *(cell D95 from Fig. 12)*
- Ethanol stock dilution volume: 100 mL *(cell E95 from Fig. 12)*
- Sample dilution volume = 5 mL *(cell C30 from Fig. 2)*

- Sample weight = 500 mg *(cell C29 from Fig. 2)*

Similarly calculate the conc. of linearity stock for methanol and MDC

Conc of methanol linearity stock in ppm wrt sample= ----------------- *x* ---------------- *x* 10^6=

Conc of MDC linearity stock in ppm wrt sample= ----------------- *x* ---------------- *x* 10^6=

Fig. 12: Excel sheet screenshot for 'preparation of linearity stock'

J95 | fx | =D95/$E$95*F95/G95*H95/I95*$C$30/$C$29*1000000

	B	C	D	E	F	G	H	I	J
91	4. RESPONSE/LINEARITY								
92									
93	LINEARITY STOCK SOLUTION								
94	Residual solvent name	Spec conc (ppm)	Solvent wt (mg)	Dil to (mL)	Pipetted (mL)	Dil to (mL)	Pipetted (mL)	Dil to (mL)	Conc in ppm (wrt sample)
95	Ethanol	5000	500		1	1	1	1	50000
96	Methanol	3000	300	100	1	1	1	1	30000
97	MDC	600	60		1	1	1	1	6000

Step 2: Calculation of expected concentration across various linearity levels:

In this example, we have chosen to study six linearity levels. Since the exact LOQ value will be determined during the method validation, the concentration for the LOQ level is currently left blank.

Let us calculate the expected impurity concentration at various linearity levels.

$$\text{Expected solvent conc. in ppm (wrt sample)} = \frac{\text{Linearity level in (\%)} \times \text{conc. of solvent at release spec. (ppm)}}{100}$$

Let us calculate the expected concentration for ethanol at 50% linearity level

$$\text{Expected ethanol conc. (ppm) at 50\% level} = \frac{50\,\% \times 5000\ \text{ppm}}{100} = 2500\ \text{ppm}$$

Linearity level in (%) for ethanol = 50 % (Refer cell B103 from Fig. 13)

Ethanol conc. at release specification = 5000 ppm (Refer cell D38 from Fig. 3)

Similarly, calculate the concentration for ethanol, methanol and MDC at other levels and tabulate below.

Table 6: Expected residual solvent concentration across various linearity levels.

	Expected residual solvent conc. in ppm		
Linearity Level	Ethanol	Methanol	MDC
LOQ			
50%	2500 ppm		
75%			
100%			
125%			
150%			

Fig. 13: Excel sheet screenshot for 'calculation of expected residual solvent conc. across levels'

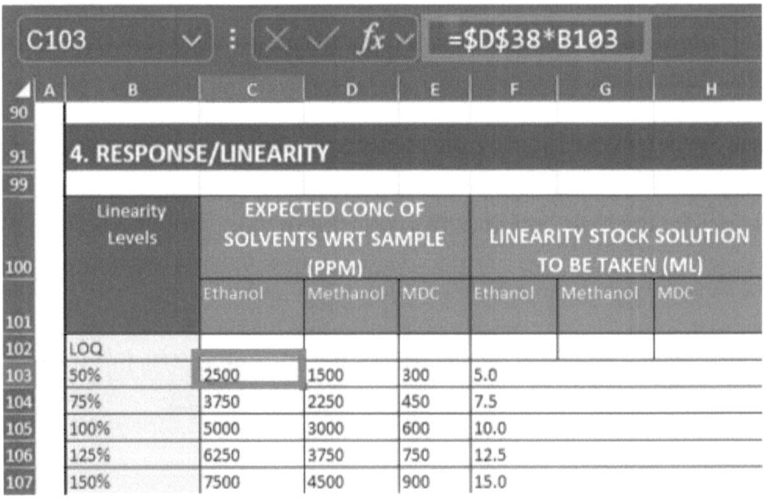

C103 =$D$38*B103

4. RESPONSE/LINEARITY

Linearity Levels	EXPECTED CONC OF SOLVENTS WRT SAMPLE (PPM)			LINEARITY STOCK SOLUTION TO BE TAKEN (ML)		
	Ethanol	Methanol	MDC	Ethanol	Methanol	MDC
LOQ						
50%	2500	1500	300	5.0		
75%	3750	2250	450	7.5		
100%	5000	3000	600	10.0		
125%	6250	3750	750	12.5		
150%	7500	4500	900	15.0		

Step 3: Preparation of linearity solutions:

Once we have identified the expected linearity concentrations, the next step is to prepare the linearity solutions. These can be prepared using the linearity stock solutions as outlined in Fig. 12.

Use the formula below to prepare the linearity solutions at the desired concentrations.

$$\text{Volume of linearity stock (mL)} = \frac{A}{B} \times \frac{C}{D} \times E$$

Where:

- A = Expected residual solvent concentration in ppm w.r.t sample
- B = Concentration of residual solvent stock in ppm (w.r.t sample)

- C = Further dilution of ethanol resulted solution in mL
- D = Further pipetted volume in mL
- E = First time dilution in mL for ethanol weight taken

Let us calculate the volume of ethanol linearity stock required for preparation of linearity level 50%

$$\text{Volume of ethanol stock (mL) for 50\% level} = \frac{2500\ ppm}{50000\ ppm} \times \frac{1\ mL}{1\ mL} \times \frac{1\ mL}{1\ mL} \times 100\ mL = 5\ mL$$

Where:
- A = Expected residual solvent conc. in ppm w.r.t sample (at 50%) = 2500 ppm (cell C103, Fig 14)
- B = Concentration of residual solvent stock in ppm (w.r.t sample) = 50000 ppm (cell J95, Fig. 12)
- C = Further dilution of ethanol resulted solution in mL = 1mL (cell M103, K103, Fig 14)
- D = Further pipetted volume in mL = 1 mL (cell L103, J103, Fig 14)
- E = First time dilution in mL for ethanol weight taken = 100 mL (cell I103, Fig 14)

Similarly calculate the volume of ethanol, methanol, and MDC linearity stock for the rest of the linearity levels and tabulate below

Table 7: Residual solvent stock volume to be taken across various linearity levels.

	Linearity stock volume to be taken in mL		
Linearity Level	Ethanol linearity stock	Methanol linearity stock	MDC linearity stock
LOQ			
50%	5 mL		
75%			
100%			
125%			
150%			

Fig. 14: Excel sheet screenshot for 'preparation of linearity solutions'

F103 `=C103/$J$95*M103/L103*K103/J103*I103`

4. RESPONSE/LINEARITY

Linearity Levels	EXPECTED CONC OF SOLVENTS WRT SAMPLE (PPM)			LINEARITY STOCK SOLUTION TO BE TAKEN (ML)			LINEARITY SOLUTION PREPARATION					RESULETD CONC OF SOLVENTS IN (PPM) WRT SAMPLE		
	Ethanol	Methanol	MDC	Ethanol	Methanol	MDC	Dil to (ml)	Pipetted (ml)	Dil. To (ml)	Pipetted (ml)	Dil. To (ml)	Ethanol	Methanol	MDC
LOQ														
50%	2500	1500	300	5.0			100	1	1	1	1	2500	1500	300
75%	3750	2250	450	7.5			100	1	1	1	1	3750	2250	450
100%	5000	3000	600	10.0			100	1	1	1	1	5000	3000	600
125%	6250	3750	750	12.5			100	1	1	1	1	6250	3750	750
150%	7500	4500	900	15.0			100	1	1	1	1	7500	4500	900

Step 4: Verification of concentration of resulted solution at various linearity levels:

The final step is to confirm whether the expected linearity concentrations are achieved using the prepared stock solutions and their respective dilutions. The resulting residual solvent concentration can be calculated using the formula below.

$$\text{Resulted conc in ppm w.r.t sample} = A \times \frac{B}{C} \times \frac{D}{E}$$

Where:

- A= Concentration of residual solvent stock in ppm w.r.t sample
- B = Volume of residual solvent linearity stock (mL)
- C = Dilution volume of residual solvent stock solution in mL
- D = Pipetted volume in mL
- E = Further dilution in mL

Let us calculate the resulted conc. of ethanol at linearity level 50%

$$\text{Resulted conc in ppm w.r.t sample of ethanol at 50\% linearity} = 50000\ ppm \times \frac{5\ mL}{100\ mL} = 2500\ ppm$$

A = Concentration of ethanol stock in ppm = 50000 ppm (Cell J95, Fig. 12)
B = Volume of ethanol linearity stock (mL) = 5 mL (Cell F103, Fig. 15)
C = Dilution volume of ethanol stock solution in mL = 100 mL (Cell I103, Fig. 15)

Conclusion:

The resulting concentration of ethanol at the 50% level matches the expected value of 2500 ppm *(Refer Cell C103, Fig. 13).*

Similarly, calculate the resulted concentration for ethanol, methanol, and MDC and tabulate below

Table 8: Residual solvent stock volume to be taken across various linearity levels.

	Resulted concentration of residual solvent in ppm		
Linearity Level	Ethanol	Methanol	MDC
LOQ			
50%	2500 ppm		
75%			
100%			
125%			
150%			

Fig. 15: Excel sheet screenshot for 'calculation of resulted residual solvent conc. across levels'

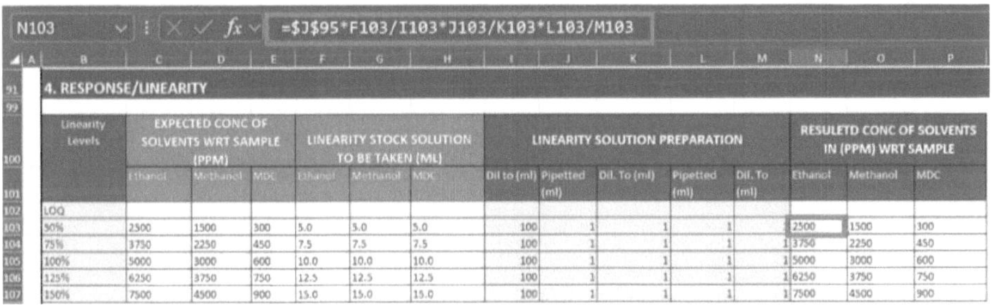

N103 =$J$95*F103/I103*J103/K103*L103/M103

4. RESPONSE/LINEARITY

Linearity Levels	EXPECTED CONC OF SOLVENTS WRT SAMPLE (PPM)			LINEARITY STOCK SOLUTION TO BE TAKEN (ML)			LINEARITY SOLUTION PREPARATION					RESULETD CONC OF SOLVENTS IN (PPM) WRT SAMPLE		
	Ethanol	Methanol	MDC	Ethanol	Methanol	MDC	Dil to (ml)	Pipetted (ml)	Dil. To (ml)	Pipetted (ml)	Dil. To (ml)	Ethanol	Methanol	MDC
LOQ														
50%	2500	1500	300	5.0	5.0	5.0	100	1	1	1		2500	1500	300
75%	3750	2250	450	7.5	7.5	7.5	100	1	1	1	1	3750	2250	450
100%	5000	3000	600	10.0	10.0	10.0	100	1	1	1	1	5000	3000	600
125%	6250	3750	750	12.5	12.5	12.5	100	1	1	1	1	6250	3750	750
150%	7500	4500	900	15.0	15.0	15.0	100	1	1	1	1	7500	4500	900

4.3 Accuracy:

We are going to prepare concentration matrix for below accuracy solutions

4.3.1 Accuracy using drug product/test sample

4.3.2 Accuracy using (API + Placebo)

4.3.1 Accuracy using drug product/test sample

To systematically design the accuracy concentration matrix using drug product, follow these key steps:

Step 1: Preparation of accuracy stock solutions

Step 2: Calculation of expected concentration across various accuracy levels

Step 3: Preparation of accuracy solutions by using test sample

Step 4: Verification of concentration of resulted solution at various accuracy levels

Let us discuss each step in detail

Step 1: Preparation of accuracy stock solutions:

Please refer to Fig. 16 for preparation of accuracy stock solution for residual solvents.

Conc. of accuracy stock in ppm (w.r.t sample) can be calculated by the formula below

$$\text{Accuracy stock conc in ppm wrt sample} = \frac{\text{Solvent wt. (mg)}}{\text{Dilution (mL)}} \times \frac{\text{Sample Dil. (mL)}}{\text{Sample Wt. (mg)}} \times 10^6$$

Let us calculate the conc. of ethanol accuracy stock in ppm w.r.t sample by using the above formula

$$\text{Conc of ethanol linearity stock in ppm w.r.t sample} = \frac{500\ mg}{100\ mL} \times \frac{5\ mL}{500\ mg} \times 10^6 = 50000\ ppm$$

Where:

- Ethanol weight for stock preparation: 500 mg *(cell C114 from Fig. 16)*
- Ethanol stock dilution volume: 100 mL *(cell D114 from Fig. 16)*
- Sample dilution volume = 5 mL *(cell C30 from Fig. 2)*
- Sample weight = 500 mg *(cell C29 from Fig. 2)*

Similarly calculate the conc. of linearity stock for methanol and MDC

$$\text{Conc of methanol accuracy stock in ppm wrt sample} = \frac{\quad}{\quad} \times \frac{\quad}{\quad} \times 10^6 =$$

$$\text{Conc of MDC accuracy stock in ppm wrt sample} = \frac{\quad}{\quad} \times \frac{\quad}{\quad} \times 10^6 =$$

Fig. 16: Excel sheet screenshot for 'preparation of accuracy stock'

I114 =C114/$D$114*E114/F114*G114/H114*$C$30/$C$29*1000000

5. ACCURACY

ACCURACY SOLUTION							
Solvent Name	Solvent wt (mg)	Dil to (mL)	Pipetted (mL)	Dil to (mL)	Pipetted (mL)	Dil to (mL)	Conc (mg/ml)
Ethanol	500	100	1	1	1	1	50000
Methanol	300		1	1	1	1	30000
MDC	60		1	1	1	1	6000

Step 2: Calculation of expected concentration across various accuracy levels

Let us now calculate the expected residual solvent concentration in ppm (w.r.t sample) at various accuracy levels.

$$\text{Expected solvent conc. in ppm (wrt sample)} = \frac{\text{Accuracy level in (\%)} \times \text{conc. of solvent at release spec. (ppm)}}{100}$$

Let us calculate the expected concentration for ethanol at 50% accuracy level

$$\text{Expected ethanol conc. (ppm) at 50\% level} = \frac{50\ \% \times 5000\ ppm}{100} = 2500\ ppm$$

Where:

- Accuracy level in (%) for ethanol = 50 % *(Refer cell B122 from Fig. 17)*

- Ethanol conc. at release specification = 5000 ppm *(Refer cell D38 from Fig. 3)*

Similarly, calculate the concentration for methanol and MDC at other levels and tabulate below.

Table 9: Expected residual solvent concentration across various accuracy levels.

	Expected residual solvent conc. in ppm (wrt sample)		
Linearity Level	Ethanol	Methanol	MDC
LOQ			
50%	2500 ppm		
75%			
100%			
125%			
150%			

Fig. 17: Excel sheet screenshot for 'calculation of expected residual solvent conc. across accuracy levels'

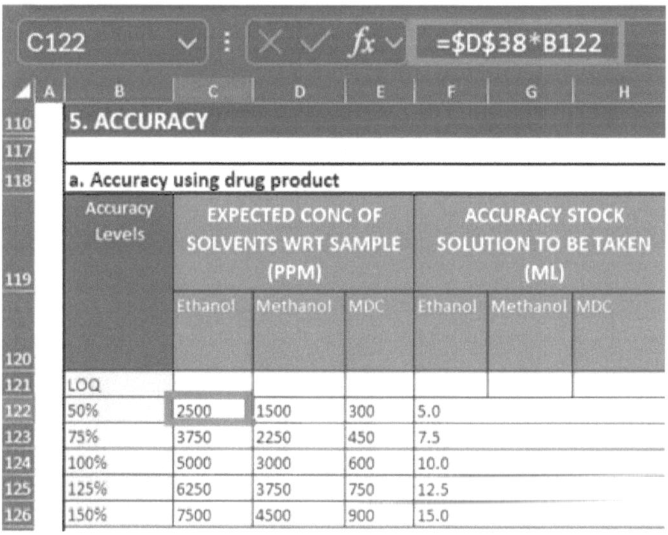

C122 fx =$D$38*B122

5. ACCURACY

a. Accuracy using drug product

Accuracy Levels	EXPECTED CONC OF SOLVENTS WRT SAMPLE (PPM)			ACCURACY STOCK SOLUTION TO BE TAKEN (ML)		
	Ethanol	Methanol	MDC	Ethanol	Methanol	MDC
LOQ						
50%	2500	1500	300	5.0		
75%	3750	2250	450	7.5		
100%	5000	3000	600	10.0		
125%	6250	3750	750	12.5		
150%	7500	4500	900	15.0		

Step 3: Accuracy using drug product/test sample:

Accuracy using the finished product can be evaluated by spiking the test solution with residual solvents at specific accuracy levels. In this example, residual solvents are spiked at their release specification levels 50%, 75%, 100%, 125%, and 150% along with the LOQ level. The required amount of residual solvent is added using the accuracy stock solution to achieve the target spiking concentration. Please ensure that all accuracy solutions are prepared by strictly following the 'test sample preparation' as defined in standard test procedure, using the exact quantity of test sample as defined.

Use the formula below to prepare the accuracy solutions at the desired concentrations by spiking accuracy stock solutions.

$$\text{Volume of accuracy stock (mL)} = \frac{A}{B} \times \frac{C}{D} \times E$$

Where:
- A = Expected residual solvent concentration in ppm (w.r.t sample)
- B = Concentration of residual solvent stock in ppm (w.r.t sample)
- C = Further dilution of ethanol resulted solution in mL
- D = Further pipetted volume in mL
- E = First time dilution in mL for ethanol weight taken

Let us calculate the volume of ethanol accuracy stock required for preparation of accuracy level 50%

$$\text{Volume of ethanol stock (mL) for 50\% level} = \frac{2500\ ppm}{50000\ ppm} \times 100\ mL = 5\ mL$$

Where:
- A = Expected residual solvent concentration in ppm w.r.t sample = 2500 ppm *(cell C122, Fig 18)*
- B = Concentration of residual solvent stock in ppm (w.r.t sample) = 50000 ppm *(cell I114, Fig. 16)*
- E = First time dilution in mL for ethanol weight taken = 100 mL *(cell I122, Fig 18)*

Similarly calculate the volume of ethanol, methanol, and MDC linearity stock for the rest of the accuracy levels and tabulate below

Table 10: Accuracy stock volume to be taken across various accuracy levels

	Accuracy stock volume to be taken in mL		
Accuracy Level	Ethanol Accuracy stock	Methanol Accuracy stock	MDC Accuracy stock
LOQ			
50%	5 mL		
75%			
100%			
125%			
150%			

Fig. 18: Excel sheet screenshot for 'volume of residual solvent stock to be spiked across accuracy levels'

F122 =C122/$J$95*O122/N122*M122/L122*I122

5. ACCURACY

a. Accuracy using drug product

Accuracy Levels	EXPECTED CONC OF SOLVENTS WRT SAMPLE (PPM)			ACCURACY STOCK SOLUTION TO BE TAKEN (ML)			ACCURACY SOLUTION PREPARATION							RESULETD CONC OF SOLVENTS IN (PPM) WRT SAMPLE		
	Ethanol	Methanol	MDC	Ethanol	Methanol	MDC	Dil to (ml)	Sample wt (mg)	Accuracy Stock Vol (ml)	Pipetted (ml)	Dil. To (ml)	Pipetted (ml)	Dil. To (ml)	Ethanol	Methanol	MDC
LOQ							100	500	5	1	1	1	1			
50%	2500	1500	300	5.0			100	500	5	1	1	1	1	2500	1500	300
75%	3750	2250	450	7.5			100	500	5	1	1	1	1	3750	2250	450
100%	5000	3000	600	10.0			100	500	5	1	1	1	1	5000	3000	600
125%	6250	3750	750	12.5			100	500	5	1	1	1	1	6250	3750	750
150%	7500	4500	900	15.0			100	500	5	1	1	1	1	7500	4500	900

Step 4: Verification of concentration of resulted solution at various accuracy levels

The final step is to confirm whether the expected accuracy concentrations are achieved using the prepared stock solutions and their respective dilutions. The resulting impurity concentration can be calculated using the formula below.

$$\text{Resulted conc in ppm w.r.t sample} = A \times \frac{B}{C} \times \frac{D}{E}$$

Where:

- A= Concentration of residual solvent stock in ppm w.r.t sample
- B = Volume of residual solvent accuracy stock (mL)
- C = Dilution volume of residual solvent stock solution in mL
- D = Pipetted volume in mL
- E = Further dilution in mL

Let us calculate the resulted conc. of ethanol at accuracy level 50%

$$\text{Resulted conc in ppm w.r.t sample of ethanol at 50\% accuracy} = 50000\ ppm \times \frac{5\ mL}{100\ mL} = 2500\ ppm$$

A = Concentration of ethanol stock in ppm = 50000 ppm (Cell I114, Fig. 16)
B = Volume of ethanol accuracy stock (mL) = 5 mL (Cell F122, Fig. 19)
C = Dilution volume of ethanol stock solution in mL = 100 mL (Cell I122, Fig. 19)

Conclusion:

The resulting concentration of ethanol at the 50% level matches the expected value of 2500 ppm (refer cell C122, Fig. 17).

Similarly, calculate the resulted concentration for ethanol, methanol, and MDC and tabulate below

Table 11: Resulted residual solvent concentration across various accuracy levels.

	Resulted concentration of residual solvent in ppm w.r.t sample		
Accuracy Level	Ethanol	Methanol	MDC
LOQ			
50%	2500 ppm		
75%			
100%			
125%			
150%			

Fig. 19: Excel sheet screenshot for 'calculation of resulted residual solvent conc. across accuracy levels'

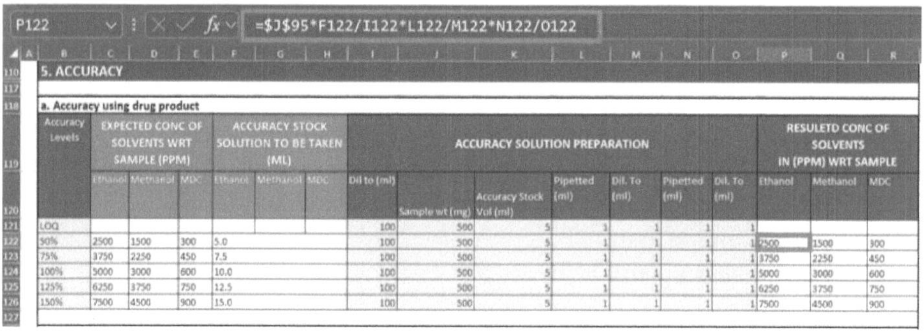

P122 =$J$95*F122/I122*L122/M122*N122/O122

5. ACCURACY

a. Accuracy using drug product

Accuracy Levels	EXPECTED CONC OF SOLVENTS WRT SAMPLE (PPM)			ACCURACY STOCK SOLUTION TO BE TAKEN (ML)			ACCURACY SOLUTION PREPARATION							RESULETD CONC OF SOLVENTS IN (PPM) WRT SAMPLE		
	Ethanol	Methanol	MDC	Ethanol	Methanol	MDC	Dil to (ml)	Sample wt (mg)	Accuracy Stock Vol (ml)	Pipetted (ml)	Dil. To (ml)	Pipetted (ml)	Dil. To (ml)	Ethanol	Methanol	MDC
LOQ							100	500	5	1	1	1	1			
50%	2500	1500	300	5.0			100	500	5	1	1	1	1	2500	1500	300
75%	3750	2250	450	7.5			100	500	5	1	1	1	1	3750	2250	450
100%	5000	3000	600	10.0			100	500	5	1	1	1	1	5000	3000	600
125%	6250	3750	750	12.5			100	500	5	1	1	1	1	6250	3750	750
150%	7500	4500	900	15.0			100	500	5	1	1	1	1	7500	4500	900

4.3.2 Accuracy using (API + Placebo):

If the test sample is unavailable or unsuitable, you can use a combination of placebo and API based on the product's composition. The first step involves accurately weighing the required quantities of placebo and API to prepare the sample. From there, the procedure follows the same steps as described earlier for "Accuracy Using Drug Product."

In the current example, the total weight of the paracetamol tablet is 700 mg, and the label claim specifies 500 mg of paracetamol. Based on this, a 500 mg portion of the sample would contain approximately 357 mg of paracetamol (API) and 143 mg of placebo.

Therefore, each accuracy solution (comprising API and placebo) should be prepared using 357 mg of paracetamol and 143 mg of placebo to accurately reflect the actual formulation.

To systematically design the accuracy concentration matrix using (API + Placebo), follow these key steps:

Step 1: Preparation of accuracy stock solutions

Step 2: Calculation of expected concentration across various accuracy levels

Step 3: Preparation of accuracy solutions by using (API + Placebo)

Step 4: Verification of concentration of resulted solution at various accuracy levels

For Steps 1 to 4, follow the same procedure as outlined in the section "Accuracy Using Drug Product."

Fig. 20: Excel sheet screenshot for accuracy using API + Placebo

B128 | b. Accuracy using (API + Placebo)

5. ACCURACY

b. Accuracy using (API + Placebo)

Accuracy Levels	EXPECTED CONC OF SOLVENTS WRT SAMPLE (PPM)			ACCURACY STOCK SOLUTION TO BE TAKEN (ML)			ACCURACY SOLUTION PREPARATION							RESULETD CONC OF SOLVENTS IN (PPM) WRT SAMPLE		
	Ethanol	Methanol	MDC	Ethanol	Methanol	MDC	Dil to (ml)	(API + Placebo) wt in mg	Accuracy Stock Vol (ml)	Pipetted (ml)	Dil. To (ml)	Pipetted (ml)	Dil. To (ml)	0.0	0	0
LOQ							100	500	5	1	1	1	1			
50%	2500	1500	300	5.0			100	500	5	1	1	1	1	2500	1500	300
75%	3750	2250	450	7.5			100	500	5	1	1	1	1	3750	2250	450
100%	5000	3000	600	10.0			100	500	5	1	1	1	1	5000	3000	600
125%	6250	3750	750	12.5			100	500	5	1	1	1	1	6250	3750	750
150%	7500	4500	900	15.0			100	500	5	1	1	1	1	7500	4500	900

Conclusion:

In this example, we learned how to create a concentration matrix for residual solvent method validation using paracetamol tablets. The same approach can be applied to other dosage forms like oral liquids, injectables, and semi-solids.

This method is also suitable for drug substances. However, since placebo is not applicable in drug substances, it should be excluded during the preparation of validation solutions.

CHAPTER: 08

PROTOCOL FORMAT

★ Objective

In the previous chapters, we discussed how to prepare the concentration matrix before drafting the protocol. In this chapter, we will talk about how to prepare the method validation protocol based on the concentration matrix.

Before we specifically discuss the preparation of the validation protocol for a specific test, it's important to first understand the general content of a method validation protocol. These components are common across all types of analytical validation whether it's for assay, related substances, dissolution, or any other parameter.

A well-drafted protocol is not just a regulatory requirement but also a critical document that outlines the entire validation strategy. It ensures consistency, defines clear responsibilities, acceptance criteria for performance characteristic, minimizes the chance of errors, and serves as a reference in case of deviations or non-conformities during execution. In short, the protocol acts as the foundation for a scientifically sound and compliant validation study.

1. Protocol Header

The header typically includes:

- Company Name (e.g., Pharma Growth Hub)
- Company Logo on the right side
- Title: Method Validation Protocol for Assay of Paracetamol Tablets 500 mg by HPLC
- Protocol Number: e.g., 001/00 (first version)
- Target Market: e.g., USA
- Test Method Number: e.g., MOA-001/01
- Specification Number: e.g., SPEC-004/02

2. Protocol Body

The protocol body is the main section of the document where the details of the method validation are specified. It includes critical information such as the product name, objective, scope, responsibilities, SOP references, site details, and most importantly, the concentration matrix and validation parameters.

This section serves as the operational roadmap for executing the validation, ensuring all stakeholders understand their roles, the methodology, and the acceptance criteria. A well-structured protocol body ensures consistency, compliance with regulatory expectations, and facilitates successful validation execution.

3. Product Name

Mention the product name (e.g., Paracetamol Tablets 500 mg). Always use proper unit formatting, such as "mg" in lowercase.

4. Prepared By / Reviewed By / Approved By

These fields should include names and designations from QC, ADL, QA, and DQA departments as per your organization's structure.

5. Footer Details

Include the format number of the control document used to prepare the protocol. Example: F-0121-01. Also mention "Confidential – For Internal Use Only."

6. Index Page

List all parameters with corresponding page numbers.

7. Objective

Your protocol must also define the objective. In current example, the objective could be "to validate the assay test procedure of Paracetamol Tablets 500 mg by HPLC."

8. Scope

Provide the scope of the protocol, such as "this protocol aims to validate the in-house developed assay test method for Paracetamol Tablets 500 mg using HPLC, as per ICH Q2(R1) guidelines."

9. Responsibilities

The protocol must clearly define the responsibilities of all departments and personnel involved. This ensures error-free execution and eliminates ambiguity, especially in the event of deviations or non-conformities.

- QC/ADL Associate: Execute and review the protocol
- HOD/Designee: Ensure execution and approval
- QA/DQA: Review and ensure compliance

10. Reference SOP

Include the SOP number used to prepare the protocol. Example: SOP-124/02.

11. Site Address

Mention the address of method validation location (e.g., Pharma Growth Hub, Pune, India).

12. Standard Test Procedure

Provide details of standard test procedure

13. Concentration Matrix/Concentration Mapping

The concentration matrix is a foundational element of the validation protocol. It provides a clear plan for the concentrations of standard and test solutions to be used for each validation parameter such as accuracy, precision, linearity, and specificity. Designing this matrix in advance helps ensure consistency, reduces errors during solution preparation, and supports scientifically sound and reproducible results throughout the validation process.

14. Specification Limits

Specification limits define the acceptable range within which a product or component must fall to be considered compliant with quality standards. These limits are typically derived from regulatory guidelines, product development data, and stability studies.

Specification limits are crucial in method validation because they guide the selection of concentration levels in the concentration matrix. For example, during accuracy or linearity testing, solutions are prepared at various percentages (e.g., 50%, 75%, 100%, 125%) of the specification limits. This ensures that the method can accurately and precisely measure within and around the expected product performance range.

Additionally, these limits are used to define acceptance criteria for assay results. For instance, if the specification is "not less than 95% and not more than 105%," the method must reliably produce results within this range for it to be considered validated.

15. Finished Product Composition

Understanding the finished product composition is essential for accurate method validation. It provides detailed information about the active pharmaceutical ingredient (API) and excipients present in the final dosage form. This knowledge helps in multiple ways:

- It ensures that the sample preparations for specificity and placebo interference studies reflect the actual formulation.
- It supports the identification of potential excipient interference during HPLC analysis.
- It assists in preparing the placebo matrix that mimics the formulation without the API, which is crucial for selectivity evaluations.

Therefore, always obtain the complete composition details from the manufacturing unit and incorporate them appropriately into the validation protocol. Get composition details from the manufacturing unit.

16. Change History / Version Control

Include a summary of changes made from previous versions. This helps in tracking modifications and supports documentation during audits.

17. Abbreviations and Definitions

List common abbreviations (e.g., API, RSD, LOQ) and their meanings to ensure clarity for all reviewers and executors.

18. Validation Strategy / Plan

Provide a brief overview of the validation approach, including which parameters will be validated, in what sequence, and using what sample types.

19. Test Equipment and Software

Mention key instruments (e.g., HPLC make and model) and software (e.g., Empower, Chromeleon) used during validation. This ensures transparency and reproducibility.

20. Deviation Handling

Provide a note on how deviations during protocol execution will be documented, investigated, and addressed. This adds a layer of robustness and traceability.

21. Annexures or Appendices

Attach any supplemental materials like:

- Chromatograms
- Data entry sheets
- Calculation worksheets
- Validation summary templates

22. Revalidation Requirements

Revalidation is a critical process undertaken to confirm that an analytical method continues to perform as intended, especially after significant changes. Revalidation ensures the ongoing reliability and compliance of the method under revised conditions.

When is Revalidation Required?

Define the situation which may necessitate revalidation:

- Change in the manufacturing process or product composition
- Change in analytical method parameters or equipment
- Transfer of method to a different laboratory
- Change in product specification
- Change in regulatory requirements or market expansion
- After a significant gap in production or analysis

23. Amending the Protocol

When revalidation is required, the existing protocol can either be:

- Amended with a version update to reflect the change, or
- Reissued as a new protocol with a new number if changes are extensive

24. Validation Parameters and Acceptance Criteria

Provide the acceptance criteria for each performance characteristic clearly.

CHAPTER: 09

PREPARATION OF PROTOCOL

★ Objective:

Protocol preparation is one of the key activities in method validation. We will develop protocols for assay, related substances, dissolution, and residual solvents using paracetamol 500 mg tablets as a reference. The concentration matrices for all these tests have already been created, and we will refer to them while preparing the protocols, especially for defining the concentrations related to each performance characteristic.

I. PROTOCOL DESIGN: SYSTEM SUITABILITY

Prepare system suitability solutions as per method of analysis.

Acceptance criteria: Follow the acceptance criteria given for system suitability such as %RSD, tailing factor, theoretical plate counts etc.

II. PROTOCOL DESIGN: SPECIFICITY/SELECTIVITY

In analytical method validation, specificity or selectivity refers to the ability of an analytical method to unambiguously assess the analyte in the presence of components that might be expected to be present, such as impurities, degradants, matrix components, or excipients. ICH Q2(R2) emphasizes specificity as a core parameter for method validation, and its evaluation ensures regulatory compliance and robustness of routine analysis.

We will describe how specificity/selectivity is demonstrated across four critical test procedures:

- Assay
- Related Substances
- Dissolution
- Residual Solvent

Note: Acceptance criteria mentioned in this chapter are provided only for reference. There are no direct regulatory guidelines prescribing fixed acceptance values for specificity.

1. Specificity for Assay by HPLC:

Purpose:

- To confirm the method's ability to measure the active pharmaceutical ingredient (API) without interference from placebo or degradation products.

Studies to be Performed:

- Blank/Diluent
- Placebo
- Standard solution
- Test solution
- Individual impurity solutions at specification levels

- Spiked test solution with impurities
- Forced degradation studies (will be discussed in separate chapter)

Execution:

- Prepare standard and test solutions as per STP.
- Prepare placebo solution using the same proportion as used in the test sample.
- Prepare individual impurity solutions at the specification levels using a validated concentration matrix.
- Prepare spiked test solution with all impurities at their respective specification levels.
- Conduct forced degradation studies under acid, base, oxidation, photolysis, thermal, humidity, and water hydrolysis conditions.
- Evaluate peak purity for API, using PDA detector.

Acceptance Criteria (only for reference):

- No peak at API retention time in blank and placebo.
- No impurity peak should elute at API retention time.
- Forced degradation: Degradation between 5% and 20% in at least one condition.
- Peak purity for standard, test, spiked test, and forced degradation sample must be spectrally pure:
  - o Empower: Purity angle < purity threshold
  - o Chromeleon: Peak purity index > 950
  - o For RI/ELSD/FID detectors: Evaluate using resolution and spiked recovery studies

2. Specificity for Related Substances by HPLC

Purpose:

- To demonstrate the method's capability to resolve and identify all known impurities and the API without cross-interference.

Studies to be Performed:

- Blank/Diluent
- Placebo interference
- Standard solution
- Test solution
- Individual known impurity solutions
- Spiked test sample with impurities
- Forced degradation studies (will be discussed in separate chapter)

Execution:

- Inject blank and diluent to verify no peaks elute at the retention times of interest.
- Perform analysis of placebo solution equivalent to test sample.
- Inject standard and test solutions.
- Inject individual impurity solutions and a spiked test solution (with known impurities).
- Extend run time (in isocratic mode) to detect late eluting impurities.
- Conduct forced degradation studies under acid, base, oxidation, photolysis, thermal, humidity, and water hydrolysis conditions.
- Evaluate peak purity for all peaks of interest, including API and impurities, using PDA detector.

Acceptance Criteria (only for reference):

- No peak at API and impurity retention time in blank and placebo.
- No impurity peak should co-elute with API.
- Forced degradation: Degradation between 5% and 20% in at least one condition. Mass balance > 95%.
- Peak purity for standard, test, individual impurity, spiked test, and forced degra dation sample must be spectrally pure:
  - o Empower: Purity angle < purity threshold
  - o Chromeleon: Peak purity index > 950
  - o For RI/ELSD/FID detectors: Evaluate using resolution and spiked recovery studies

•**Note:** Interference from diluent or placebo below the detection limit (DL) may be accepted on a case-by-case basis, with proper justification and documentation.

3. Specificity for Dissolution by HPLC

Purpose:

- To confirm that dissolution of the drug is measured accurately in the presence of excipients and placebo components.

Studies to be Performed:

- Blank media
- Placebo preparation
- Standard solution
- Test solution

Execution:

- Perform dissolution on test and placebo equivalent to actual test sample weight.
- Prepare and analyze blank dissolution media.

Acceptance Criteria (only for reference):

- No peak at API retention time in blank and placebo.
- Use of PDA detector preferred for confirmation of peak purity.

4. Specificity for Residual Solvents by GC

Purpose:

- To verify the method can detect and quantify residual solvents (e.g., ethanol, methanol, methylene dichloride) without interference from placebo or other excipients.

Studies to be Performed:

- Blank (diluent)
- Placebo solution
- Standard solution
- Test solution
- Residual solvent identification solutions
- Spiked test sample with residual solvents

Execution:

- Inject diluent and placebo solution to ensure no interfering peaks at retention times of residual solvents.

- Analyze standard solutions and test solution.
- Prepare residual solvent identification solutions by diluting each reference standard to match specification levels.
- Inject test sample spiked with all solvents at specification levels.

Acceptance Criteria (only for reference):

- No interference at retention time of each residual solvent from placebo, API, and diluent.
- Baseline resolution between solvents if co-eluting.
- Peak purity cannot be evaluated using FID; therefore, resolution and comparison of spiked and unspiked samples are critical (e.g. recovery).

•**Note:** Interference from diluent or placebo below the detection limit (DL) may be accepted on a case-by-case basis, with appropriate scientific justification.

Summary

The specificity parameter must be tailored to each method based on its objective, detection technique, and formulation matrix. While PDA detectors offer spectral tools to evaluate peak purity, non-UV detectors demand alternative criteria like resolution and system suitability or recovery.

III. PROTOCOL DESIGN: PRECISION

1. Precision for Assay by HPLC

Purpose:

- To evaluate the closeness and reproducibility of assay results when performed under repeat and varied conditions.

Studies to be Performed:

- Repeatability (intra-assay precision)
- Intermediate Precision (ruggedness)
- Reproducibility (if applicable)

Execution:

Overview:

- Precision should be evaluated using either:
  - o 9 determinations covering the reportable range (e.g., 3 concentrations × 3 replicates)
  - o Or 6 determinations at 100% of the test concentration

The following concentration matrix is applicable for all three levels of precision.

Preparation of Repeatability Solutions Using Finished Product:

- Prepare six individual assay test preparations from the actual product as per the STP.
- The amount of API in the sample is 250 mg and placebo is 100 mg.

Sample Preparation Table – Repeatability (Finished Product):

Preparation No.	Sample Weight (mg)	Initial Dilution Volume (mL)	Pipetted Volume (mL)	Further Dilution Volume (mL)
1 to 6	350 mg	1000 mL	10 mL	50 mL

Preparation of Repeatability Solutions Using (API + Placebo):

- If test product is unavailable, prepare sample using 250 mg of API and 100 mg of placebo to mimic the formulation matrix.
- Proceed with sample preparation steps similar to the STP.

Sample Preparation Table – Repeatability (API + Placebo):

Preparation No.	API Weight (mg)	Placebo Weight (mg)	Initial Dilution Volume (mL)	Pipetted Volume (mL)	Further Dilution Volume (mL)
1 to 6	250 mg	100 mg	1000 mL	10 mL	50 mL

C. Intermediate Precision:

- Conduct the same experiment on a different day, by a different analyst, using a different instrument and column (same or equivalent type).

D. Reproducibility (If Applicable):

- Study to be performed in a different laboratory to assess inter-lab variation using the same concentration matrix.

Acceptance Criteria (only for reference):

- Each assay value: Within 95.0%–105.0% of label claim.
- % RSD (Repeatability): NMT 2.0%
- % RSD (Intermediate Precision and Overall): NMT 2.0%

2. Precision for Related Substances by HPLC

Purpose:

- To evaluate the consistency of the method in detecting and quantifying known and unknown impurities across replicates under repeat and varied conditions.

Studies to be Performed:

- Repeatability (using finished product and API + placebo)
- Intermediate Precision (ruggedness)
- Reproducibility (if applicable)

Execution:

Precision is evaluated at the impurity release specification levels. The variability is expected to be higher at lower concentrations (release spec) and hence proving precision at this level builds confidence in method performance across a broader range.

Impurity Specification Table:

Impurity Name	Limit in (%) - Release	Limit in (%) - Stability	Limit in (ppm) - Release	Limit in (ppm) - Stability
Impurity A	0.5%	1.0%	2.5 ppm	5.0 ppm
Impurity B	0.3%	0.6%	1.5 ppm	3.0 ppm
HUI	0.2%	0.2%	1.0 ppm	1.0 ppm

Preparation of Impurity Stock Solutions:

- Prepare separate impurity A and B stock solutions at 200 ppm by dissolving 20 mg of each in 100 mL diluent.

Preparation of Repeatability Solutions Using Finished Product:

- Weigh test sample equivalent to 500 mg paracetamol.
- Spike impurity A and B stock solutions to achieve respective release specifications.
- Final spiked solution should match 2.5 ppm (impurity A) and 1.5 ppm (impurity B), adjusted based on impurity content in unspiked test.

Sample Preparation Table – Repeatability (Finished Product):

Preparation No.	Sample Weight (mg)	Volume of Impurity A Stock (mL)	Volume of Impurity B Stock (mL)	Initial Dilution Volume (mL)	Pipetted Volum (mL)	Final Dilution Volume (mL)
1 to 6	700 mg (eq. to 500mg API)			100 mL	5 mL	50 mL

Preparation of Repeatability Solutions Using API + Placebo:

- Repeatability using API + Placebo can be done in case if sample is not suitable on not available.
- Weigh 500 mg API + 200 mg placebo.
- Spike impurity A and B stock solutions to achieve respective release specifications.
- Final solution should match 2.5 ppm (impurity A) and 1.5 ppm (impurity B), adjusted based on impurity content in API.

Sample Preparation Table – Repeatability (API + Placebo):

Preparation No.	API Weight (mg)	Placebo Weight (mg)	Volume of Impurity A Stock (mL)	Volume of Impurity B Stock (mL)	Initial Dilution Volume (mL)	Pipetted Volum (mL)	Final Dilution Volume (mL)
1 to 6	500mg	200mg			100 mL	5 mL	50 mL

Preparation of Repeatability Solutions for Unknown Impurity:

- Use API as surrogate for unknown impurity.
- Target 1.0 ppm (release spec conc.).
- Prepare 500 ppm API stock (50 mg in 100 mL).
- Spike 2 mL of this stock into 200 mg placebo and dilute to 100 mL.

Sample Preparation Table – Max Unknown Impurity:

Preparation No.	Placebo Weight (mg)	Volume of API Stock Spiked (mL)	Initial Dilution Volume (mL)	Pipetted Volume (mL)	Further Dilution Volume (mL)
1 to 6	200 mg	2 mL	100 mL	5 mL	50 mL

Intermediate Precision:

- Repeat all the above on a different day, with different analyst, instrument, and column.

Reproducibility (If Applicable):

- Repeat the entire study in a different laboratory.

Acceptance Criteria (only for reference):

- % RSD of individual impurities and total impurities: NMT 15.0%

3. Precision for Dissolution by HPLC

Purpose:

- To evaluate the repeatability and ruggedness of the HPLC method for quantifying dissolution.

Studies to be Performed:

- Repeatability
- Intermediate Precision (ruggedness)
- Reproducibility (if applicable)

Execution:

Repeatability:

- Prepare six individual test solutions of the product as per STP.
- Conduct the dissolution test, calculate % dissolution for each, and determine % RSD.

Alternate Approach (if test product is unavailable):

- Prepare solution using 500 mg of API (Paracetamol) and 200 mg of placebo.
- Add to six dissolution vessels each containing 900 mL of dissolution medium pre-equilibrated at 37 ± 0.5°C.
- Proceed with dissolution test as per STP.

Sample Preparation Table – Repeatability (API + Placebo):

Preparation No.	API Weight (mg)	Placebo Weight (mg)	Dissolution Medium Volume (mL)	Temperature (°C)	RPM
1 to 6	500 mg	200 mg	900 ml	37 ± 0.5	As per STP

Precautions (if using API + Placebo):

- If the API does not settle properly, it may float on the surface.
- In such cases, dissolve the API in a suitable diluent to form a liquid concentrate.
- Spike the liquid API solution into dissolution vessels to ensure uniform dispersion.

Intermediate Precision:

- Perform the same procedure on a different day, with a different analyst, using different apparatus and HPLC column/system.
- Evaluate % dissolution and % RSD of each set.
- Calculate overall % RSD from all 12 results (6 from repeatability and 6 from intermediate precision).

Acceptance Criteria (only for reference):

- % RSD of dissolution results: NMT 5.0%
- Each value must meet product dissolution specification.
- Overall % RSD from 12 units: NMT 5.0%

Reproducibility (If Applicable):

- Conduct the entire study in another laboratory using different equipment and team.

4. Precision for Residual Solvents by GC

Purpose:

- To evaluate the repeatability and ruggedness of the GC method for quantifying residual solvents (ethanol, methanol, and methylene dichloride).

Studies to be Performed:

- Repeatability
- Intermediate Precision (ruggedness)
- Reproducibility (if applicable)

Execution:

Repeatability:

- Prepare six individual test solutions of the product as per STP.
- Spike ethanol, methanol, and MDC in each preparation to reach their respective release specification concentrations.

Residual Solvent Specification Table:

Solvent Name	Release Spec (ppm)
Ethanol	5000 ppm
Methanol	3000 ppm
Methylene Chloride	600 ppm

Preparation Table – Repeatability (Residual Solvent Precision):

Preparation No.	Sample Weight (mg)	Conc. Of Ethanol in Stock (ppm)	Conc. Of Methanol in Stock (ppm)	Conc. Of MDC in Stock (ppm)	Volume of Stock (mL)
1 to 6	500 mg	To be calculated	To be calculated	To be calculated	5 mL

Note: Concentration of ethanol, methanol, and MDC in stock solution should be calculated after determining the amount of solvent already present in the unspiked sample. Target concentration in spiked sample should match the release specification.

Preparation Table – Repeatability Using API + Placebo (Residual Solvent Precision):

- Repeatability using API + Placebo can be done in case if sample is not suitable on not available.
- Weigh 357 mg API + 143 mg placebo.
- Spike ethanol, methanol, MDC to achieve respective release specifications.
- Final solution should match 5000 ppm ethanol, 3000 ppm methanol, 600 ppm MDC, adjusted based on residual solvent content in API.

Preparation No.	API Weight (mg)	Placebo Weight (mg)	Conc. Of Ethanol in Stock (ppm)	Conc. Of Methanol in Stock (ppm)	Conc. Of MDC in Stock (ppm)	Volume of Stock (mL)
1 to 6	357 mg	143 mg	To be calculated	To be calculated	To be calculated	5 mL

Note: Concentration of ethanol, methanol, and MDC in stock solution should be calculated after determining the amount of solvent already present in the unspiked sample.

Target concentration in spiked sample should match the release specification.

Intermediate Precision:

- Repeat the procedure on a different day, using a different GC system and analyst.
- Ensure column type remains consistent (e.g., same dimensions and stationary phase).

Reproducibility (If Applicable):

- Conduct the precision study in another laboratory with different instrumentation.

Acceptance Criteria (only for reference):

- % RSD for each solvent should not exceed 15.0%

IV. PROTOCOL DESIGN: DETECTION LIMIT (DL) AND QUANTITATION LIMIT (QL)

Purpose:

To outline the protocol for determining the lowest concentration of impurity or residual solvent that can be reliably detected (DL) and quantified (QL) using the respective chromatographic method.

Applicable To:

- Related Substances (HPLC)
- Residual Solvents (GC)

1. DL and QL for Related Substances by HPLC:

Method: HPLC with UV/PDA Detector

Approach:

DL and QL will be evaluated using:

- Signal-to-noise ratio method (preferred approach)

A. Procedure – Signal-to-Noise Method:

1. Prepare a series of increasingly dilute solutions of known impurities (e.g., Impurity A and Impurity B) containing placebo.
2. Inject each dilution into the HPLC system.
3. Observe the signal-to-noise ratio for each solution.
4. Identify:

o The dilution giving an S/N ratio of approximately 3:1 (DL)

o The dilution giving an S/N ratio of approximately 10:1 (QL)

Sample Preparation Table – DL/QL Protocol (HPLC):

Impurity Name	Stock Concentration (ppm)	Dilution Scheme	Final Conc. (ppm)	S/N Ratio	Observation
Impurity A	To be defined	To be defined	To be determined	To be recorded	DL/QL determination point
Impurity B	To be defined	To be defined	To be determined	To be recorded	DL/QL determination point

Note: S/N ratio will be measured using chromatographic software. Adjust dilution volumes as required.

Acceptance Criteria (for reference):
- DL: Signal-to-noise ratio ~3:1
- QL: Signal-to-noise ratio ~10:1

B. Procedure – Standard Deviation and Slope Method:
1. Draw calibration curve (with not less than 5 concentrations) for impurity A, impurity B and API in the range of linear response.
2. Calculate the slope (S) of the calibration curve.
3. Prepare and measure the response for impurity and API solutions containing placebo in the range of expected DL and QL concentration.
4. Calculate the standard deviation (SD) of residuals for impurity and API for the above solution.
5. Determine:
   - o DL = (3.3 × SD) / S
   - o QL = (10 × SD) / S

2. DL and QL for Residual Solvents by GC:

Method: Headspace GC with FID Detector

A. Procedure – Signal-to-Noise Method:
1. Prepare serial dilutions of ethanol, methanol, and methylene dichloride (MDC) standards containing placebo.
2. Inject each solution into the GC system.
3. Record the S/N ratio for each solvent.
4. Identify:
   - o DL: Concentration giving ~3:1 S/N
   - o QL: Concentration giving ~10:1 S/N

Sample Preparation Table – DL/QL Protocol (GC):

Solvent Name	Stock Conc. (ppm)	Dilution Scheme	Final Conc. (ppm)	S/N Ratio	Observation
Ethanol	To be defined	To be defined	To be determined	To be recorded	DL/QL determination point
Methanol	To be defined	To be defined	To be determined	To be recorded	DL/QL determination point
Methylene Chloride	To be defined	To be defined	To be determined	To be recorded	DL/QL determination point

Note: Ensure no interference near the solvent peaks. Include blank and placebo injections.

Acceptance Criteria (for reference):
- DL: Signal-to-noise ratio ~3:1
- QL: Signal-to-noise ratio ~10:1

B. Procedure – Standard Deviation and Slope Method:
1. Draw calibration curve (with not less than 5 concentrations) for ethanol,

methanol, and MDC in the range of linear response.
2. Calculate the slope (S) of the calibration curve.
3. Prepare and measure the response for residual solvents containing placebo in the range of expected DL and QL concentration.
4. Calculate the standard deviation (SD) of residuals for residual solvents for the above solution.
5. Determine:
   - o DL = (3.3 × SD) / S
   - o QL = (10 × SD) / S

V. PROTOCOL DESIGN: RESPONSE/LINEARITY

1. Linearity for Assay (by HPLC):

Purpose:

To evaluate the relationship between analyte concentration and detector response for the assay method, ensuring the method is linear across the reportable range as per ICH Q2(R2).

Studies to be Performed:

- Preparation of five linearity levels (50% to 150% of test concentration)
- Recording detector response (peak area) at each level
- Construction of calibration curve and statistical analysis

Execution:

- Determine reportable range based on ICH Q2(R2):

Use of analytical procedure	Low end of reportable range	High end of reportable range
Assay of a product (1)	80% of declared content or 80% of lower specification acceptance criterion	120% of declared content or 120% of the upper specification acceptance criterion

- o Actual sample concentration is 50 ppm
- o Assay limit is (95% to 105%)
- o Lower range: 40 ppm (80% of 50 ppm) or 38ppm (80% of lower spec-95%)
- o Upper range: 60 ppm (120% of declared content) or 63 ppm (120% of upper spec.- 105%)

- Prepare linearity stock: 50 mg of paracetamol in 100 mL → 500 ppm stock solution
- Prepare solutions as per concentration matrix at least covering 38 ppm to 63 ppm (76 % to 126%) to meet ICH Q2(R2) requirements.
- Linearity levels include 50%, 75%, 100%, 125%, and 150%, ensuring coverage of ICH Q2(R2) requirements and extending beyond for added robustness

Linearity Level Preparation Table – Assay Linearity:

Linearity Level (%)	Expected Concentration (ppm)	Volume from Stock (mL)	Final Dilution Volume (mL)
50%	25 ppm	5.0 mL	100.0 mL
75%	37.5 ppm	7.5 mL	100.0 mL
100%	50 ppm	10.0 mL	100.0 mL
125%	62.5 ppm	12.5 mL	100.0 mL
150%	75 ppm	15.0 mL	100.0 mL

Acceptance Criteria (only for reference):

- Correlation coefficient (r): Not less than 0.999
- Bias at 100% concentration: ±2.0% max
- Report slope, residual sum of squares, y-intercept

Note: In case of not meeting the acceptance criteria of linearity, narrow the range and establish the range in which it is linear.

2. Linearity for Related Substances (by HPLC):

Purpose:

To demonstrate that the analytical method provides a linear response for known impurities over a specified concentration range, typically from the LOQ to 300% of the impurity release specification.

Studies to be Performed:

- Preparation of at least five impurity levels (e.g., LOQ, 50%, 75%, 100%, 125%, 150%, 300%)
- Individual injections of each impurity level
- Recording detector responses (peak areas)
- Construction of individual calibration curves for each impurity

Impurity Specification Table:

Impurity Name	Limit in (%) - Release	Limit in (%) - Stability	Limit in (ppm) - Release	Limit in (ppm) - Stability
Impurity A	0.5%	1.0%	2.5	5.0
Impurity B	0.3%	0.6%	1.5	3.0
HUI	0.2%	0.2%	1.0	1.0

Execution:

- Determine reportable range on ICH Q2(R2)

Use of analytical procedure	Low end of reportable range	High end of reportable range
Impurity (1)	Reporting threshold	120% of specification acceptance criterion

o Actual sample concentration is 500 ppm
o Reporting threshold can be found based on maximum daily dose
o Low end of the linearity solution should be less than or equal to QL
o High end of the linearity shall be 120% of stability specification (6ppm, 3.6 ppm, 1.2 ppm for impurity A, impurity B, and HUI)

- Preparation of impurity and drug substance linearity stock solution: Weigh accurately 12.5 mg of Impurity A, 7.5mg of Impurity B and 5mg of Paracetamol standard and transfer into 100 mL volumetric flask, add 70 mL of diluent and sonicate it to dissolve and dilute it up to the mark with diluent.
- Prepare linearity solutions using linearity stock solution
- Prepare solutions as per concentration matrix at least covering QL to 120% of stability specification to meet ICH Q2(R2) requirements.
- Linearity levels selected are QL, 50%, 75%, 100%, 125%, 150%, and 300%.

Linearity Level Preparation Table – Related Substances Linearity:

Linearity	Expected conc. (ppm)			Volume of linearity stock to be taken (mL)	Final vol (mL) (L1)
	Imp. A	Imp. B	Paracetamol		
LOQ					
50%	1.25 ppm	0.75 ppm	0.50 ppm	5.0 mL	100 mL
75%	1.88 ppm	1.13 ppm	0.75 ppm	7.5 mL	100 mL
100%	2.50 ppm	1.50 ppm	1.00 ppm	10.0 mL	100 mL
125%	3.13 ppm	1.88 ppm	1.25 ppm	12.5 mL	100 mL
150%	3.75 ppm	2.25 ppm	1.50 ppm	15.0 mL	100 mL
300%	7.50 ppm	4.50 ppm	3.00 ppm	30.0 mL	100 mL

Further, dilute 10 mL of each L1 solution to 50 mL with diluent.

Note: While preparing the linearity stock solution, ensure that the total volume is adequate to prepare all required linearity levels. For example, in the current case, we have prepared 100 mL of the linearity stock solution, which is sufficient since the total volume needed to prepare all linearity solutions (excluding QL/LOQ) is 80 mL.

Acceptance Criteria (only for reference):

- Correlation coefficient (r): Not less than 0.997
- Bias at 100% response should be not more than 5%.
- Report slope, residual sum of squares, y-intercept

Note: In case of not meeting the acceptance criteria of linearity, narrow the range and establish the range in which it is linear.

3. Linearity for Dissolution (by HPLC):

Purpose: To evaluate the linearity of the analytical method used for dissolution samples to ensure detector response is proportional to concentration over the required range.

Studies to be Performed:

- Preparation of standard solutions across 25% to 150% levels
- Analysis of detector response at each level
- Evaluation of calibration curve and correlation

Execution:

- Determine reportable range on ICH Q2(R2)

Use of analytical procedure	Low end of reportable range	High end of reportable range
Dissolution:	Q-45% of the lowest strength	
Immediate release • one point specification • multiple point specification	Lower limit of reportable range (as justified by the specification) or QL, as appropriate.	130% of declared content of the highest strength
Modified release	Lower limit of reportable range (as justified by the specification) or QL, as appropriate.	

o Actual sample concentration is 56 ppm

o For immediate release dosage forms:

- Q-45% of the lowest strength. Dissolution specification is 75% Q, so Q vale is 75%
- Hence Q-45 = 30%
- Low end of reportable range is 30%

o High end of reportable range is 130% of declared content of highest strength.

o Expected linearity as per ICH Q2(R2) is between 30% to 130%

- **Stock solution:** 56 mg paracetamol in 100 mL = 560 ppm

Linearity Preparation Table – Dissolution Linearity:

Table: Linearity

Linearity level	Expected Conc. (ppm)	Volume taken from Linearity stock solution (mL)	Diluted to volume with diluent (mL)
25%	14 ppm	2.5 mL	100 mL
75%	42 ppm	7.5 mL	100 mL
100%	56 ppm	10.0mL	100 mL
125%	70 ppm	12.5 mL	100 mL
150%	84 ppm	15.0 mL	100 mL

Acceptance Criteria (only for reference):

- Correlation coefficient (r): Not less than 0.999
- Bias at 100% response should be not more than 2%.
- Report slope, residual sum of squares, y-intercept

Note: In case of not meeting the acceptance criteria of linearity, narrow the range and establish the range in which it is linear.

4 Linearity for Residual Solvents (by GC):

Purpose:

To establish the proportionality between detector response and concentration of residual solvents (ethanol, methanol, MDC) over a defined range.

Studies to be Performed:

- Preparation of standard solutions from LOQ to 150% of the specification

- Analysis by GC with FID
- Calibration curve construction for each solvent

Execution:

- Determine reportable range on ICH Q2(R2)
- Low end of the linearity solution should be less than or equal to QL
- High end of the linearity shall be 120% of release specification (6000 ppm ethanol, 3600 ppm methanol, and 720 ppm MDC)
- Preparation of linearity stock solution: Transfer accurately about 500 mg ethanol, 300 mg methanol, and 60 mg MDC into a 100-mL volumetric flask containing about 30 mL of diluent, dilute to volume with diluent and mix well.
- Prepare linearity solutions as per concentration matrix at least covering QL to 120% of release specification to meet ICH Q2(R2) requirements.
- Linearity levels selected are QL, 50%, 75%, 100%, 125%, and 150%.

Linearity	Expected conc. (ppm)			Volume of linearity stock to be taken (mL)	Final vol (mL) (L1)
	Ethanol	Methanol	MDC		
LOQ					
50%	2500 ppm	1500 ppm	300 ppm	5.0 mL	100 mL
75%	3750 ppm	2250 ppm	450 ppm	7.5 mL	100 mL
100%	5000 ppm	3000 ppm	600 ppm	10.0 mL	100 mL
125%	6250 ppm	3750 ppm	750 ppm	12.5 mL	100 mL
150%	7500 ppm	4500 ppm	900 ppm	15.0 mL	100 mL

Acceptance Criteria (only for reference):

- Correlation coefficient (r): Not less than 0.995
- % Bias at 100%: ±5.0%

Note: In case of not meeting the acceptance criteria of linearity, establish the range in which it is linear.

V. PROTOCOL DESIGN: ACCURACY

1. Accuracy for assay (by HPLC):

Purpose: To validate, the assay method can accurately quantify active ingredient in product by spiking active ingredient in placebo at various concentrations ranging from 50% to 150% of the target test concentration.

Studies to be Performed:

- Prepare accuracy sample solutions at five concentration levels: 50%, 75%, 100%, 125%, and 150% of target assay concentration.
- For lowest (50%) and highest (150%) levels, prepare six replicate solutions.
- For other levels (75%, 100%, 125%), prepare three replicate solutions each.
- Calculate % recovery and mean % recovery at each level.

Rationale: Six replicates at 50% and 150% levels help fulfil the requirement of "range" studies under ICH guidelines without requiring additional sample preparation. The first three replicates from these can be considered for accuracy evaluation, while all six can be used for range assessment. Perform recovery study for lowest and highest concentrations six times and for other concentrations in triplicate. Calculate % recovery and mean of % recovery of individual levels.

Execution:

Weigh accurately 100mg of placebo and suitable amount of Paracetamol API/working standard as per specified accuracy level given in below table and transfer it to 1000 mL volumetric flask. Add 500 ml of diluent, sonicate it for 10 minutes and make up to volume with Diluent. Mix well and centrifuge a portion of solution at 5000 rpm for 10 minutes. Dilute 10 mL of centrifuged portion of above sample solution to 50 mL with diluents and mix well.

Table: Preparation of Accuracy solution

Accuracy level (%)	Expected Initial Conc. in (ppm)	Placebo Wt. (mg)	API Wt. (mg)	Dilution Vol (mL)	Pipetted Vol (mL)	Final Dilution (mL)	Final Conc. (ppm)	No. of measurements
50%	125 ppm	100 mg	125 mg	1000 mL	10 mL	50 mL	25 ppm	06
75%	187.5 ppm	100 mg	187.5 mg	1000 mL	10 mL	50 mL	37.5 ppm	03
100%	250 ppm	100 mg	250 mg	1000 mL	10 mL	50 mL	50 ppm	03
125%	312.5 ppm	100 mg	312.5 mg	1000 mL	10 mL	50 mL	62.5 ppm	03
150%	375 ppm	100 mg	375 mg	1000 mL	10 mL	50 mL	75 ppm	06

Acceptance criteria (for information only):

Individual recovery of API should be between 97.0% to 103.0%.

2. Accuracy for related substances (by HPLC):

Purpose:

To validate that the related substances (RS) test method can accurately quantify known impurities and potential unknown impurities within the drug product matrix and placebo across a defined concentration range.

Studies to be Performed:

- For known impurities (Impurity A & B): Prepare accuracy solutions by spiking impurity stock solution into test preparation at six levels: 50%, 75%, 100%, 125%, 150%, and 300% of the shelf-life specification level.
- For unknown impurity surrogate (API): Spike API into placebo matrix at five levels: 50% to 300% of the target concentration (typically the single unknown impurity limit).
- Prepare six replicates for the highest level (300%), and three replicates for all other levels.
- Calculate % recovery for each spiked level.

Execution:

Preparation of un-spiked test sample:

Weigh accurately 20 tablets of Paracetamol. Determine average weight and crush tablets to fine powder. Weigh accurately and transfer tablets powder equivalent to 500mg of Paracetamol into 100 mL volumetric flask. Add 70 mL of diluent, sonicate it for 10 minutes, cool to room temperature and make up to volume with diluent.

Mix well and centrifuge a portion of solution at 5000 rpm for 10 minutes, then pipette out and transfer 5ml centrifugate into a 50ml volumetric flask, make up to volume with diluent.

Preparation of impurity stock solution:

Weigh accurately 12.5 mg of Impurity A, 7.5mg of Impurity B standard and transfer into 50 mL volumetric flask, add 30 mL of diluent and sonicate it to dissolve and dilute it up to the mark with diluent.

Preparation of accuracy test solution:

Weigh accurately 20 tablets of Paracetamol. Determine average weight and crush tablets to fine powder. Weigh accurately and transfer tablets powder equivalent to 500mg of Paracetamol into 100 mL volumetric flask. Add suitable volume of impurity stock solution as per accuracy levels and add 70 mL of diluent, sonicate it for 10 minutes, cool to room temperature and make up to volume with diluent. Mix well and centrifuge a portion of solution at 5000 rpm for 10 minutes, then pipette out and transfer 5ml centrifugate into a 50ml volumetric flask, make up to volume with diluent.

Preparation of API stock solution:

Weigh accurately 25mg of API and transfer into 50 mL volumetric flask, add 30 mL of diluent and sonicate it to dissolve and dilute it up to the mark with diluent.

Preparation of unknown impurity (drug substance) accuracy solution:

Weigh accurately 200mg of placebo and transfer into 100 mL volumetric flask. Add suitable volume of API stock solution as per accuracy levels and add 70 mL of diluent, sonicate it for 10 minutes, cool to room temperature and make up to volume with diluent. Mix well and centrifuge a portion of solution at 5000 rpm for 10 minutes, then pipette out and transfer 5ml centrifugate into a 50ml volumetric flask, make up to volume with diluent

Table: Expected impurity concentration in sample stock solution

Accuracy Level	Expected Impurity conc. in sample stock solution (ppm)		
	Impurity A	Impurity B	HUI
LOQ			
50%	12.5 ppm	7.5 ppm	5.0 ppm
75%	18.8 ppm	11.3 ppm	7.5 ppm
100%	25.0 ppm	15.0 ppm	10.0 ppm
125%	31.3 ppm	18.8 ppm	12.5 ppm
150%	37.5 ppm	22.5 ppm	15.0 ppm
300%	75.0 ppm	45.0 ppm	30.0 ppm

Table: Preparation of Accuracy solution for Impurities

Accuracy level (%)	Expected Impurity conc. in final accuracy solution (ppm)		Sample Wt (mg)	Impurity stock vol (mL)	Dilution Volume (mL)	Pipetted Volume (mL)	Final Dilution Volume (mL)	No. of measurements
	Imp A	Imp B						
LOQ								06
50%	1.25 ppm	0.75 ppm	700mg	5.0 mL	100 mL	5 mL	50 mL	03
75%	1.88 ppm	1.13 ppm	700mg	7.5 mL	100 mL	5 mL	50 mL	03
100%	2.50 ppm	1.50 ppm	700mg	10.0 mL	100 mL	5 mL	50 mL	03
125%	3.13 ppm	1.88 ppm	700mg	12.5 mL	100 mL	5 mL	50 mL	03
150%	3.75 ppm	2.25 ppm	700mg	15.0 mL	100 mL	5 mL	50 mL	03
300%	7.50 ppm	4.50 ppm	700mg	30.0 mL	100 mL	5 mL	50 mL	06

Table: Preparation of Accuracy solution for Unknown Impurity (Drug Substance)

Accuracy level. (%)	Expected Drug Substance Conc. in (ppm)	Placebo Weight (mg)	Vol of API stock (ml)	Dilution Volume a(mL)	Pipetted Volume (mL)	Final Dilution Volume mL)	No. of measurements
LOQ							06
50%	0.50 ppm	200mg	1.0 mL	100 mL	5 mL	50 mL	03
75%	0.75 ppm	200mg	1.5 mL	100 mL	5 mL	50 mL	03
100%	1.00 ppm	200mg	2.0 mL	100 mL	5 mL	50 mL	03
125%	1.25 ppm	200mg	2.5 mL	100 mL	5 mL	50 mL	03
150%	1.50 ppm	200mg	3.0 mL	100 mL	5 mL	50 mL	03
300%	3.00 ppm	200mg	6.0 mL	100 mL	5 mL	50 mL	06

Acceptance criteria (for information only):

The individual recovery of impurity and drug substance should be not less than 85.0% and not more than 115.0%.

3. Accuracy for dissolution (by HPLC):

Purpose

To validate that the dissolution method can accurately quantify the active ingredient in the product by spiking the drug substance (API) into placebo across a range of concentrations, typically from 25% to 150% of the target test concentration.

Note: For controlled-release drug products, the lowest accuracy level should be determined based on the QL. In such cases, accuracy should be studied from QL to 150% of the target.

Studies to be Performed:

- Prepare accuracy solutions by spiking API into placebo within dissolution medium at five different levels: 25%, 75%, 100%, 125%, and 150% of target test concentration.
- For lowest (25%) and highest (150%) levels, prepare six replicates each.
- For other levels (75%, 100%, and 125%), prepare three replicates each.

• Calculate % recovery and mean % recovery at each level.

Execution:

Preparation of accuracy sample solutions:

Transfer 200mg of placebo and suitable amount of API as described in below table as per the specific accuracy level into dissolution bowl containing 900ml of the dissolution medium, pre-equilibrated to 37 ± 0.5 °C. Start the dissolution apparatus and withdraw 10ml of the sample after 30 minutes. Centrifuge the sample and further dilute 5ml of the centrifuged sample to 50ml with dissolution medium.

Table: Preparation of Accuracy solution

Accuracy level. (%)	Placebo Weight (mg)	API Weight (mg))	Dissolution medium Volume (mL)	Expected Initial conc. (ppm)	Pipetted Volume (mL)	Final Dilution Volume (mL)	Expected Final Conc. (ppm)	No. of measurements
25%	200mg	125 mg	900 mL	139 ppm	5 mL	50 mL	14 ppm	06
75%	200mg	375 mg	900 mL	417 ppm	5 mL	50 mL	42 ppm	03
100%	200mg	500 mg	900 mL	556 ppm	5 mL	50 mL	56 ppm	03
125%	200mg	625 mg	900 mL	694 ppm	5 mL	50 mL	69 ppm	03
150%	200mg	750 mg	900 mL	833 ppm	5 mL	50 mL	83 ppm	06

Acceptance criteria (for information only): Individual recovery of API should be between 95.0% to 105.0%.

4. Accuracy for Residual Solvents (by GC):

Purpose

To validate that the gas chromatographic method can accurately quantify residual solvents (ethanol, methanol, and methylene dichloride) in the pharmaceutical product by spiking known concentrations of these solvents into the product matrix across a specified range.

Studies to be Performed

• Prepare accuracy solutions by spiking ethanol, methanol, and MDC into the sample or placebo matrix at six levels: QL, 50%, 75%, 100%, 125%, and 150% of the residual solvent specification limits (generally based on ICH Q3C guidelines or internal shelf-life specifications).

• Prepare six replicates at the lowest level (QL) and highest level (150%) and three replicates at all other levels.

•Calculate % recovery for each residual solvent at each spiked level.

Execution

Preparation of accuracy stock solution: Transfer accurately about 500 mg ethanol, 300 mg methanol, and 60 mg MDC into a 100 mL volumetric flask containing about 60 mL of diluent, dilute to volume with diluent and mix well. Prepare accuracy standard solutions (to be used for preparation of accuracy samples) as per below table

Table: Preparation of accuracy standard solutions

Accuracy Level	Accuracy Stock Volume (mL)	Dilution to (mL)
QL		
50%	5.0 mL	100 mL
75%	7.5 mL	100 mL
100%	10.0 mL	100 mL
125%	12.5 mL	100 mL
150%	15.0 mL	100 mL

Preparation of accuracy solutions:

Accurately weigh about 500 mg of crushed tablet powder into a head space vial, add exactly 5 mL of the specified accuracy standard solution and seal immediately with septum using crimper.

Accuracy Level	Expected conc. (ppm) wrt sample			Sample weight in (mg)	Volume of accuracy standard solution (mL)
	Ethanol	Methanol	MDC		
QL				500 mg	5 mL
50%	2500	1500	300	500 mg	5 mL
75%	3750	2250	450	500 mg	5 mL
100%	5000	3000	600	500 mg	5 mL
125%	6250	3750	750	500 mg	5 mL
150%	7500	4500	900	500 mg	5 mL

Acceptance criteria (for information only):

The individual recovery of residual solvent should be not less than 85.0% and not more than 115.0%.

VI. PROTOCOL DESIGN: RANGE

The range of the method is defined by the concentration level over which acceptable linearity, accuracy and precision are obtained.

Note: For range, the data shall be considered from linearity and accuracy sections. The precision shall be calculated for LOQ and highest concentration calculated in accuracy section.

1.Range for assay (by HPLC):

Acceptance criteria (for information only):

Linearity	Coefficient of correlation(r) should be not less than 0.999. The bias at 100% response shall not be more than 2%.
Precision	The relative standard deviation of six replicate preparations made in accuracy section at highest level and at lowest level should not be more than 2.0%
Accuracy	Individual recovery at highest and lowest level should be between 97.0% to 103.0%

2. Range for related substances (by HPLC):
Acceptance criteria (for information only):

Linearity	Coefficient of correlation(r) should be not less than 0.997. The bias at 100% response shall not be more than 5%.
Precision	The relative standard deviation of six replicate preparations made in precision at LOQ and accuracy section at highest level should not be more than 15.0%
Accuracy	Individual recovery at LOQ and highest and lowest level should be between 85.0% to 115.0%

3. Range for dissolution (by HPLC):
Acceptance criteria (for information only):

Linearity	Coefficient of correlation(r) should be not less than 0.999. The bias at 100% response shall not be more than 2%.
Precision	The relative standard deviation of six replicate preparations made in accuracy section at highest level and at lowest level should not be more than 5.0%
Accuracy	Individual recovery at highest and lowest level should be between 95.0% to 105.0%

4. Range for residual solvent (by GC):
Acceptance criteria (for information only):

Linearity	Coefficient of correlation(r) should be not less than 0.997. The bias at 100% response shall not be more than 5%.
Precision	The relative standard deviation of six replicate preparations made in precision at LOQ and accuracy section at highest level should not be more than 15.0%
Accuracy	Individual recovery at LOQ and highest and lowest level should be between 85.0% to 115.0%

VII. PROTOCOL DESIGN: ROBUSTNESS

1. Robustness for assay (by HPLC):

i. Filter Validation

Purpose

To evaluate the robustness of the assay method by performing a filter validation study using two different membrane filters:

- 0.45 µm PVDF (Polyvinylidene fluoride) membrane filter
- 0.45 µm Nylon membrane filter

Studies to be Performed

- Prepare the test solution in duplicate as per the assay test method.
- Use a sample from the accuracy (100% level) or precision study for the filter validation.

Execution

1.Centrifuge approximately 10 mL of the test solution at 5000 rpm for 10 minutes.
2.Filter the remaining test solution separately through:
 o 0.45 µm PVDF membrane filter
 o 0.45 µm Nylon membrane filter
 Discard the first 3–5 mL of each filtrate before collecting the sample for analysis.
3.Inject the following into the HPLC system under the test conditions:

o Unfiltered standard solution
o Centrifuged test solution
o Filtered test solutions (both filters)
4.Calculate the % assay of centrifuged and filtered test solutions against the unfiltered standard.
5.Determine the difference in % assay between the filtered and centrifuged test solutions.

Acceptance Criteria (for information only)

- The difference in % assay between the centrifuged and filtered test solutions should be NMT 2.0%

ii. Effect of Variation in Mobile Phase Composition

Purpose:

To evaluate the robustness of the analytical method by assessing the effect of variations in the organic phase composition of the mobile phase (±10%) on system suitability parameters and assay results.

Studies to be Performed:

- Prepare two mobile phases:
  - o One containing 110% of the method-defined organic phase.
  - o Another containing 90% of the method-defined organic phase.
- Inject the standard preparation using both mobile phases and evaluate system suitability parameters.
- Analyze the test sample in duplicate using each mobile phase and calculate the % difference in assay compared to the result obtained with the original method composition.

Execution:

Mobile Phase Preparation

- Mobile phase preparation as per STP: Mix buffer and acetonitrile in 68: 32 v/v ratio
- 90% Organic Phase Composition:
  Mix buffer and acetonitrile in a 68:28.8 (v/v) ratio. Sonicate and degas for 10 minutes.
- 110% Organic Phase Composition:
  Mix buffer and acetonitrile in a 68:35.2 (v/v) ratio. Sonicate and degas for 10 minutes.

Analysis Procedure

1. Inject the standard preparation with each mobile phase and assess system suitability.
2. Analyze the test sample in duplicate using both modified compositions.
3. Compare the % assay results with those obtained under standard (as such) method conditions.

Acceptance Criteria (for information only)

- All system suitability parameters must meet the established method criteria.
- The difference in % assay between original and modified compositions should be NMT 2.0%.

Note: If system suitability or assay variation fails to meet acceptance criteria, narrow the range of organic phase variation and report the acceptable range at which system suitability and assay variation passes.

iii. Effect of Variation in Flow Rate

Purpose:

To assess the robustness of the analytical method by evaluating the impact of ±10% variation in the HPLC flow rate on system suitability parameters and assay results.

Studies to be Performed

Analyze the standard preparation using flow rates set at ±10% of the method-defined value.

Evaluate system suitability parameters at each flow rate condition.

Analyze the test sample in duplicate and calculate the % difference in assay compared to results obtained under the original flow rate.

Execution

Set the HPLC flow rate to +10% and –10% of the specified method flow rate.

Inject the standard solution and verify system suitability at each flow rate.

Analyze the test sample in duplicate using both altered flow rates.

Compare the assay results with those from the original method conditions.

Acceptance Criteria (for information only)

All system suitability parameters should meet the established criteria.

The % difference in assay between the original and varied flow rates should be NMT 2.0%.

Note: If system suitability or assay variation fails to meet criteria, narrow the flow rate range and report the range at which the system suitability criteria are satisfied.

iv. Effect of variation in column oven temperature:

Purpose:

To evaluate the robustness of the test method by assessing the impact of ±5°C variation in column oven temperature on system suitability parameters and assay results.

Studies to be Performed

Analyze the standard solution using the HPLC system at column oven temperatures ±5°C from the method-defined condition.

Evaluate system suitability parameters at each temperature condition.

Analyze the test sample in duplicate and calculate the % difference in assay results compared to those obtained under the original method conditions.

Execution

Set the column oven temperature to +5°C and –5°C relative to the method-defined temperature.

Inject the standard preparation and assess system suitability at each temperature setting.

Analyze the test sample in duplicate at both temperature conditions.

Compare the assay results with those obtained using the as such method parameters.

Acceptance Criteria (for information only)

System suitability should comply with predefined criteria.

The difference in % assay between the original and varied temperature conditions should be NMT 2.0%.

Note: If any system suitability parameter fails, narrow the column oven temperature variation range and define the acceptable temperature range within which the system suitability criteria are consistently met.

v. Effect of variation in buffer pH of mobile phase:

Purpose:

To evaluate the robustness of the analytical method by assessing the effect of slight variations in buffer pH (±0.2 units) on the system suitability parameters and assay results.

Studies to be Performed:

Prepare mobile phase with buffer pH adjusted to +0.2 and –0.2 units from the method-defined pH.

Analyze the standard solution and verify system suitability parameters.

Analyze the test sample in duplicate using each modified pH condition.

Calculate the % difference in assay compared to results obtained using the original (as such) method parameters.

Execution:

Prepare two mobile phases with buffer pH at ±0.2 from the specified method pH.

Inject the standard solution to assess system suitability for each pH condition.

Analyze the test sample in duplicate under both modified pH conditions.

Compare assay results with those obtained using the original mobile phase..

Acceptance criteria (for information only):

All system suitability parameters should comply with the predefined method criteria.

The % difference in assay results between original and modified pH conditions should be NMT 2.0%.

Note: If system suitability or assay variation fails to meet acceptance criteria, narrow the buffer pH variation and report the acceptable range at which the system suitability and assay variation passes.

vi. Bench top stability of standard and test preparation:

Purpose:

To evaluate the stability of standard and test sample preparations when stored at bench top conditions (room temperature) over a defined period.

Studies to be Performed:

Perform the assay of the product in duplicate using freshly prepared standard and test solutions.

Keep both standard and test preparations on the bench (room temperature) and analyze at 1-day intervals up to 2 days.

On each day, analyze against a freshly prepared standard to determine the stability.

Execution:

On Day 0 (initial), prepare and analyze the standard and test sample as per method.

Store the remaining standard and test solutions at room temperature.

On Day 1 and Day 2, prepare a fresh standard and analyze:

The bench top standard vs. fresh standard → calculate similarity factor.

The bench top test solution → determine % assay and calculate the difference from the initial (Day 0) result.

Note: If either the standard or test solution shows instability on Day 1, perform hourly bench top stability assessment on the day of preparation to determine usable holding time.

Acceptance criteria (for information only):

The difference in % assay from Day 0 to Day 1/Day 2 should be NMT 2.0%.

The similarity factor for the standard solution should be between 0.98 and 1.02.

vii. Refrigerator Stability of Standard and Test Preparation

Purpose:

To evaluate the stability of standard and test solutions when stored under refrigerated conditions (2–8°C) for up to 2 days, by assessing their performance against freshly prepared standards.

Execution:

1. Perform the assay of the product in duplicate using freshly prepared standard and test solutions (Day 0).
2. Store the remaining standard and test preparations in the refrigerator (2–8°C).
3. On Day 1 and Day 2, analyze the stored solutions against a freshly prepared standard.
4. Evaluate the following for each day:
   - oSimilarity factor of the refrigerated standard vs. freshly prepared standard.
   - o % assay of refrigerated test solution.
   - o % difference in assay from initial (Day 0) to Day 1 and Day 2.

Important Notes

1. Do not perform refrigerator stability if bench top stability of both standard and test solution is established and found acceptable for 2 days.
2. If instability is observed on Day 1, perform refrigerator stability on an hourly basis on the day of preparation to determine suitable holding time.
3. The duration of the solution stability study may vary depending on practical circumstances; however, the minimum evaluation period shall not be less than 2 days.

Acceptance Criteria (for information only)

1. The difference in % assay from initial to Day 1 and Day 2 should be NMT 2.0%.
2. The similarity factor for the standard should be in the range of 0.98 to 1.02.

viii. Bench Top Stability of Mobile Phase

Purpose:

To evaluate the stability of the mobile phase when stored at bench top (room temperature) for up to 2 days, by assessing its effect on system suitability and assay results.

Execution:

1. Prepare the standard solution and test solution as per the test method and inject using the same lot of mobile phase stored on the bench top:
   - o At initial (Day 0)
   - o After 1 day
   - o After 2 days
2. Perform the assay of the product in duplicate on each day using the same mobile phase lot.
3. For each time point (Day 0, 1, and 2):

o Evaluate system suitability parameters

o Determine the % assay of the test solution

o Calculate the difference in % assay from the initial value

Note: If the mobile phase shows instability on Day 1, conduct the study at shorter time intervals (e.g., every 2–4 hours) and report the maximum duration for which the mobile phase remains stable at room temperature.

Acceptance Criteria (for information only)

1. System suitability must comply with the predefined criteria.
2. The difference in % assay of the test sample from the initial (Day 0) result should be not more than 2.0%.

2. Robustness – Related Substances (by HPLC)

i. Filter Validation

Purpose

To evaluate the robustness of the method by assessing the impact of different filter types on the quantification of impurities.

Studies to be Performed

- Prepare test solution in duplicate by spiking impurities at target concentration (refer method precision).
- Filter separate portions of the solution through 0.45 µm PVDF and 0.45 µm Nylon membrane filters.
- Centrifuge a portion of the same solution and compare impurity results.

Execution

Inject centrifuged and filtered test solutions into the HPLC system. Compare the % of individual and total impurities between centrifuged and filtered samples.

Acceptance Criteria (for information only)

- Meets system suitability requirements
- In impurity spiked test, % difference in individual and total impurities: NMT 10.0%
- Impurities below LOQ need not be compared.

ii. Effect of Variation in Mobile Phase Composition

Purpose

To assess method robustness against deliberate ±10% variation in the organic content of the mobile phase.

Studies to be Performed:

- Prepare two mobile phases:
  - o One containing 110% of the method-defined organic phase.
  - o Another containing 90% of the method-defined organic phase.
- Inject the standard preparation using both mobile phases and evaluate system suitability parameters.
- Analyze the impurity spiked test sample in duplicate using each mobile phase and calculate the % difference in assay compared to the result obtained with the original method composition.

Execution:

Mobile Phase Preparation

- Mobile phase preparation as per STP: Buffer pH 2.0 : Methanol = 60:40 (v/v).
- 90% organic: Buffer pH 2.0 : Methanol = 60:36 (v/v)
- 110% organic: Buffer pH 2.0 : Methanol = 60:44 (v/v)

Acceptance Criteria (for information only)

- Meets system suitability requirements
- In impurity spiked test, % difference in individual and total impurities: NMT 10.0%
- Impurities below LOQ need not be compared.

iii. Effect of Variation in Flow Rate

Purpose

To evaluate method robustness against ±10% change in HPLC flow rate.

Studies to be Performed

- Adjust flow rate to ±10% of the method-specified value.
- Inject standard solution and impurity-spiked test solution in duplicate.
- Compare impurity values with standard condition.

Execution

Analyze solutions at varied flow rates. Evaluate system suitability and calculate % difference in impurity levels.

Acceptance Criteria (for information only)

Refer: Effect of Variation in Mobile Phase Composition

iv. Effect of Variation in Column Oven Temperature

Purpose

To assess the robustness of the method with respect to ±5°C variation in column oven temperature.

Studies to be Performed

- Vary column temperature by ±5°C from the method-defined setting.
- Inject standard solution and impurity-spiked test solution in duplicate.
- Compare impurity values with those under standard conditions.

Execution

Analyze test and standard preparations under both temperature variations. Monitor system suitability and impurity content.

Acceptance Criteria (for information only)

Refer: Effect of Variation in Mobile Phase Composition

v. Effect of Variation in Buffer pH of Mobile Phase

Purpose

To evaluate robustness against ±0.2 unit variation in the pH of mobile phase buffer.

Studies to be Performed

- Prepare mobile phase with buffer pH adjusted by +0.2 and –0.2 units.
- Inject standard and impurity-spiked test solution in duplicate.
- Compare impurity data with the original method.

Execution

Analyze solutions with both altered buffer pH conditions. Assess impurity profiles and system suitability.

Acceptance Criteria (for information only)

Refer: Effect of Variation in Mobile Phase Composition

vi. Bench Top Stability of Standard and Test Preparation

Purpose

To verify the stability of standard and test solutions when stored at bench top (room temperature) for up to 2 days.

Studies to be Performed

- Store standard and impurity-spiked test solutions at room temperature.
- Analyze at initial, Day 1, and Day 2.
- Calculate difference in impurity results and similarity factor for standard.

Execution

Analyze solutions each day using fresh standard. Compare % of individual and total impurities with Day 0. Calculate similarity factor for standard solution.

Acceptance Criteria (for information only)

- % difference in individual and total impurities: NMT 10.0%
- Similarity factor for standard: 0.95–1.05
- Ignore impurities below LOQ.

vii. Refrigerator Stability of Standard and Test Preparation

Purpose

To assess the stability of standard and test solutions when stored under refrigerated conditions (2–8°C) for 2 days.

Studies to be Performed

- Store impurity-spiked test and standard solutions in the refrigerator.
- Analyze at initial, Day 1, and Day 2.
- Calculate % difference in impurity content and similarity factor.

Execution

Analyze solutions daily. Compare impurity levels with Day 0. Determine similarity factor for standard.

Acceptance Criteria (for information only)

Refer: Bench Top Stability of Standard and Test Preparation

viii. Bench Top Stability of Mobile Phase

Purpose

To evaluate the stability of mobile phase when stored at room temperature for up to 2 days.

Studies to be Performed

- Store a batch of mobile phase at bench top.
- Use the same batch to analyze standard and impurity-spiked test solution at initial, Day 1, and Day 2.
- Assess system suitability and impurity recovery.

Execution

Analyze standard and test solutions each day using stored mobile phase. Compare impurity values with initial. Determine similarity factor.

Acceptance Criteria (for information only)

- System suitability must comply with STP requirements.
- % difference in impurities: NMT 10.0%
- Similarity factor: 0.95–1.05

3.Robustness – Dissolution (by HPLC):

i. Filter Validation

Purpose

To evaluate the robustness of the dissolution method by verifying the impact of different filter types on dissolution results.

Studies to be Performed

- Prepare test solution in duplicate as per test method (use 100% accuracy or precision sample).
- Filter aliquots through 0.45 μm PVDF and 0.45 μm Nylon filters.
- Centrifuge a portion of the same solution.

Execution

Centrifuge 10 mL of test solution at 5000 rpm for 10 minutes.

Filter the remaining solution using each filter, discarding the first 3 mL, 5mL etc.

Analyze filtered and centrifuged solutions by HPLC.

Calculate % dissolution for each and determine the difference.

Acceptance Criteria (for information only)

- Difference in % dissolution between filtered and centrifuged solutions: NMT 2.0%

ii. Effect of Variation in Mobile Phase Composition

Purpose

To assess method robustness against ±10% variation in organic solvent content of the mobile phase.

Studies to be Performed:

- Prepare two mobile phases:
  - o One containing 90% of the method-defined organic phase.
  - o Another containing 110% of the method-defined organic phase.
- Analyze standard and test solution in duplicate using each mobile phase

Execution:

Mobile Phase Preparation

- Mobile phase preparation as per STP: Buffer and acetonitrile in the ratio 70: 30 (v/v).
- 90% organic: Buffer : Acetonitrile = 70:27 (v/v)
- 110% organic: Buffer : Acetonitrile = 70:33 (v/v)
- Inject standard and test solutions prepared under standard conditions using both varied mobile phases.
  Evaluate system suitability and compare % dissolution with standard mobile phase results.

Acceptance Criteria (for information only)

1. System suitability should meet method-defined criteria
2. Difference in % dissolution from standard condition: NMT 2.0%

iii. Effect of Variation in Flow Rate

Purpose

To evaluate the effect of ±10% variation in HPLC flow rate on dissolution test results.

Studies to be Performed

- Vary flow rate by ±10% from method-specified value.
- Analyze standard and test solution in duplicate at each flow rate.

Execution

Inject standard and test solutions at modified flow rates.
Compare system suitability and % dissolution with original condition.

Acceptance Criteria (for information only)

1. System suitability must comply with STP
2. Difference in % dissolution: NMT 2.0%

iv. Effect of Variation in Column Oven Temperature

Purpose

To evaluate the robustness of the method to ±5°C variation in column oven temperature.

Studies to be Performed

- Analyze standard and test solution in duplicate at ±5°C from method-defined column temperature.

Execution

Inject solutions at modified temperatures and compare results with original condition.

Acceptance Criteria (for information only)

1. System suitability must meet STP

2. Difference in % dissolution: NMT 2.0%

v. Effect of Variation in Buffer pH of Mobile Phase

Purpose

To assess the impact of ±0.2 pH unit variation in mobile phase buffer on dissolution performance.

Studies to be Performed

- Prepare mobile phases with buffer pH at ±0.2 units from standard.
- Analyze standard and test solutions in duplicate under each condition.

Execution

Evaluate system suitability and compare % dissolution results with original condition.

Acceptance Criteria (for information only)

1. System suitability must pass
2. Difference in % dissolution: NMT 2.0%

vi. Bench Top Stability of Standard and Test Preparation

Purpose

To assess the stability of standard and test solutions at room temperature for up to 2 days.

Studies to be Performed

- Store standard and test solutions on bench top.
- Analyze at initial, Day 1, and Day 2 against freshly prepared standard.

Execution

Evaluate % dissolution of test solution and similarity factor for standard each day. Compare results with Day 0.

Acceptance Criteria (for information only)

1. Difference in % dissolution: NMT 2.0%
2. Similarity factor for standard: 0.98–1.02

Note: If instability is seen on Day 1, perform the study at shorter intervals.

vii. Refrigerator Stability of Standard and Test Preparation

Purpose

To assess the stability of standard and test solutions under refrigerated conditions (2–8°C) for 2 days.

Studies to be Performed

- Store test and standard solutions in the refrigerator.
- Analyze at initial, Day 1, and Day 2.

Execution

Compare % dissolution of test solutions and similarity factor for standards with Day 0 values.

Acceptance Criteria (for information only)

1. Difference in % dissolution: NMT 2.0%
2. Similarity factor for standard: 0.98–1.02

viii. Bench Top Stability of Mobile Phase

Purpose

To evaluate the impact of mobile phase storage at room temperature for up to 2 days on method performance.

Studies to be Performed

- Use the same lot of mobile phase stored at bench top for 0, 1, and 2 days.
- Analyze standard and test solutions at each time point.

Execution

Compare % dissolution and system suitability at each interval.
Calculate similarity factor for standard.

Acceptance Criteria (for information only)

1. System suitability should comply with STP
2. Difference in % dissolution: NMT 2.0%

Note: If instability is observed, test at shorter intervals and define stable duration.

ix. Effect of Deaeration of Dissolution Medium

Purpose

To assess the impact of deaeration on dissolution performance.

Studies to be Performed

- Perform dissolution using deaerated and non-deaerated medium on six units each.
- Compare average % dissolution and RSD.

Execution

Analyze both sets as per STP. Calculate % dissolution, average, and RSD.

Acceptance Criteria (for information only)

1. Product must meet dissolution specification
2. RSD of % dissolution: NMT 5.0%
3. Difference in average % dissolution: NMT 5.0%

x. Effect of Variation in Dissolution Medium Volume

Purpose

To evaluate the robustness of dissolution with ±1% variation in medium volume.

Studies to be Performed

- Perform dissolution on six units each using standard and varied medium volume.

Execution

Calculate % dissolution, average, and RSD of both sets.

Acceptance Criteria (for information only)

1. Product must meet dissolution specification
2. RSD: NMT 5.0%
3. Difference in average % dissolution: NMT 5.0%

xi. Effect of Apparatus Speed

Purpose

To evaluate the effect of ±4% change in dissolution apparatus speed on test results.

Studies to be Performed

- Perform dissolution on six units at ±4% of defined apparatus speed.
- Compare with standard condition.

Execution

Determine % dissolution, average, and RSD for both sets.

Acceptance Criteria (for information only)

1. Product must meet dissolution specification
2. RSD: NMT 5.0%
3. Difference in average % dissolution: NMT 5.0%

4. Robustness – Residual Solvents (by GC)

i. Filter Validation (if applicable, for direct injection technique)

Purpose

To evaluate the robustness of the GC method by assessing the impact of different filter types on the quantification of residual solvents.

Studies to be Performed

- Prepare test solution in duplicate by spiking placebo with known levels of ethanol, methanol, and methylene dichloride (MDC).
- Filter portions of the solution using 0.45 μm PVDF and 0.45 μm Nylon filters.
- Centrifuge a portion of the same solution.

Execution

Centrifuge ~10 mL of test solution at 5000 rpm for 10 minutes.
Filter the remaining solution, discarding the first 1,2,3 mL of each filtrate.
Inject filtered and centrifuged samples into the GC system.
Compare % recovery of each solvent.

Acceptance Criteria (for information only)

- Difference in % recovery for each solvent between filtered and centrifuged solutions: NMT 10.0%

ii. Effect of Variation in Carrier Gas Flow Rate

Purpose

To assess the impact of ±10% variation in carrier gas flow rate on system suitability and residual solvent content.

Studies to be Performed

- Prepare spiked test solution (refer accuracy at 100%) and standard solution.
- Adjust GC carrier gas flow rate by ±10% from the method-defined value.
- Analyze standard and test solutions under each condition.
- Use precision data for comparison.

Execution

Inject test and standard solutions using modified flow rates.
Compare residual solvent content and system suitability with original conditions.

Acceptance Criteria (for information only)

- System suitability must meet method-defined limits
- Difference in residual solvent content: NMT 10.0%

Note: If results exceed limits, narrow the flow rate variation range and define acceptable range.

iii. Effect of Variation in Column Oven Temperature

Purpose

To evaluate robustness of the method with respect to ±5°C change in column oven temperature.

Studies to be Performed

- Prepare spiked test solution (refer accuracy at 100%) and standard solution.
- Set column oven temperature to +5°C and –5°C from method-defined value.
- Compare residual solvent content and system suitability.

Execution

Inject standard and test solutions at varied temperatures.

Compare results to original method conditions.

Acceptance Criteria (for information only)

Follow Effect of Variation in Carrier Gas Flow Rate

Note: Narrow the oven temperature range if needed and define allowable limits.

iv. Effect of Variation in Head Space Vial Equilibration Time

Purpose

To assess the method robustness against ±5 minutes variation in vial equilibration time.

Studies to be Performed

- Prepare spiked test solution (refer accuracy at 100%) and standard solution.
- Set vial equilibration time to +5 min and –5 min from the method-defined value.
- Evaluate ethanol recovery and system suitability.

Execution

Analyze samples at both varied equilibration times.

Compare results with precision data and standard condition.

Acceptance Criteria (for information only)

Follow Effect of Variation in Carrier Gas Flow Rate

Note: Define acceptable equilibration time range if deviation is observed.

v. Effect of Variation in Vial Incubation Temperature

Purpose

To evaluate the impact of ±5°C change in vial incubation temperature on residual solvent recovery.

Studies to be Performed

- Prepare ethanol-spiked test solution (refer accuracy at 100%) and standard solution.
- Analyze using vial temperatures ±5°C from the method-defined value.
- Compare ethanol content and system suitability.

Execution

Inject samples under each modified temperature condition.

Compare results to original condition.

Acceptance Criteria (for information only)

Follow Effect of Variation in Carrier Gas Flow Rate

Note: Define acceptable vial incubation temperature range if deviation is observed.

vi. Bench Top Stability of Standard and Test Solution

Purpose

To evaluate the stability of standard and test solutions when stored at room temperature for up to 2 days.

Studies to be Performed

- Prepare ethanol/mixed solvent-spiked test solution and standard.
- Store at room temperature.
- Analyze at initial, Day 1, and Day 2.

Execution

Analyze stored solutions using fresh standard each day.

Compare % recovery of solvents and similarity factor for standard.

Acceptance Criteria (for information only)

- Difference in % recovery: NMT 10.0%
- Similarity factor for standard: 0.95–1.05

Note: If instability is observed, conduct hourly study and define usable time.

vii. Refrigerator Stability of Standard and Test Solution

Purpose

To evaluate the stability of residual solvent solutions when stored under refrigerated conditions (2–8°C) for 2 days.

Studies to be Performed

- Store test and standard solutions at 2–8°C.
- Analyze at initial, Day 1, and Day 2.

Execution

Evaluate % recovery of residual solvents and similarity factor at each interval.

Acceptance Criteria (for information only)

- Difference in % recovery: NMT 10.0%
- Similarity factor for standard: 0.95–1.05

Note: If instability is observed, conduct hourly study and define usable time.

CHAPTER: 10

REPORT FORMAT

★ Objective

The primary objective of this chapter is to provide a clear and structured framework for drafting a comprehensive Method Validation Report. It aims to guide professionals in accurately documenting the outcomes of analytical method validation studies in alignment with regulatory expectations such as those from ICH, USFDA, and EMA.

This chapter will help readers understand the essential elements that must be captured in a validation report, including methodology, results, observations, deviations (if any), and conclusions. It emphasizes the importance of clarity, completeness, and consistency in reporting to ensure that the data presented is scientifically sound and compliant with global regulatory standards.

Let us discuss the content of well-structured report

Title:

Method Validation Report for [Test Name] of [Product Name] by [Technique (e.g., HPLC, GC, UV)]

1. Objective

To summarize and conclude the analytical method validation conducted as per protocol number [Protocol No.], for the estimation of [Analyte] in [Product Name] using [Instrument/Technique], in accordance with ICH Q2 (R2), pharmacopoeial standards, and internal SOPs.

2. Scope

Applicable to the analytical method developed for [Product Name, Dosage Form, Strength] intended for use in [QC release / stability studies / regulatory submission, etc.].

3. Responsibilities

Role	Name Department
Executed By	QC / ADL
Reviewed By	QA
Approved By	QA / Head

4. Summary of Validation Parameters

Validation Parameter	Protocol Ref	Outcome	Conclusion
System Suitability	Sec. 7.1	Passed	Accepted
Specificity	Sec. 7.2	Passed	Accepted
Linearity	Sec. 7.3	Passed	Accepted
Accuracy	Sec. 7.4	Passed	Accepted

Precision	Sec. 7.5	Passed	Accepted
Robustness	Sec. 7.6	Passed	Accepted
LOD / LOQ	Sec. 7.7	Passed	Accepted

5. Product Information

- Product Name: [e.g., Paracetamol Tablets 500 mg]
- API: [e.g., Paracetamol]
- Dosage Form: [Tablet / Capsule / Injectable]
- Specification Reference: [SPEC No.]
- Batch Number(s): [Insert]
- Manufacturing Site: [Insert site name]

6. Standard Test Procedure and Specification Information

- STP Number
- Detailed STP
- Specification No.
- Specification for validated test

7. Detailed Validation Summary (For Each Parameter)

Each parameter section should include:

- Reference to Protocol Section
- Summary of Approach
- Key Observations & Data
- Acceptance Criteria
- Conclusion (Pass/Fail)

Include visuals like chromatograms, graphs for linearity, tables for accuracy, precision, and robustness.

8. Deviations (if any)

Clearly mention any deviations from the protocol, with:

- Reason
- Impact assessment
- CAPA (if required)
- QA justification

9. Overall Conclusion

Confirm whether the method has met the pre-defined acceptance criteria and whether it is suitable for its intended purpose.

"All validation parameters met the acceptance criteria as outlined in the protocol. The method is deemed validated and fit for use in the routine analysis of [Product Name]."

10. Version Control and Document History

Version	Change Description	Prepared By	Approved By	Date
00	Initial Issue			

11. Optional Enhancements

a) Cross-reference with Protocol

Mention the exact section numbers from protocol for traceability.

b) Glossary of Abbreviations

- API – Active Pharmaceutical Ingredient
- LOQ – Limit of Quantitation
- LOD – Limit of Detection
- RSD – Relative Standard Deviation
- STP – Standard Test Procedure

c) Visual Summaries

- Linearity plots
- Overlay chromatograms for specificity
- Accuracy recovery plots
- Bar graphs for robustness data comparison

d) Reviewer Checklist (Internal Use Only)

- Protocol followed?
- Data complete and traceable?
- Acceptance criteria clearly referenced?
- Raw data attached?
- Calculations verified?
- Deviations documented and justified?

e) Statement of Intended Use

"This method is validated and intended for use in [release / stability / regulatory filing] testing of [Product Name]."

f) Digital Integration

Ensure the format is compatible with electronic signing tools or 21 CFR Part 11 compliant systems if applicable.

12. Annexures (Attach as Needed)

- Raw data sheets
- Chromatograms
- System suitability results
- Calibration curves
- Worksheets for accuracy, precision
- Final concentration matrix

This guidance is intended to ensure consistency, clarity, and regulatory readiness for all analytical method validation reports generated under Pharma Growth Hub or partner institutions.

CHAPTER: 11

FORCED DEGRADATION STUDIES

★ 1. Introduction to Forced Degradation Studies in Pharmaceutical Development

Forced degradation studies are conducted to simulate the types of stress a pharmaceutical product might encounter during its manufacturing, storage, and distribution. These studies help us understand how a product behaves under different environmental conditions, including exposure to heat, light, humidity, oxidation, and hydrolytic environments. The results guide formulation scientists and quality control teams to design products that remain stable throughout their intended shelf life.

A pharmaceutical product can undergo degradation when exposed to high temperatures (thermal degradation), intense light (photolytic degradation), oxidative environments (oxidative degradation), or the presence of moisture (hydrolytic degradation). Even small amounts of free radicals or impurities can catalyze these degradation reactions, leading to product deterioration.

Hence, it is important to design stress conditions that are realistic and scientifically justified. Conditions must be severe enough to generate meaningful degradation products but should not cause total destruction of the drug substance. The goal is to produce degradation in a controlled manner, typically targeting a 5% to 20% degradation of the active pharmaceutical ingredient (API).

Understanding the stability of a product under such conditions allows scientists to:

- Predict the potential degradation pathways.
- Identify likely degradation products.
- Develop stability-indicating analytical methods.
- Design protective packaging.
- Select appropriate manufacturing and storage conditions

The selection of stress conditions is done carefully. For example:

i. Acid Hydrolysis

Acid hydrolysis is typically conducted by exposing the drug sample to an acidic medium under controlled temperature and time conditions. Following the reaction, the sample is neutralized and analyzed. This helps evaluate whether the analytical method can maintain resolution and purity of the API and impurity peak in the presence of acid-induced degradation products.

ii. Base Hydrolysis

In this study, the sample is subjected to an alkaline environment to simulate degradation under basic conditions. The process is similar to acid hydrolysis, involving exposure to base, followed by neutralization and analysis. It is essential that the method distinguishes the API from any degradation products formed under these conditions.

iii. Oxidation

To simulate oxidative stress, the sample is treated with an oxidizing agent such as hydrogen peroxide and stored under controlled conditions, usually protected from light. This test evaluates the method's capacity to detect and resolve oxidation products that may form during manufacturing or storage.

iv. Photolytic Degradation

Photostability testing involves exposing the sample to defined light intensity, covering both UV and visible spectra, in accordance with ICH Q1B guidelines. After exposure, the sample is analyzed to ensure the method can detect any degradants resulting from light exposure. This is particularly important for APIs or formulations known to be photosensitive.

For confirmatory studies, samples should be exposed to light providing an overall illumination of not less than 1.2 million lux hours and an integrated near ultraviolet energy of not less than 200 watt hours/square meter to allow direct comparisons to be made between the drug substance and drug product. Samples may be exposed side-by-side with a validated chemical actinometric system to ensure the specified light exposure is obtained, or for the appropriate duration of time when conditions have been monitored using calibrated radiometers/lux meters. An example of an actinometric procedure is provided in the Annex. If protected samples (e.g., wrapped in aluminum foil) are used as dark controls to evaluate the contribution of thermally induced change to the total observed change, these should be placed alongside the authentic sample.

v. Thermal Degradation

Thermal degradation is assessed by exposing the drug substance or product to elevated temperatures for a specified duration. Once the stress period is complete, the sample is prepared and analyzed. The objective is to determine whether the method remains capable of resolving the API from thermally induced degradation products.

vi. Humidity Stress

In humidity stress studies, the sample is exposed to high relative humidity commonly 90% RH under controlled temperature for a designated time. Following exposure, the material is processed and analyzed. This condition helps to evaluate the impact of moisture on the stability of the product and the adequacy of the analytical method to detect any resulting degradation.

Each condition aims to simulate potential real-world exposures that the product may face.

Moreover, forced degradation is not only limited to assessing the stability of the final drug product. It also plays a crucial role during analytical method validation. A stability-indicating method must demonstrate its ability to separate the API from its degradation products, ensuring the method's specificity.
It is equally important to recognize that excessive degradation is not desirable.

Careful selection of stress intensity and duration ensures that degradation remains within acceptable limits. If degradation is too low, it may not reveal all potential pathways. If it is too high, it may not be reflective of real-world scenarios and could lead to meaningless or misleading results.

Additionally, the degradation profiles obtained help in setting proper specifications for impurities and degradation products, which are critical for regulatory submissions and overall product safety.

Forced degradation studies provide critical information needed for developing robust, stable, and safe pharmaceutical products. They help in understanding the intrinsic stability of drug substances and offer insights that are invaluable for ensuring product quality throughout its lifecycle.

2. Understanding Mass Balance in Forced Degradation Studies

Mass balance is one of the most important and critical parameters in forced degradation studies, particularly during the analysis of related substances. Without a careful assessment of mass balance, it becomes extremely difficult to ascertain whether all degradation products have been suitably quantified or detected. That is precisely why mass balance holds such significant importance in any forced degradation study.

In an ideal world, one would expect a perfect mass balance of 100%. However, in practical scenarios, achieving an exact 100% is often challenging. There may be situations where the observed mass balance is lower than 100%, or even cases where it exceeds 100%. Understanding these deviations is essential for accurately interpreting forced degradation results and for confidently presenting scientific justifications where needed.

To begin, it is important to first understand the concept and definition of mass balance. Mass balance is evaluated during the forced degradation study of related substances, where the principle expectation is that the amount of API (Active Pharmaceutical Ingredient) before degradation should be equal to the sum of the amount of API remaining after degradation plus the amount of degradation products formed. Ideally, the total mass present at the beginning and the end of the study should match. The calculation formula for mass balance is:

$$\%\,\text{Mass Balance} = \frac{\%\,\text{Assay of API after degradation} + \%\,\text{Total degradants}}{\%\,\text{Assay of API before degradation}} \times 100$$

When it comes to acceptance criteria, regulatory guidelines such as ICH or FDA do not specify any strict numerical limit. However, in industry practice, a mass balance of not less than 95% and not more than 105% is widely accepted across many organizations as a reasonable threshold.

Understanding the potential reasons behind lower or higher mass balance outcomes is equally important. There are several causes that can lead to lower mass balance results:

• Degradants with Lack of UV Response: In cases where degradants do not possess chromophores, they may not respond to UV detectors during HPLC analysis, leading to an apparent loss of mass.

- Early Eluting Degradants: Highly polar degradants may elute too early in reversed-phase chromatography, potentially co-eluting with solvent or reagent peaks, making them undetectable.
- Degradants with Low Relative Response Factors (RRFs): If the degradants have significantly lower detector response compared to the API, their quantities may be underestimated.
- Non-Eluting Degradants: Degradants with strong affinity to the stationary phase may not elute from the column, leading to undetected losses.
- Volatile Degradants: Thermal treatment may cause volatile degradants to escape from the sample, leaving no trace in the chromatographic analysis.
- Poor Recovery of Degradation Products: Complex sample matrices may bind degradants, preventing them from being dissolved and analyzed.
- Precipitation of Degradation Products: Insoluble degradants may precipitate out during sample preparation, particularly if the chosen diluent system does not adequately dissolve them.
- Poor Method Sensitivity: Analytical methods that lack sufficient sensitivity may fail to detect and quantify small degradant peaks.

While lower mass balance scenarios are common and expected in some cases, situations where higher mass balance is observed are also possible. These can arise due to:

- Degradants with Higher Relative Response Factors: If a degradant has a detector response much higher than that of the API, a small quantity may appear dispro portionately large during quantification.
- Formation of Adducts or Complexes: APIs may form adducts with excipients or degradation reagents, adding extra mass that was not originally part of the API.
- Degradant Co-elution with API in Assay Methods: If degradants co-elute with the main API peak during assay testing, their contribution may be counted twice once during related substances analysis and again during assay quantificatio artificially inflating the calculated mass balance.

Thus, a comprehensive understanding of mass balance is not just limited to its calculation, but extends to the careful evaluation of practical challenges and their scientific justifications. Whether facing lower or higher mass balances, it is important to analyze the situation thoughtfully and prepare appropriate scientific rationales supported by experimental data.

3. Understanding Peak Purity and its Evaluation

In forced degradation (HPLC by UV), achieving an excellent separation of analytes from potential interferences such as impurities or excipients is a remarkable accomplishment. However, an important question still remains: how do we confirm that there is no hidden interference within the analyte peak? How do we ensure that no impurity or matrix component is co-eluting along with the analyte?

This is precisely where the concept of peak purity becomes vital.

Peak purity assessment verifies whether a chromatographic peak represents a single component or a mixture of co-eluting compounds. The measurement of peak purity fundamentally depends on two parameters: the purity angle and the purity threshold. Here, we will explore these concepts step by step, helping you develop a deep and practical understanding.

i. What is Peak Purity?

Imagine observing a chromatogram with several peaks. A peak is formed by plotting detector response over time, with each point reflecting the absorbance at that specific moment. If we are using a Photodiode Array (PDA) detector, the chromatogram not only records the absorbance response but also collects the UV spectra across the entire peak from its beginning to its end.

Now, how can we guarantee that the spectra throughout the peak belong to the same analyte and not to any impurity?

Peak purity is essentially the assessment of spectral homogeneity across the chromatographic peak. If the UV spectra are consistent across the entire peak, it indicates that the peak likely belongs to a single component. Conversely, dissimilarities in spectra may suggest the presence of co-eluting impurities.

ii. Evaluating Peak Purity

The general workflow to assess peak purity involves:

- Recording spectra across the chromatographic peak using a PDA detector.
- Extracting and normalizing these spectra.
- Overlaying them for comparison.

While visual inspection offers an initial idea, it is not reliable when handling multiple spectra. For precise evaluation, mathematical tools are used, notably vector analysis.

iii. Concept of Vectors in Spectral Analysis

Just like geometric figures (circle, square, triangle) are defined using formulas, complex UV spectra are uniquely characterized using vector mathematics. A vector is a quantity with both magnitude and direction. The intensity of the spectra defines the magnitude and shape of the spectra defines the direction.
When two spectra are similar, their corresponding vectors are closely aligned, resulting in a small angle between them. If the spectra are dissimilar, the angle between the vectors is larger.

Thus, the angle between vectors provides a quantitative measure of spectral similarity.

iv. Purity Angle and Purity Threshold

- The Purity Angle (also called the Spectral Contrast Angle) is the maximum angular difference observed between vectors derived from spectra across a peak.
- A smaller purity angle indicates high spectral homogeneity; a larger angle

suggests possible co-elution.

However, we must recognize that even in the absence of impurities, small variations in spectra can occur due to factors such as detector noise and solvent background. Hence, to account for these unavoidable variations, we define a reference limit known as the Purity Threshold.

The Purity Threshold is determined by analyzing the noise and solvent baseline regions areas of the chromatogram where no actual peaks are present, only system noise. It represents the maximum expected variability due to system noise.

v. Decision Criteria: Confirming Peak Purity

Once the purity angle and purity threshold are measured, the peak purity decision is made:

- If the purity angle is less than the purity threshold, the peak is considered spectrally pure. Dispersion in purity angle is within the noise of the system & hence peak is spectrally homogeneous or pure
- If the purity angle exceeds the purity threshold, the peak is suspected to be spectrally impure, indicating potential co-elution. There is something within the peak that cannot be explained by solvent & noise alone & hence peak is not spectrally pure

This logical approach ensures that the assessment is scientific, reproducible, and less prone to subjective interpretation.

It is important to remember that absolute spectral homogeneity is rare in practical scenarios due to minor fluctuations caused by instrumentation and environmental conditions. Therefore, a structured evaluation using purity angle and purity threshold becomes essential.

vi. Factors Affecting Peak Purity Measurements

Several factors can influence spectral homogeneity:

- Detector noise (electronic disturbances in the detector response)
- Solvent effects (background absorbance variations)
- Baseline drift or pressure fluctuations in the chromatographic system
- Electrical impedance variations

These factors reinforce why measuring both the purity angle and purity threshold is necessary to accurately judge peak purity.

CHAPTER: 12

FORCED DEGRADATION AND DEGRADATION PROFILING AS PER ANVISA

★ Forced degradation is more than just a regulatory requirement it is a critical scientific approach that helps establish the robustness and specificity of an analytical method. Developing a stability-indicating method goes far beyond routine quality checks; it involves a deep understanding of how a drug substance and product respond under various stress conditions. This knowledge empowers us, as pharmaceutical professionals, to ensure the consistent quality, safety, and efficacy of medicines throughout their intended shelf life.

1. The Purpose of Degradation Profiling

Resolution-RDC n. 53/2015 is a Brazilian regulatory document issued by the National Health Surveillance Agency (ANVISA) that outlines requirements for forced degradation studies (FDS) on pharmaceuticals. These studies, also known as "stress tests," are crucial for identifying potential degradation products and ensuring the stability and quality of drug products.

This guideline applies to new drug registrations, generic and branded generics, and products already registered in Brazil.

ANVISA encourages us to recognize three distinct types of degradation profiles:

- **Potential degradation profile** – This is obtained through forced degradation (also called stress testing) and represents the broadest possible set of degradation products that may arise under exaggerated conditions. It serves as a predictive tool.
- **Accelerated stability degradation profile** – This is obtained by storing the product under elevated temperature and humidity conditions for a defined period, as per ICH Q1A(R2). It gives early insights into degradation trends and stability.
- **Real degradation profile** – This is the most representative of actual product behavior, derived from long-term stability studies conducted under recommended storage conditions over the product's shelf life.

In the real world, a product may degrade slowly over a span of several months or even years. But during method development, we can't afford to wait that long. That's why we use stress testing exposing the product to harsh conditions like acid, base, oxidation, light, heat, and humidity to accelerate the degradation process.

This strategy allows us to visualize degradation pathways and assess whether our method can accurately distinguish the active pharmaceutical ingredient (API) from its degradation products. In doing so, we confirm that our method is truly stability-indicating.

So yes, while regulatory bodies like ANVISA require these studies, it's not just about checking a box. It's about adopting a scientific mindset, being proactive, and ensuring that the medicines we develop remain safe and effective from the first tablet to the last.

Figure 1 – Relationship between "potential" degradation profile, obtained in stress study, and the "real" degradation profile, obtained in the long term stability study

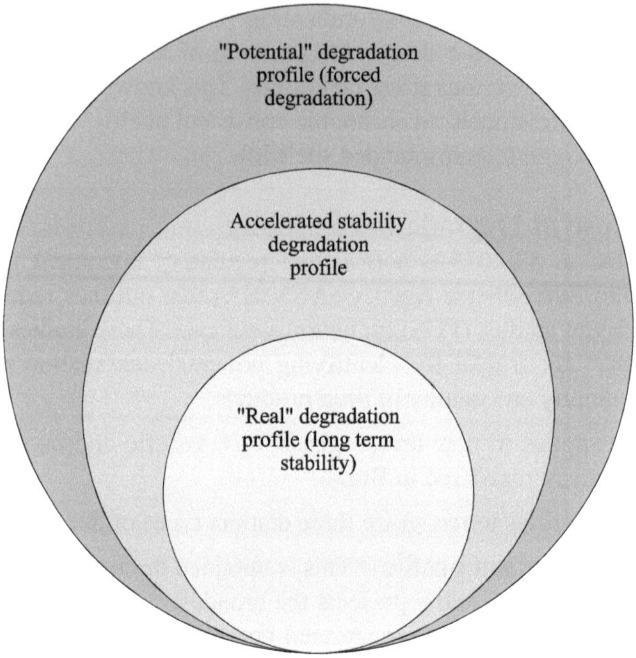

2. When is the Study Needed?

According to ANVISA, a degradation profile study is essential during:

• **New drug registration** – for every strength and dosage form.

• **Post-approval changes** – including formulation changes or modifications in the synthesis route.

• **Method re-validation** – especially when changes in selectivity or formulation might impact degradation behavior.

Even if a forced degradation study was already conducted, a reassessment is needed if any change might alter the degradation pathway or product profile.

3. Degradation profile experimental section

The degradation profile study has two components: a critical part and an experimental part.

The critical part includes background research:

• Known degradation pathways of the API,

• Excipient interactions,

• Functional groups susceptible to hydrolysis or oxidation,
• Reports of toxic or genotoxic impurities.

The experimental part involves actual forced degradation studies under conditions such as:

Table: ANVISA's Recommended Forced Degradation Conditions

Stress Condition	ANVISA Recommendations
Heating (Thermal)	Apply dry heat without increasing humidity or dissolving the product.
Humidity (Wet Thermal)	Expose the product to controlled relative humidity (without dissolution) above ambient RH.Applicable to liquid and semi-solid forms.
Acidic Conditions	Use a buffer solution with pH < 7.0 or mineral acid (e.g., HCl).
Basic Conditions	Use a buffer solution with pH > 7.0 or alkali metal hydroxide (e.g., NaOH).
Oxidative Stress	Use oxidizing agents such as hydrogen peroxide (H_2O_2) or equivalent.
Photolytic Exposure	Expose to variable light intensity (lux hours and/or watt hours per square meter).
Metal Ion Exposure	Use transition metal ion solutions, typically Iron (III) or Copper (II).

ANVISA mandates that each forced degradation study (FDS) condition must result in a degradation level greater than 10%, but not so extensive that it leads to complete degradation of the sample or compromises the integrity of the analysis. This threshold is technically significant, as it ensures that the degradation is sufficient to allow meaningful evaluation of potential degradation products.

Achieving this target degradation approximately 10% of the initial active content requires careful selection of parameters such as exposure time, temperature, and the type and concentration of stress-inducing agents.

In instances where degradation remains below the 10% threshold under any given condition, ANVISA expects the sponsor to provide a clear technical justification. This justification must confirm that more aggressive or extended conditions were evaluated and ruled out based on scientific rationale.

This requirement introduces the concept of FDS "endpoints." While ANVISA has not prescribed fixed endpoint criteria beyond the general guidance of avoiding both under- and over-degradation, it acknowledges that some compounds may inherently resist degradation under certain stress conditions. In such cases, the study may yield minimal or no degradation, despite extended or intensified exposure.

Therefore, it becomes the responsibility of each sponsor to clearly define and justify the chosen endpoints in their regulatory submission. These justifications should be supported with scientific references and rationale, thereby demonstrating the robustness and relevance of the FDS approach adopted.

4. Analytical Method Requirements

High-Performance Liquid Chromatography (HPLC) remains the technique of choice for degradation studies, particularly when equipped with a Diode Array Detector (DAD). ANVISA strongly recommends the use of DAD, as it allows spectral comparison of peaks, thereby ensuring the specificity of the analytical method. Once the method is validated using DAD, it is acceptable to use a UV detector for routine analysis.

To ensure the reliability and reproducibility of results, several system suitability parameters must be assessed. These include resolution between the active pharmaceutical ingredient (API) and its degradation products, peak purity (for example, Chromeleon scores ≥950 or Empower peak purity angle < threshold), peak asymmetry, and column efficiency (measured as the number of theoretical plates). All chromatograms those of the API, placebo, and finished product—should be reviewed together, preferably side-by-side. Any additional peak present in the product chromatogram but absent in the API or placebo must be carefully evaluated as a potential degradation product.

a. Data Interpretation and Reporting

Mass balance is a key expectation from a regulatory standpoint. The sum of the assay value and all detected degradation products should be close to 100%, taking into account reasonable analytical variability. This helps confirm that the method accurately accounts for all chemical changes occurring in the product.

Each chromatogram included in the report must contain critical data such as retention time, peak area, resolution, theoretical plates (column efficiency), and peak purity information. Alongside chromatographic results, the study should also document the percentage degradation of the API, the total impurity levels detected, and the "potential" degradation profile of the product. If any peaks are excluded from consideration or thresholds applied to ignore low-level impurities, a scientific justification must be clearly provided.

b. Degradation Profile Study: Conclusions

At the conclusion of the Degradation Profile Study (DPS), a well-reasoned scientific discussion is essential to interpret the findings and assess their implications for product stability and control strategy. Three primary aspects must be addressed.

First, the study must confirm that the analytical method is indeed stability-indicating. It should demonstrate the capability to detect and quantify degradation products both under stress conditions and during routine stability monitoring. Second, the discussion should identify specific vulnerabilities of the product such as sensitivity to heat, light, pH, or oxidation. These factors may be influenced by the manufacturing process and the nature of excipients used in the formulation. Third, the key degradation products that are likely to form during storage must be clearly identified, and their inclusion in the routine stability monitoring plan should be justified.

It is important to note that the appearance of a degradation product in forced degradation studies alone does not mandate its identification or qualification. These requirements are determined by the results of long-term stability studies and must align with the thresholds and criteria outlined in ANVISA's resolution on degradation products.

5. Documentation Requirements for a Degradation Profile Study

When submitting a Degradation Profile Study (DPS) to ANVISA, it is essential to include well-organized scientific documentation that supports the evaluation of a product's stability and its associated degradation products.

The introduction to the DPS report should briefly explain the scientific rationale behind the study. It must identify the functional groups within the drug molecule that are most susceptible to degradation, supported by literature or structural analysis. Additionally, the analytical method(s) used especially those that are stability-indicating must be clearly described to demonstrate their ability to detect and quantify degradation products.

The experimental section presents the design and results of the forced degradation study. This includes a detailed account of the stress conditions applied such as type and concentration of degrading agents, temperature, and duration. Each condition should be assessed for whether it achieved meaningful degradation, typically above 10%. If this threshold is not met, a scientific justification supported by references must be provided.

Chromatographic data play a central role in this section. Chromatograms should be submitted for the API, placebo, and drug product under each degradation condition, especially for those showing significant breakdown. In fixed-dose combinations, chromatograms of each active ingredient and the final formulation must also be included. If degradation is not observed, data from samples exposed to maximum justified conditions should be provided. For better interpretation, it is advisable to present chromatograms in two scales one to clearly display the main peak (typically 125% of peak height) and another to highlight smaller peaks (suggested at 5% of the main peak height).

Each chromatogram must include key system suitability parameters such as retention time, peak area, resolution, theoretical plates (efficiency), asymmetry, and peak purity. Additionally, purity and threshold values for API peaks should be reported across all test conditions. Tabular comparisons should also be provided to show the extent of API degradation and the corresponding rise in impurity levels. The section should conclude with a brief discussion on mass balance and, where possible, propose degradation mechanisms supported by the observed data.

Finally, the conclusion of the report should summarize the product's potential degradation profile based on the study. It should discuss how the formulation and manufacturing process may influence degradation pathways and identify environmental factors such as light, humidity, and temperature that could impact long-term product stability.

This streamlined yet detailed documentation approach ensures alignment with regulatory expectations while providing valuable scientific insight into product behavior, ultimately helping to ensure consistent quality and safety throughout its shelf life.

6. Identification of a Degradation Product

The identification of degradation products is a critical component of impurity profiling and must be conducted in accordance with the provisions outlined in the relevant ANVISA resolution on degradation impurities.

Degradation product identification becomes essential when impurity levels exceed predefined identification thresholds or when there is a regulatory requirement based on safety concerns. The goal is to confirm the chemical structure of the impurity to support risk assessment, safety evaluation, and control strategies.

7. Acceptable Methods for Degradation Product Identification

ANVISA outlines specific methodologies that are considered scientifically acceptable for the identification of degradation products. These approaches are designed to ensure confidence in structural confirmation and support appropriate impurity risk assessments.

One of the most straightforward and commonly applied methods involves the use of a characterized reference standard. When a known substance whether pharmacopoeial or in-house matches the degradation product in both retention time and UV spectral profile under a validated stability-indicating method, its identity can be reasonably confirmed. This approach is especially practical when suitable reference materials are available.

In cases where a reference standard is not available, a second approach involves mechanistic and spectroscopic confirmation. Here, a plausible degradation pathway is proposed based on the chemical structure and known reactivity of the molecule. The hypothesized degradation product is then structurally confirmed using spectroscopic techniques such as mass spectrometry (MS), nuclear magnetic resonance (NMR), or infrared (IR) spectroscopy. This method combines theoretical and experimental insights to support identification.

For conclusive identification, it is advisable to apply at least two complementary spectroscopic techniques. For example, the combined use of MS and NMR, or MS and IR, increases the confidence in structural assignment. This multi-technique strategy not only enhances the accuracy of identification but also aligns with international best practices for impurity characterization.

By following these accepted approaches, sponsors can ensure that degradation product identification is thorough, scientifically justified, and aligned with ANVISA's regulatory expectations.

8. Degradation Product Qualification

Qualification of degradation products (DPs) is a regulatory requirement under specific conditions, as outlined in the applicable ANVISA Resolution concerning degradation impurities. The qualification process must be preceded by a risk assessment that categorizes the degradation products based on their potential for genotoxicity and carcinogenicity. This classification can be guided by established international regulatory frameworks and scientific literature.

a. Safety Studies for Qualification

When qualification of a degradation impurity is warranted, it should be supported by safety studies that take into account:

- The intended patient population
- The daily dosage of the drug
- The duration of drug administration

The following study types are recommended:

i. Assessment of Genotoxic Potential

This involves evaluating the degradation product's potential to cause genetic mutations or chromosomal abnormalities. Tests for point mutations and structural chromosome damage are commonly employed.

ii.General Toxicity Studies

These studies should be conducted in an animal species that is most sensitive to the suspected toxicity of the degradation product. The duration of the studies should typically range from a minimum of 14 days to a maximum of 90 days, depending on the risk level and intended duration of drug use in humans.

The selection of the most appropriate type of study should be scientifically justified. As a standard approach, screening for genotoxic potential is considered highly relevant. Additionally, Quantitative Structure-Activity Relationship (QSAR) models may be used to support and supplement experimental findings. These computational toxicology assessments should follow internationally accepted modeling standards and validation criteria.

Studies may be conducted either:

- Using the isolated degradation product, or
- Using the active pharmaceutical ingredient (API) spiked with the degradation product at concentrations reflective of those observed during stability testing.

b. Conclusion of Qualification Studies

Upon completion of the safety evaluation, the sponsor must provide a scientific discussion addressing the following key points:

i.Clinical Relevance of Observed Effects

- Was there any indication of adverse effects that are clinically significant?
- Is there a need to revise the impurity specification limits to ensure patient safety?

ii.Safety of Proposed Thresholds

- Based on the study outcomes, can the established thresholds for the degradation product be considered safe?

These conclusions form a critical component of the overall impurity risk assessment and must be included in the regulatory submission dossier as part of the impurity qualification strategy.

9. Study Report: From Forced Degradation to Degradation Profile

ANVISA emphasizes that a Forced Degradation Study (FDS) is only one component of a broader and more comprehensive assessment known as the Degradation Profile Study (DPS). While the FDS represents the experimental phase, the DPS encompasses a critical analysis of the degradation behavior of a drug substance or drug product throughout its lifecycle.

As such, ANVISA's expectations for an FDS report extend beyond simply documenting stress condition results. Instead, the focus is on presenting a holistic discussion of the degradation profile of the product. The FDS results are to be considered as supportive evidence within this broader degradation assessment framework.

In line with this approach, the FDS/DPS report should also capture preliminary evaluations those made following the bibliographic research and prior to initiating the FDS itself. These evaluations should explore how the compound's degradation sensitivity could influence formulation, manufacturing, and storage conditions.

10. Final Takeaway

ANVISA's guidance reminds us that forced degradation is not just about ticking a regulatory checkbox. It's about building scientific confidence in the method. It's about anticipating problems, preventing surprises, and protecting the patient.

As you develop methods for assay or related substances, always remember this simple principle:

A well-executed degradation study is a window into the future stability of your product.

CHAPTER: 13

COMMON CHALLENGES & WAY FORWARD

★ Introduction:

No matter how well-planned and well-executed an analytical method validation strategy may be, real-world scenarios often present unforeseen hurdles. From unexpected variability in system response to overlooked details like filter saturation or impurity stock traceability, challenges can emerge at every stage of validation. These challenges, if not addressed proactively, can compromise the integrity of the data, delay regulatory submissions, or even lead to failed audits.

This chapter brings together a collection of commonly encountered issues during analytical method validation gathered from industry experiences, regulatory observations, and practical implementation. More importantly, for each challenge, offered a clear and actionable 'way forward', helping professionals not only recognize potential pitfalls but also take informed steps to overcome them.

1.Accuracy at QL for Impurity in Drug Product with High Impurity Content
2.Precision at QL in Presence of High Impurity Levels
3.Lower Mass Balance Observed During Forced Degradation in Related Substances Study
4.Higher Mass Balance During Forced Degradation in Related Substances Study
5.Failure in peak purity during specificity
6.Unavailability of Test Sample (Drug Product) During Method Validation
7.Impurity standard not available for impurity method validation
8.Very Limited Quantity of Impurity Standards
9.Theoretical DL/QL Too Low for Practical Use
10.Challenges in Performing Forced Degradation Studies for Combination Products
11.Non-Homogeneous Drug Product Samples
12.Impurity Supplied in Salt Form vs. Non-Salt Form in Sample
13.Consideration of Impurity Purity During Impurity Solution Preparation
14.Unverified Stability of Analytical Solutions
15.Alignment of Instrument Operating Ranges with Method Requirements
16.Validating an R&D-Developed Method in the QC Laboratory
17.Preparation of Placebo: Manual vs. Processed
18.Use of Validated Spreadsheets or Chromatography Software for Result Calculation
19.Inaccurate or Poorly Designed Validation Protocol:
20.Untrained Analyst in Method Validation
21.Incomplete Method Transfer Documentation
22.Unjustified Stress Conditions in Forced Degradation
23.Variability in Chromatographic Columns

24.Impact of Uncontrolled Environmental Conditions
25.Undefined Integration Parameters
26.Method Not Fit for Multi-Site Implementation
27.Rushed, Checklist-Driven Validation Approach
28.Inappropriate Selection of Validation Ranges
29.Incomplete/Unsuitable Range for Immediate Release Product Dissolution Method
30.Wrong Concentration of Sample for Filter Saturation during Dissolution
31.Response and Retention Time Variation Across Different HPLC Systems (During Intermediate Precision)
32.Inadequate Traceability for the Impurity Stock Used Across Validation Studies
33.Response Affected by pH Change
34.Different Response Factor for Impurities
35.Blank Interference Near LOD/LOQ
36.Ambiguity in Acceptance Criteria
37.Not Capturing Method Changes or Deviations
38.Failing to Identify Critical Validation Gaps
39.Incomplete Validation Protocol or Report
40.Discrepancy in Version-Controlled Documents
41.Inadequate Sample Tracking During Validation
42.Not Updating Standard Test Procedure (STP) After Method Changes or Validations
43.Statistical Tools Not Validated or Controlled
44.Validation Being Treated as a Checklist Activity, not a Scientific Exercise
45.No Internal System for Continuous Method Performance Review
46.Pseudo Dose-Proportionate Formulation with Same Test and Standard Concentrations
47.Pseudo Dose-Proportionate Formulation with Different Test and Standard Concentrations:
48.Dose-Proportionate Formulation with Same Test and Standard Concentration
49.Dose-Proportionate Formulation with Different Test and Standard Concentration
50.Same analytical method for different dosage forms
51.Cross Specificity in Case of Combination Drug Products
52.Placebo for Residual Solvents
53.A Precise Method May Not Be Accurate
54.Understanding QL Requirement as per ICH Q3A and Q3B

1.Accuracy at QL for Impurity in Drug Product with High Impurity Content:

Performing accuracy at the quantitation limit (QL) can be particularly challenging when the sample already contains a high level of the impurity. For example, consider a case where the drug product sample contains 0.50% of impurity A, while the QL for impurity A is established at 0.02%. In such a situation, any small variation such as a spiked recovery resulting in 0.48% or 0.52% would be well within the acceptable range of variability at the 0.50% level.

However, this 0.02% change actually represents a 100% difference at the QL level, making it impossible to meaningfully assess recovery or accuracy at such a low concentration.

The recommended approach in such cases is to use an API batch containing impurity A near the QL level, and then spike impurity A into a placebo + API matrix to simulate the sample for recovery studies. However, if such API batch is not available, an alternative strategy is to dilute the drug product sample in such a way that the absolute concentration of impurity A matches the QL level (in terms of µg/mL or ppm). The impurity A standard can then be spiked at the QL level, and recovery can be assessed with better sensitivity and meaning.

Here's an example to illustrate how you can dilute a drug product sample to bring impurity A concentration close to the QL (0.04%) for an accurate recovery study. Let's say the test concentration is 1000 ppm of the active ingredient. The impurity A level in the sample is 0.5%, which means its concentration in test is: 1000 ppm×0.5/100=5 ppm

Now, assume the Limit of Quantitation (LOQ) for impurity A is 0.04%, which corresponds to:

1000 ppm×0.04/100=0.4 ppm impurity A in test sample.

To bring impurity A content in test close to the LOQ level (0.4ppm), the test solution should be diluted by a factor of 10: 5 ppm÷10=0.5 ppm

This brings impurity A very close to the LOQ (0.4 ppm), allowing you to spike the diluted sample at the QL and assess recovery more accurately.

2.Precision at QL in Presence of High Impurity Levels:

Similar to the challenge faced in accuracy assessment, establishing precision at the QL becomes difficult when the drug product already contains impurity levels significantly above the QL. For example, if impurity A is present at 0.50% and its QL is 0.02%, the sample cannot be used directly to demonstrate precision at the QL level.

To overcome this, the preferred approach is to use an API batch with impurity A content near the QL, and prepare a placebo-spiked matrix for precision study. However, if such API batch is not available, the sample can be diluted to reduce the absolute concentration of impurity A to the QL level. This diluted samples can then be used to perform precision at QL.

3.Lower Mass Balance Observed During Forced Degradation in Related Substances Study:

This is one of the common challenges encountered with mass balance assessment. While there is no official acceptance criterion defined for mass balance, a range of 95.0% to 105.0% is widely accepted in practice. However, in some instances, mass balance values lower than 95.0% may be observed. What could be the potential reasons for such lower mass balance?

i.Degradant with lower response:

This is one of the potential reasons for mass balance failure during forced degradation studies.

When a degradation product has a lower detector response compared to the API, it results in underestimation of its actual content. For example, if a degradant has half the response of the API and is present at 10%, it may be reported as only 5%, due to the lower response factor. This leads to an apparent loss of 5% mass, thereby reducing the overall mass balance.

The way forward in such situations is to determine the response factor or relative response factor (RRF) for the degradant. To achieve this, the degradation product should be isolated using preparative HPLC or synthesized, and then purified to the desired level. Once purified, the RRF can be established by comparing its detector response to that of the API. After determining the RRF, the mass balance should be recalculated using the corrected values. For routine stability or release testing, it may become necessary to identify major degradants and establish their respective RRFs, especially when they significantly impact mass balance results.

ii.Loss of Degradation Products During Forced Degradation Studies:

Another possible reason for lower mass balance is the loss of degradation products during forced degradation (FD) treatment. Certain degradation products may be volatile, and if the degradation involves high-temperature conditions, these volatiles may evaporate and escape, resulting in a loss of measurable content. In other cases, the degradation product may be insoluble in the diluent system used for sample preparation. This can lead to precipitation and separation during sample handling, making it unavailable for chromatographic analysis.

Such losses during the FD process lead to underestimation of degradants, thereby contributing to lower mass balance. The way forward in such situations is to avoid open high-temperature treatments or to carry out thermal degradation under closed conditions, using condensation or sealed systems, so that volatile degradants are retained.

For insoluble or precipitating degradants, the loss is often harder to detect. In such cases, it is recommended to explore solvents with varying polarity or strength to dissolve the degradation products effectively. Additionally, this challenge may necessitate a discussion on the adequacy of the sample diluent system, especially if insoluble degradants are observed during stability studies. If such degradants are identified as part of the product's degradation profile, a revision of the diluent composition may be required to ensure consistent recovery and accurate mass balance throughout the product's shelf life.

iii.Degradation Product Eluting Beyond the Specified Chromatographic Run Time:

This is another common and often overlooked reason for the loss of degradants during forced degradation studies. If the chromatographic run time is insufficient, and a degradation product elutes after the final programmed time point, the analyst may miss detecting and quantifying it. As a result, the impurity content appears lower than it actually is, leading to an artificially low mass balance.

The way forward is to ensure that the chromatographic run time is adequately extended, allowing complete elution of late-eluting degradants. This helps in capturing and quantifying any previously missed impurities and improves the accuracy of mass balance calculations. Method development and forced degradation protocols should always be designed to cover sufficient runtime beyond the last known peak.

iv. Degradant Eluting in the Void Volume:

A degradation product that elutes in or near the void volume of the chromatographic run may go undetected or remain unquantified, especially if it overlaps with system peaks or baseline noise. Such non-retained degradants are often missed, leading to underestimation of impurity content and resulting in a lower mass balance.

The way forward is to carefully examine the chromatograms of both the blank and degradation samples, paying close attention to the void volume region. If a peak or abnormal response is observed near the void, the sample should be re-analyzed using a modified method with a weaker mobile phase composition, allowing the degradant to retain longer on the column and improve its peak shape and detectability. If the degradant is later confirmed in stability samples, the test procedure should be revised accordingly to enhance its retention and ensure reliable quantification in routine analysis.

v.Loss of Degradant Due to Poor Extraction or Adsorption onto Excipients:

Another potential cause of lower mass balance is the incomplete extraction of degradation products during sample preparation. This can occur if the degradant is either poorly soluble in the diluent or adsorbs onto excipients, leading to partial or total loss during sample processing.

To address this issue, various extraction techniques such as shaking, vortexing, or sonication should be explored to determine the most effective condition for maximizing the recovery of the degradant. In addition, it is important to evaluate different diluents, including variations in organic solvent content or buffer pH, to identify the most suitable extraction medium for the specific degradation profile.

However, if the optimal extraction conditions or diluent system differ from those used in the proposed analytical method, the method parameters must be revised and revalidated accordingly. This ensures that when the degradant appears particularly during stability studies it is adequately extracted and reliably quantified, thereby improving the overall accuracy of the mass balance assessment

vi.Degradant Co-eluting with API:

Although less common, the possibility of a degradant co-eluting with the API cannot be ruled out, and it can contribute to loss of mass balance. When a degradant elutes at the same retention time as the API, it may remain undetected as a separate peak, leading to underestimation of the total degradant content.

To identify such cases, especially when using HPLC with UV detection, it is advisable to compare the UV spectra of the API standard with that of the degradation sample. If the spectra differ, it may indicate spectral merging due to co-elution. This suggests that an impurity is present under the API peak, compromising both specificity and mass balance accuracy.

In such cases, it is essential to re-optimize the chromatographic conditions with the goal of separating the degradant from the API. This may involve changes in mobile phase composition, gradient program, pH, or column chemistry. A new or revised analytical method should then be proposed and validated to ensure that all degradants, including those previously hidden under the API peak, are properly resolved and quantified.

vii.API Adduct Formation with Low Response:

Similar to degradants, if the forced degradation conditions lead to the formation of an adduct of the API and the resulting adduct exhibits a poor detector response it may go underreported or undetected, thereby contributing to lower mass balance. These adducts can form through interaction with stress agents, excipients, or solvents under degradation conditions, and their low response can cause them to appear in smaller quantities than they actually are.

In such cases, the approach is similar to that described in Point i: efforts should be made to isolate or synthesize the adduct, determine its relative response factor (RRF), and use this correction to recalculate the mass balance accurately.

viii.Poor Peak Height and Broad Peak Shape for Late-Eluting Impurities:

In chromatographic analysis, late-eluting impurities often suffer from broad peak shapes, tailing, and reduced peak height. These poorly resolved peaks may blend into the baseline or fall below the reporting threshold, resulting in missed quantification and ultimately contributing to a lower mass balance.

To address this, analysts should carefully inspect the baseline, especially toward the end of the chromatographic run, for low-height, wide peaks that may represent significant degradants. Additionally, chromatographic conditions should be optimized to improve retention, resolution, and peak symmetry for these late-eluting species. This may include modifications to the mobile phase composition, gradient slope, column type, or flow rate to enhance detectability and quantification.

ix.Degradants with No Detector Response:

In some cases, degradation products may not respond to the detector used in the original related substances (RS) method particularly if the method relies on UV detection and the degradant lacks a chromophore. As a result, such degradants remain undetected and unquantified, contributing to an unexplained loss in mass balance.

If this situation is suspected, the sample should be analyzed using a universal detection technique, such as Refractive Index (RI) detection, Evaporative Light Scattering Detection (ELSD), or Charged Aerosol Detection (CAD). These techniques can help identify non-chromophoric compounds that elude UV-based methods. Once the pres]nce of such a degradant is confirmed, it may be necessary to develop or supplement the existing method using an alternative detector to enable accurate quantification and mass balance correction.

x.Degradants Present Below the Detection or Quantitation Limit:

Consider a scenario where multiple degradants, each present at 0.03%,]are formed during forced degradation. If the quantitation limit (QL) of the method is 0.05%, none of these degradants will be reported individually, despite their collective contribution being significant. As a result, a substantial portion of degradation products may go undetected, leading to a notably lower mass balance.

To avoid such outcomes, it is essential to develop a related substances method with optimum sensitivity, ensuring that even low-level degradants can be reliably detected and quantified. Additionally, care should be taken to avoid excessively harsh degradation conditions, which can lead to the formation of numerous low-level degradants, complicating analysis and increasing the risk of under-reporting. A balanced approach to forced degradation, combined with a method that offers sufficient sensitivity, will help ensure more accurate impurity profiling and improved mass balance recovery.

xi. Degradants Detectable Only by Alternate Analytical Methods:

In some cases, a specific impurity or degradant may not be detected, retained, or quantified under the conditions of the primary related substances method, due to poor UV absorbance, lack of retention, or incompatibility with the detector used (e.g., UV detection). If such an impurity is known and routinely analyzed using an alternative method (e.g., HPLC-ELSD, CAD, or MS-based method), it will not be accounted for in the forced degradation study conducted with the primary HPLC-UV method. This results in an underreporting of the total impurity content and may contribute to lower mass balance.

To avoid this oversight, it is important to identify such impurities in advance, especially if they are known to form under stress conditions. The same forced degradation samples should be analyzed using the alternative method validated for that specific impurity. For example, if impurity A is quantified using an HPLC-ELSD method due to poor UV response, then the forced degradation samples generated for HPLC-UV should also be run on the ELSD method to ensure impurity A is captured in the overall degradation profile. This ensures a more comprehensive and accurate mass balance assessment.

xii. Degradants Formed as Volatile or Solvent-Type Compounds:

In some degradation pathways, the API may break down into volatile degradants, such as solvent-type by-products. A classic example is the hydrolysis of Aspirin, which yields salicylic acid (UV-active) and acetic acid. While the related substances method may successfully detect and quantify salicylic acid, acetic acid may go undetected, especially if the method is based on HPLC-UV detection. This results in an underestimation of total degradants and contributes to lower mass balance.

In such cases, it is critical to identify the possibility of solvent-type degradant formation during method development or forced degradation planning. These components should be measured using a suitable complementary method, such as GC with headspace. Once quantified, these components should be factored into the overall mass balance calculation to provide a complete picture of the degradation pathway.

4.Higher Mass Balance During Forced Degradation in Related Substances Study:

While lower mass balance is more commonly discussed, there are also instances where the mass balance exceeds 100% during forced degradation studies. This can raise concerns about analytical accuracy, method reliability, or system-related interferences. A higher-than-expected mass balance typically indicates that more impurity content is being reported than what is actually degraded, suggesting potential overestimation of degradation products or misinterpretation of analytical signals. Some of the key reasons for higher mass balance during forced degradation in related substances testing include:

i.Degradant with Higher Detector Response:

One of the potential reasons for observing higher mass balance during forced degradation is when a degradation product exhibits a higher detector response than the API. In such cases, even though the actual amount of degradant formed may be low, its strong detector response leads to an overestimation of its content, thereby pushing the overall mass balance beyond 100%.

The way forward in such situations is to identify the response factor or relative response factor (RRF) of the degradant in comparison to the API. Once the RRF is established either through isolation, synthesis, or by using a structurally similar standard the impurity quantification can be corrected using the RRF, and the mass balance recalculated accordingly.

ii.Loss of API During Forced Degradation Study:

A loss of API during forced degradation can lead to a false appearance of higher mass balance, especially when degradants are reported using area normalization or % area approach. If the API undergoes precipitation, adsorption, or volatilization during the stress treatment, its detector response may decrease significantly. As a result, the relative percentage of degradants appears artificially high, even if their absolute quantity remains unchanged.

The way forward is to compare the detector response of the API in the untreated (as such) sample and the forced degradation sample. If a noticeable reduction in API response is observed, it may indicate API loss due to solubility issues, chemical degradation, or volatility under the applied stress conditions. In such cases, it is advisable to modify the diluent system or degradation conditions to prevent the loss ensuring the API remains solubilized and stable enough for accurate quantification. This correction helps restore a more accurate mass balance calculation.

iii.API Adduct with Higher Detector Response:

Similar to degradants, API adducts formed during forced degradation may exhibit a higher detector response than the API itself. These adducts can form through interactions with excipients, degradation agents, or solvents under stress conditions. If such an adduct is not accounted for with its correct response factor, it may lead to an overestimation of impurity content and result in a mass balance exceeding 100%.

In this situation, the approach is similar to what is described in Point i: the relative response factor (RRF) of the adduct should be determined by isolating or synthesizing the adduct and comparing its detector response to the API. Once the RRF is established, it should be applied to correct the quantification, and the mass balance should be recalculated accordingly to reflect the true degradation profile.

iv.Leachables and Extractables from the Container Closure System:

Although relatively uncommon, leachables and extractables from the container-closure system used during forced degradation studies can sometimes contribute to artificially elevated impurity levels, resulting in a higher mass balance. These foreign components may be extracted from plasticware, rubber stoppers, or sample containers, especially when harsh degradation reagents or elevated temperatures are used. Such extractables can appear as additional peaks in the chromatogram, mistakenly counted as degradation products.

To avoid this, it is recommended to use recently prepared samples and avoid storing them in containers for extended periods, particularly under stress conditions. Glassware should be preferred over plastic, as plastic materials are more prone to leaching additives or stabilizers. Additionally, harsh reagents that could extract leachables from the container should be either avoided or substituted with milder alternatives when possible. Proper controls (blank container and reagent runs) should also be included to help identify and exclude such contributions from the impurity profile.

v.Degradants Originating from the Sample Matrix (Non-API Components):

Related substances methods are primarily designed to detect degradation products related to the API or drug substance. However, during forced degradation, excipients or other components of the sample matrix may also degrade under stress conditions. If these degradation products are detectable by the selected detection technique (e.g., UV, ELSD, CAD), they may appear as additional peaks in the chromatogram and be mistakenly attributed to the API, leading to an inflated impurity profile and higher mass balance.

To avoid such misinterpretation, it is essential to subject the placebo or excipient matrix to the same forced degradation conditions. This allows for the identification of any degradation products arising from the matrix itself. Such degradants, once confirmed to originate from excipients and not the API, should be excluded from the mass balance calculation. This distinction ensures that the degradation profile accurately reflects API-related changes, maintaining the scientific integrity of the study.

vi.Water Loss During Dry Thermal Treatment:

During thermal degradation studies such as treating a crushed tablet powder at 105°C there is often a significant loss of water content from the sample. This water loss reduces the overall sample weight; for instance, if 10% of the sample is moisture, heating will lead to a 10% reduction in weight. If this water loss is not accounted for and the sample is weighed as per the standard test procedure (without adjustment), you may unintentionally use 10% more active pharmaceutical ingredient (API) than intended. This happens because the sample, post-thermal treatment, is now drier and more concentrated in API. As a result, the assay value may appear falsely elevated, and the mass balance can exceed expected limits. To prevent such discrepancies, either perform the thermal treatment after weighing the exact required amount of sample, or apply a correction factor to the assay result to compensate for the loss of water.

5.Failure in peak purity during specificity:

Peak purity is one of the essential evaluations to define the absence co-elution or spectral purity. Peak purity assessment is possible with UV detector and can be a surrogate of spectral peak purity. Peak purity helps to assess specificity/selectivity or interference.

i.Co-elution of impurities:

Co-elution of impurities is a common challenge in peak purity assessment, especially when two or more compounds elute very closely or overlap. This can lead to false assumptions about purity. The way forward is to enhance chromatographic resolution by optimizing parameters such as mobile phase composition, pH, column selection, and gradient. Additionally, orthogonal methods like LC-MS or changing the column chemistry can help confirm the presence or absence of co-eluting components.

ii.Similar UV absorbance spectra among related compounds or isomers:

Similar UV absorbance spectra among related compounds or isomers can mislead the purity check, as a DAD may not differentiate between them. To overcome this, it's advisable to use complementary detection techniques such as LC-MS, apply derivatization methods where applicable, or test separation using alternative columns with different selectivity to ensure adequate resolution of such closely related substances.

iii.Low-level impurities below the detection:

Low-level impurities below the detection capability of a UV detector (typically <0.1–0.2%) pose a risk of undetected contamination. The solution is to conduct spiking studies to determine the detection capability, optimize the wavelength to increase response, or use more sensitive detectors such as MS or ELSD, especially during development and validation stages.

iv.Misinterpretation of peak purity results:

Misinterpretation of peak purity results from software tools like purity angle and purity threshold is another challenge, often due to lack of understanding of how these parameters are calculated. The best approach is to train analysts thoroughly, manually compare spectral overlays at different parts of the peak (start, apex, end), and treat borderline purity results with caution by confirming them using alternative methods.

v.Baseline noise and peak tailing:

Baseline noise and peak tailing can interfere with spectral clarity and lead to incorrect purity conclusions. This issue can be resolved by improving sample preparation, degassing the mobile phase properly, maintaining the HPLC system to reduce baseline drift, and optimizing the method to produce sharp, symmetrical peaks.

vi.Incorrect selection of baseline start and end points:

Incorrect selection of baseline start and end points during peak purity assessment is a critical challenge, especially in DAD systems where the purity threshold is influenced by baseline noise. If a segment of the chromatogram with high noise is chosen as the baseline region, the calculated purity threshold becomes artificially high, which may lead to a false pass of an impure peak. Conversely, if a very low-noise segment is selected, the threshold may be too stringent, causing a false fail of a pure peak. The way forward is to carefully select representative baseline regions on either side of the peak that reflect normal system noise levels neither overly noisy nor artificially flat and ensure that the baseline is stable, away from interfering peaks or drift. Training analysts to understand the impact of these selections and cross-verifying with manual spectral overlay can significantly improve the reliability of the assessment.

vii.False pass in cases of exact or near-exact coelution:

False pass in cases of exact or near-exact coelution is a serious limitation of DAD-based peak purity assessment. When two compounds coelute perfectly and have nearly identical UV spectra, the purity tool may still indicate the peak is pure because spectral differences are minimal or undetectable. This creates a false sense of security, especially in the case of critical quality attributes like related substances. The way forward is to recognize the limitations of DAD for such scenarios and never rely solely on peak purity results. Instead, use orthogonal techniques such as LC-MS to detect coelution at a molecular level, perform spiking studies to intentionally introduce known impurities, and always validate separation robustness during method development. A visually good peak with a "pass" purity result does not guarantee chemical purity spectral similarity is not chemical identity.

viii.False failure of peak purity due to photometric effects:

False failure of peak purity due to photometric effects is a known issue when peak height exceeds the optimal absorbance range of the detector, typically around 1.0 AU. At higher concentrations, especially when the peak apex absorbs beyond this level, the spectral shape may become slightly flattened or distorted due to non-linearity or detector saturation. This distortion causes the software to read the apex spectrum as different from that at the start or end of the peak, resulting in a false purity failure despite the peak being truly pure. The practical way forward is to keep the peak height below 1.0 AU, which helps maintain spectral integrity. This can be achieved by diluting the sample, optimizing injection volume, or adjusting detector settings, ensuring the detector operates well within its linear response range for accurate spectral comparisons.

ix.Wrong Selection of Start and End Wavelength for Spectral Comparison:

Improper selection of the wavelength range used for spectral analysis in DAD can lead to inaccurate purity results. If the start wavelength falls within the UV cutoff range of the mobile phase (e.g., below 210 nm for ACN or below 220 nm for MeOH), high background absorbance or noise may distort the spectra. Similarly, if the end wavelength extends beyond the actual absorbance range of the compound (where it no longer absorbs), it can introduce irrelevant spectral data and reduce the reliability of comparison. The result can be either false passes or false failures in peak purity. So, always select the start wavelength above the UV cutoff of the mobile phase to avoid background interference. For the end wavelength, analyze the compound's absorbance spectrum carefully and stop just after the last significant absorbance peak avoiding flat, non-informative tail regions.

x. Baseline Drift Especially in Gradient Runs:

Baseline drift is a critical challenge in DAD-based peak purity assessment, particularly during gradient elution, where shifting solvent composition leads to gradual changes in baseline absorbance. The challenge becomes more significant when defining the baseline segments used for calculating the purity threshold a key metric in peak purity evaluation.

In the first scenario, if the peak elutes in a flat and stable baseline region, but the analyst mistakenly selects a drifted or noisy baseline segment (e.g., from earlier or later in the run), the calculated purity threshold becomes artificially high, potentially causing a false pass where co-eluting impurities go undetected.

In the second scenario, if the peak elutes on a drifted or sloped baseline, but the baseline for purity threshold calculation is selected from a very flat and clean region (e.g., pre-gradient section), the threshold becomes too low, increasing the chances of false failure where minor spectral variations within a pure peak are flagged unnecessarily.

The key is to select a representative baseline one that truly reflects the actual baseline behavior near the peak. It should not be artificially clean or excessively noisy, but rather consistent with the chromatographic environment at the time of peak elution. Choosing baseline points just before and after the peak within the same gradient composition zone improves the accuracy of purity threshold calculation. Supporting this with blank gradient injections can help visualize baseline behavior and guide better segment selection. Proper method development, gradient optimization, and system equilibration further minimize baseline variability and improve overall purity assessment reliability.

6. Unavailability of Test Sample (Drug Product) During Method Validation:

In some cases, especially during early development, the required quantity of drug product may not be available to complete all validation parameters such as accuracy, precision, linearity, and robustness. This shortage can slow down or delay the validation process. A practical solution is to use a matrix-based simulation, combining API with placebo to mimic the actual formulation. This helps in performing parameters like recovery, specificity, and matrix interference without consuming full drug product batches. Additionally, design combined validation sets for example, use the same dilution series for linearity, accuracy, and precision.

7.Impurity standard not available for impurity method validation:

A critical challenge arises when an impurity standard is not available at all meaning it has not yet been synthesized, isolated, or procured. This situation is common during early-stage development, in cases of unknown degradants, new process impurities, or impurities detected during stress studies. In such cases, performing key validation parameters specificity, precision, and accuracy becomes particularly difficult. The real challenge here lies in how to scientifically justify and perform these parameters without the actual impurity standard:

i.Specificity:

Specificity can still be established using forced degradation studies, where the impurity of interest appears under known stress conditions and is shown to be well separated from the main peak and other components. DAD-based peak purity or LC-MS can be used to confirm resolution.

ii.Precision& Accuracy:

Precision and Accuracy can be addressed using a spiking strategy with degraded samples. Prepare a co-blended or cocktail degradation sample by combining different stress condition samples (acid, base, oxidative, thermal, etc.) to ensure the presence of all possible degradants in one solution. Then, spike this cocktail sample into an undegraded matrix (API or placebo) at target impurity levels. This composite sample mimics a worst-case scenario and can be used to perform repeatability (precision) by analyzing multiple replicates and calculating %RSD of the impurity peak(s). Perform recovery (accuracy) by comparing spiked vs. unspiked samples and evaluating the added impurity response.

This method enables validation to proceed without delay while staying within a scientifically sound and risk-based framework. Be sure to clearly document the approach, limitations, and commitment to complete full validation when the impurity standard becomes available.

8.Very Limited Quantity of Impurity Standards:

One of the common and practical challenges encountered during impurity method validation is the very limited availability of impurity standards. This issue is especially relevant during early phases of development, when impurity reference materials are either newly synthesized, in small amounts, or extremely expensive. In such cases, performing a full-scale validation with independent sets of samples for accuracy, precision, linearity, and system suitability can quickly exhaust the available quantity.

A smart and scientifically sound approach to tackle this challenge is to draw multiple validation parameters from a single set of samples. One of the most effective strategies is to design the accuracy study in such a way that it simultaneously supports linearity and precision. For instance, the five or six concentration levels used for spiking during the accuracy study (e.g., QL, 50%, 100%, 125%, and 150% of impurity specification limit) can also be used to construct the calibration curve for linearity. By injecting replicates at key levels (especially 100%), the same dataset can also provide repeatability (precision) data.

To further conserve material, minimizing the number of dilution steps is critical. Start by preparing a high-concentration stock solution of the impurity standard and dilute it just enough to reach the target working concentrations. This reduces wastage and ensures maximum utilization of the available impurity.

Another efficient approach is to perform validation on two chromatographic systems, ideally involving two different analysts to address intermediate precision requirements. In this scenario, both analysts can use the same stock solution of the impurity standard but should prepare their working dilutions independently. This introduces variability due to analyst technique while conserving the impurity stock. Such an approach satisfies regulatory expectations related to intermediate precision including variation due to analysts, instruments, and possibly columns without duplicating the consumption of limited resources.

Where applicable, reuse prepared samples for system suitability, or robustness provided the sample stability is established. This ensures that the limited quantity of impurity standards is used judiciously, while still achieving scientifically valid and regulatorily acceptable validation outcomes.

9. Theoretical DL/QL Too Low for Practical Use:

In impurity method validation, it is common to calculate the Limit of Detection (DL) and Limit of Quantitation (QL) using theoretical approaches such as the signal-to-noise ratio (S/N = 3:1 for QL and 10:1 for QL) or the standard deviation of response and slope method (using the ICH Q2 formula: $3.3\times\sigma/S$ for DL and $10\times\sigma/S$ for QL). However, in many practical situations, these theoretically calculated values turn out to be too low to generate consistent, reliable results in real-world conditions.

This becomes particularly problematic in impurity methods, where trace-level quantification is required. When DL/QL solutions are prepared in pure diluent, the background noise is artificially low, and signal-to-noise ratios may appear acceptable. However, this does not account for matrix effects such as baseline drift, interference from excipients, or system noise in real samples. As a result, the method may appear sensitive on paper but fail precision and accuracy criteria when tested with actual formulation samples.

To overcome this, it is essential to prepare DL and QL solutions by spiking impurities into placebo, rather than using diluent alone. This mimics the real sample matrix and provides a more realistic picture of method performance. The spiked placebo solution should then be used to determine signal-to-noise ratio or to calculate slope and standard deviation for the statistical approach. This ensures that matrix-related variability is accounted for during method sensitivity determination.

Furthermore, the calculated QL must always be verified experimentally. Inject six replicates at the proposed QL concentration (in matrix), and assess both precision (RSD%) and accuracy (recovery). If these do not meet acceptance criteria, then the QL should be adjusted upward to the level at which acceptable results are obtained. This practical QL becomes the validated reporting threshold. Please note that the QL shall be equal to or less than reporting threshold (refer ICH guideline Q3A for drug substance and Q3B for drug product).

10.Challenges in Performing Forced Degradation Studies for Combination Products:

Forced degradation (FD) studies are essential for understanding the stability profile of pharmaceutical products. However, when it comes to combination products containing two or more active pharmaceutical ingredients (APIs), the complexity of degradation studies increases significantly. These formulations often present unique analytical and interpretational challenges, owing to the interactions between APIs, excipients, and degradation pathways.

Below are the key challenges commonly encountered during FD studies for combination products, along with strategies to address them effectively:

i.Overlapping Degradation Profiles:

In combination products, multiple APIs and their respective degradation products may elute at similar retention times, leading to peak overlap and difficulties in distinguishing individual degradants. This challenge complicates both identification and quantification. The possible way forward is to develop chromatographic methods with enhanced resolution, possibly using gradient optimization, column chemistry variation, or orthogonal techniques like LC-MS or UV spectral overlay to differentiate co-eluting peaks.

ii.Differential Degradation Behavior:

Each API may respond differently to stress conditions. For example, one API may be sensitive to acidic hydrolysis, while the other degrades under oxidative conditions. Applying a single stress condition may fail to degrade all components adequately. The possible way forward is to perform individual FD studies for each API first to establish their unique degradation behavior. Then, conduct combined FD studies to observe any potential interactions. This staged approach ensures comprehensive coverage.

iii.API–API and API–Excipient Interactions:

In the presence of other APIs or excipients, an API may degrade differently than it would alone. These interactions can lead to novel degradation products that may not appear in as such API degradation studies. The possible way forward is to include FD studies on placebo formulations and individual APIs to distinguish degradation patterns unique to the combination. Carefully evaluate any new or unknown degradants through structural characterization.

iv.Analytical Method Development Complexity:

Designing a single analytical method that is selective, sensitive, and robust enough to monitor multiple APIs and all possible degradants is inherently difficult. Some APIs may require different detection techniques or mobile phases for optimal analysis. Hence consider using multi-detector approaches (UV, ELSD, CAD, MS) or validate multiple analytical methods if a single method is insufficient.

Ensure that each API and its degradants are appropriately monitored under validated conditions.

v.Solubility and Diluent Challenges:

Finding a common diluent that provides adequate solubility for all APIs and their degradants can be problematic. Poor solubility may result in incomplete extraction and reduced recoveries. Optimize the diluent composition based on solubility studies for each API and expected degradants. Ensure the selected diluent system provides effective extraction and compatibility without interfering with peak shapes or detector response.

vi.Complexity in Mass Balance Interpretation:

In a combination product, mass balance calculations become more complicated due to the presence of multiple APIs, their degradants, and potential cross-reactivity. This may lead to unclear or misleading conclusions during mass balance assessment. Calculate and interpret mass balance individually for each API. Utilize peak purity analysis, MS characterization, and placebo subtraction to accurately assign peaks and ensure comprehensive profiling.

vii.Regulatory Expectations and Documentation:

Regulatory agencies expect a detailed understanding of the degradation pathways for each API both individually and in combination. This includes degradant identification, method suitability, and stability data. So, design FD studies with scientific justification, covering all relevant stress conditions for each API. Document all observations, decisions, and deviations thoroughly. Where necessary, consult regulatory guidelines (e.g., ICH) and provide risk-based reasoning.

11.Non-Homogeneous Drug Product Samples:

One of the critical prerequisites for successful method validation is the use of a homogeneous drug product sample. If the sample is non-homogeneous due to poor mixing, stratification of API, or uneven distribution of excipients it can lead to significant variability in test results. This directly impacts the ability to demonstrate precision and accuracy, as replicate preparations may not truly represent the same sample composition. To ensure meaningful and reproducible validation outcomes, it is essential to confirm sample uniformity before initiating analytical testing. Adequate mixing, blending, or dispersion techniques must be applied based on the dosage form. For complex matrices such as suspensions, semisolids, or multi-layer tablets, special care must be taken during sampling and preparation. The use of validated sampling and homogenization procedures becomes critical to ensure that the analytical method is being evaluated on a representative and reproducible sample.

12.Impurity Supplied in Salt Form vs. Non-Salt Form in Sample:

Another critical consideration during impurity quantification is the form of the impurity standard used for method validation or routine analysis. In some cases, the impurity is supplied as a salt form (e.g., hydrochloride, sodium salt), while in the actual drug product or degradation pathway, the impurity is present in its free base or non-salt form. If this difference is not accounted for, it can lead to incorrect estimation of impurity content due to the difference in molecular weight between the salt and non-salt forms.

To ensure accurate quantification, it is essential to apply a molecular weight correction factor when weighing and preparing impurity standards. This correction ensures that the calculated concentration reflects the free form of the impurity the form that exists in the actual sample. Failing to do so can compromise the accuracy of results and impact the interpretation of both method validation and routine release data.

13.Consideration of Impurity Purity During Impurity Solution Preparation:

When preparing solutions of impurities for method validation (e.g. linearity), it is essential to account for the actual purity of the impurity reference standard. Impurities are often supplied with less than 100% purity due to the presence of residual solvents, moisture, or other unidentified components. If this is not considered during weighing, the final concentration of the solution will be lower than intended, leading to inaccurate quantification.

For instance, if Impurity A has a reported purity of 90%, and the goal is to prepare a 100 ppm solution, then simply weighing 10 mg and diluting to 100 mL will result in only 90 ppm of the active impurity. To achieve the desired 100 ppm concentration, the weighed quantity must be adjusted for purity, i.e., Required weight = (100 ppm × 100 mL) ÷ 0.90 = 11.11 mg. Therefore, when preparing impurity solutions, always correct for the purity.

14.Unverified Stability of Analytical Solutions:

The stability of test and standard solutions plays a critical role in ensuring the reliability of analytical results, particularly during long analytical runs or method validation sequences. If a solution degrades, precipitates, or undergoes chemical change over time, it can significantly affect the accuracy and precision of the results potentially leading to incorrect conclusions about method performance.

Before planning long-duration sequences such as those required for precision, linearity, robustness, or batch analysis it is essential to verify the solution stability under intended storage and usage conditions. This includes assessing stability at room temperature, under autosampler conditions, and over the expected run time. If the solution is found to be unstable, it may become a limiting factor in evaluating the parameter under study.

15.Alignment of Instrument Operating Ranges with Method Requirements:

Before initiating method validation particularly for parameters such as robustness it is essential to ensure that the operating ranges of the analytical instruments are fully aligned with the test procedure requirements. A mismatch between the method's defined operating conditions and the instrument's qualified range can compromise the validity of the study and may result in non-compliance.

For example, consider a gas chromatography (GC) method where robustness testing involves varying the oven temperature between 30°C and 40°C. If the GC system is only qualified down to 40°C, it would not be appropriate to operate it at 30°C without first extending the qualification range. Conducting robustness testing outside the instrument's qualified range introduces an unverified variable, rendering the data scientifically and regulatory questionable.

To address this, a gap assessment should be performed during method planning. If such discrepancies are identified, the instrument should be re-qualified or calibrated to include the required range (e.g., calibrating the GC oven to operate reliably at 30°C) before proceeding with validation. This proactive step ensures that method validation is conducted within scientifically controlled and compliant conditions.

16.Validating an R&D-Developed Method in the QC Laboratory:

When a method developed in the Research and Development (R&D) laboratory is transferred to the Quality Control (QC) laboratory for validation, several important considerations must be addressed to ensure its suitability for routine use in a regulated environment. While R&D methods are often designed with flexibility and experimental needs in mind, QC laboratories require methods that are robust, rugged, and practically executable under routine conditions with strict adherence to SOPs and regulatory guidelines.

Before initiating validation, the QC team should conduct a thorough method review and feasibility assessment, ensuring that all critical parameters such as system suitability, sample preparation, diluent compatibility, injection volume, detection settings, and instrument capability are aligned with QC expectations. Often, minor optimizations or adjustments are required to make the method more robust and reproducible in a QC setting without altering its intended purpose.

It is also essential to confirm that all instruments and reagents in the QC lab are suitable and qualified to support the method as developed. Method performance characteristics such as precision, accuracy, robustness, and solution stability must be rigorously validated under real-time, real-use conditions. Furthermore, any gaps identified during the review (e.g., missing system suitability criteria, unclear integration parameters, or unverified sample stability) should be addressed collaboratively between R&D and QC before formal validation begins.

17.Preparation of Placebo: Manual vs. Processed:

The preparation of placebo plays a vital role in analytical method validation, especially when evaluating specificity, interference, and degradation behavior in formulations. Placebos can be prepared either as a manual blend of excipients or as a processed placebo manufactured using the same unit operations as the actual drug product (e.g., granulation, compression, coating). Each approach has its own implications and should be selected based on the objective of the study.

Manual placebo preparation involves physically mixing the excipients in their raw form without subjecting them to manufacturing processes. While this method is quick and convenient, it may not fully represent the physical or chemical state of the excipients as they exist in the finished product. Interactions formed during processing such as thermal degradation during drying or compression-related stress may be missed, leading to incomplete or misleading conclusions, especially in forced degradation or specificity studies.

In contrast, a processed placebo, manufactured through the same process as the final drug product (minus the API), more accurately simulates the true matrix environment. This approach is particularly valuable when evaluating matrix effects, potential degradation of excipients, or adsorption behavior, and is often preferred in stability studies and method validation for impurity profiling.

Therefore, while manual placebos may suffice for basic interference checks, processed placebos are recommended for studies requiring matrix simulation under actual processing conditions. The choice should be justified based on the risk level and intended analytical outcome, and clearly documented in the validation protocol or study design.

18.Use of Validated Spreadsheets or Chromatography Software for Result Calculation:

In modern pharmaceutical laboratories, the reliance on manual calculations for analytical results is discouraged due to the potential for human error, transcription mistakes, and lack of traceability. Instead, the use of validated calculation tools such as custom field functions in chromatography data systems like Empower or Chromeleon, or validated Excel spreadsheets is strongly recommended for method validation and routine analysis.

Custom field programming within chromatography software enables automated, consistent, and traceable calculations directly linked to the raw data, such as peak areas, retention times, weight, response factors, or impurity percentages. These systems also support audit trails, version control, and electronic signatures, making them fully compliant with data integrity and regulatory requirements (e.g., 21 CFR Part 11, ALCOA+ principles).

When chromatography software is not equipped to handle specific calculations,validated Excel spreadsheets can be used as an alternative provided they are version-controlled, locked for editing, and tested for accuracy and robustness. These spreadsheets must undergo documented validation, including verification of formulas, data protection, and change control.

By transitioning from manual to validated electronic calculation systems, laboratories not only improve efficiency and reduce error rates but also ensure regulatory compliance, audit readiness, and data integrity critical components in pharmaceutical quality systems.

19.Inaccurate or Poorly Designed Validation Protocol:

An inaccurate or poorly constructed validation protocol can compromise the entire validation exercise, leading to ambiguous results, incomplete data, and regulatory non-compliance. Common issues include incorrect parameter definitions, unrealistic acceptance criteria, missing system suitability criteria, or mismatched experimental design. Such protocols may cause confusion during execution and hinder data interpretation.

To ensure scientific and regulatory robustness, validation protocols must be technically accurate, clearly written, and thoroughly reviewed by cross-functional teams before approval. Any errors or inconsistencies should be identified and resolved prior to execution. A well-prepared protocol ensures that the study meets its objectives and withstands scrutiny during internal or external audits.

20. Untrained Analyst in Method Validation:

Assigning an untrained analyst for method validation poses a significant risk to data integrity, scientific accuracy, and regulatory compliance. Validation requires more than just routine analytical skills it demands a thorough understanding of each parameter, precise execution, and strict adherence to documentation standards.

Errors such as incorrect sample preparation, poor system suitability handling, or incomplete records are common when analysts lack proper training, and may invalidate the entire study. Therefore, only trained and qualified personnel familiar with the method, technique, and validation protocol should perform validation. Validation is not a training exercise; it is a critical quality activity that must be handled with technical rigor and accountability.

21. Incomplete Method Transfer Documentation:

When a method is transferred from R&D to QC, incomplete documentation such as missing chromatograms, undefined system suitability criteria, or unclear integration settings can lead to confusion during execution and impact the success of validation. The way forward is to ensure the method is accompanied by a comprehensive transfer package, including all essential parameters, representative chromatograms, and a joint review meeting between R&D and QC teams to ensure clarity and alignment before validation begins.

22. Unjustified Stress Conditions in Forced Degradation:

Forced degradation conditions are sometimes selected without considering the chemical nature of the API, leading to either insufficient or excessive degradation, which in turn results in a poor representation of the molecule's degradation pathways. This can affect the reliability of the stability-indicating method and may fail to uncover relevant degradants. The way forward is to design stress studies based on the functional groups present in the API and the formulation matrix, ensuring that each condition whether acidic, basic, oxidative, photolytic, or thermal is scientifically justified. The goal should be to achieve meaningful degradation (typically 5–20%) that allows for the identification and resolution of degradants, thereby confirming the method's capability to indicate stability under real-time conditions. However, in some cases, an API may inherently resist degradation even under harsh conditions, and that is scientifically acceptable. In such instances, it should be clearly documented that the API does not undergo significant degradation under the applied stress conditions.

23. Variability in Chromatographic Columns:

Using different column lots or brands can introduce variability in retention times, resolution, and peak shape, potentially compromising method reproducibility and robustness. The way forward is to define minimum acceptable column characteristics in the method (e.g., L1, particle size, plate count) and qualify at least two column lots during method validation, maintaining a list of acceptable alternatives supported by equivalency data.

24. Impact of Uncontrolled Environmental Conditions:

Uncontrolled lab conditions such as high humidity or temperature fluctuations may impact sample integrity, peak shape, or system suitability, particularly for hygroscopic or thermally sensitive substances. The way forward is to perform validation under representative environmental conditions, monitor and control lab environments during runs, and define sample handling precautions to minimize environmental influence on results.

25. Undefined Integration Parameters:

Lack of defined integration settings can lead to inconsistent results across analysts, especially in impurity analysis where integration choices significantly impact quantification. The way forward is to document integration parameters within the chromatographic method and, where possible, lock the method in the software. If manual integration is permitted, establish clear rules and require justification with audit trail documentation.

26. Method Not Fit for Multi-Site Implementation:

Methods developed and validated at one site may not perform equivalently at another due to differences in instruments, columns, water quality, reagents, or analyst interpretation. The way forward is to conduct inter-lab transfer studies and qualify the method on representative instruments and setups across intended locations, ensuring robustness in diverse operating environments.

27. Rushed, Checklist-Driven Validation Approach:

Focusing solely on regulatory checklists without scientific understanding can result in superficial validations that miss critical risks. The way forward is to adopt a science- and risk-based approach, ensuring each parameter is justified by method criticality and product quality impact, and involving cross-functional teams in protocol development and review.

28. Inappropriate Selection of Validation Ranges:

One commonly overlooked challenge in method validation is the inappropriate selection of validation ranges, particularly when they do not fully cover the actual specification limits or potential variability of the product. For example, validating an assay method over a range of 80–120% may seem acceptable, but if the product specification allows assay between 90% to 110%, the 80% to 120% range fails to meet the range requirement as per ICH Q2(R2). So, select the range as per ICH Q2(R2).

29.Incomplete/Unsuitable Range for Immediate Release Product Dissolution Method:

Dissolution testing for immediate release (IR) products is widely recognized as a surrogate for in vivo bioavailability and is often used to justify biowaivers. Typically, even though the product specification may be defined at a single Q point such as NLT 75% at 30 minutes the dissolution study is conducted at multiple time points (e.g., 10, 15, 30, and 45 minutes) to capture the release profile and enable statistical comparisons such as similarity factor (f_2).

According to ICH Q2(R2), the lower end of the reportable range for dissolution should be defined as Q – 45%. For instance, if the Q point is 75%, the calculated lower limit becomes 30%. Many validations start their reportable range from this 30% value. However, this approach can be problematic in real-world multipoint dissolution studies.

If the dissolution at early time points such as 10 minutes yields values below 30% (e.g., 25%), the preselected range fails to cover the actual observed data. This misalignment compromises the validity of the method and may raise questions during regulatory assessment or biowaiver justification. Therefore, it is crucial to determine the lowest expected dissolution value based on actual multipoint data during method development and ensure the chosen validation range fully encompasses this value. Doing so enhances method robustness and ensures that it reflects real product behavior, especially in pivotal studies.

30.Wrong Concentration of Sample for Filter Saturation during Dissolution:

A frequently overlooked challenge during dissolution method validation is incorrect estimation of the filter saturation volume particularly when dealing with time-dependent sample concentrations in multipoint dissolution studies. Many commonly used filters, such as nylon, can adsorb a portion of the drug substance during sample filtration. This leads to an artificial reduction in the measured concentration of API in the filtrate, resulting in under-reported dissolution values.

To mitigate this, filter saturation studies are typically conducted to determine the minimum volume of test solution required to saturate the filter. Once the filter is saturated, further filtrate is expected to pass through without significant drug loss. However, a common error is conducting this study using only a single time point usually the Q-point like 30 minutes, where drug release is high (e.g., 80%). For such a time point, it might be determined that 3 mL of the solution is needed to saturate the filter.

But here's the critical flaw: the same dissolution method is often used for multipoint analysis, including earlier time points like 10 or 15 minutes. If the drug release at 10 minutes is only 40%, the concentration of drug in the test solution is half of that at 30 minutes. Consequently, the saturation volume should be adjusted accordingly potentially requiring 6 mL instead of 3 mL to achieve full saturation at the lower concentration.

If this adjustment is not made and only 3 mL is passed through the filter, some of the API may still be adsorbed, leading to falsely low values at early time points. This misrepresentation can affect critical parameters like similarity factor (f2) during pivotal bio-batch comparisons.

Therefore, it's essential that filter saturation studies are conducted using sample solutions representative of all relevant time points, especially the lowest expected drug concentrations. This ensures accuracy and consistency across the entire dissolution profile.

31.Response and Retention Time Variation Across Different HPLC Systems (During Intermediate Precision):

A common challenge observed during intermediate precision studies in HPLC is the variation in peak response (area) and retention time when analyses are performed on different HPLC systems even when using the same method, column type, and sample. These variations may arise due to several factors:

i.Differences in system dwell volume (gradient delay):

Each HPLC system has a unique dwell volume, which can affect gradient delivery timing and result in shifts in retention times particularly for gradient methods. (Way forward: Always compare system dwell volumes during method development and adjust gradient delay where needed.)

ii.Differences in detector lamp intensity or age:

Slight differences in UV lamp performance or alignment across systems can lead to changes in peak area. (Way forward: Use well-maintained and calibrated systems.)

iii.Pump calibration and flow accuracy:

Even minor deviations in actual vs. set flow rates or gradient formation can impact both response and retention time. (Way forward: Standardize critical system parameters and conditions as much as possible.)

iv.Column oven temperature control accuracy:

Inconsistent temperature control between systems may alter analyte interaction with the stationary phase, causing retention time shifts. (Way forward: Incorporate system suitability criteria with realistic limits considering inter-system variability.)

v.Tubing and connection dead volume:

Different internal diameters or extra dead volumes may lead to peak broadening or shifting. (Way forward: Include multiple systems in validation to demonstrate robustness.)

If not properly accounted for, such variations can exceed acceptable limits during intermediate precision, causing a method to fail validation. Recognizing and planning for such variability ensures the method is truly reproducible across different instruments and laboratories.

32.Inadequate Traceability for the Impurity Stock Used Across Validation Studies:

In analytical method validation, especially for impurity, it is common practice to prepare a single batch of impurity stock solution and use it across multiple validation parameters such as specificity, linearity, accuracy, and precision due to the limited quantity or high cost of impurity standards. However, a frequent oversight is the lack of proper traceability for these stock solutions.

If the impurity stock is used over several days or across different validation runs, but the preparation date, storage conditions, or expiry/retest period are not clearly documented, it becomes difficult to verify the reliability and stability of that stock. This can raise questions during regulatory inspections or audits regarding the integrity of the validation data. To ensure traceability and compliance:

i.Maintain a stock solution preparation log, clearly stating the impurity name, lot number, purity, weight taken, diluent used, final volume, concentration, date of preparation, and analyst initials.

ii.Include storage conditions and expiry/retest date as per impurity stability data or general guidance (e.g., ICH).

iii.Document the usage history, specifying for which validation parameters and on which dates the stock was used.

iv.If long-term use is expected, validate or verify the stability of the impurity stock solution under defined storage conditions.

Ensuring complete traceability of impurity stock solutions enhances the credibility of the validation study and supports data integrity throughout the method lifecycle.

33.Response Affected by pH Change:

In some cases, the UV response of a compound is highly sensitive to the pH of the diluent. The UV absorbance characteristics, including the intensity and wavelength of maximum absorbance, can vary significantly with changes in pH. This becomes particularly relevant when forced degradation studies are conducted under extreme pH conditions (acidic or alkaline), as these conditions may alter the ionization state of the analyte or its impurities, leading to different UV responses.

If such pH-induced shifts are not corrected before sample analysis, the resulting chromatograms may show altered peak responses potentially affecting impurity quantification and API assay. To avoid this discrepancy, it is recommended to adjust the pH of the sample solution back to the original diluent pH before injecting into the HPLC system. This ensures that all analytes are measured under consistent conditions, maintaining the accuracy and comparability of results.

34.Different Response Factor for Impurities:

When using a pharmacopoeial (monograph) method for related substances testing, the method may specify Relative Response Factors (RRFs) for known impurities. However, in practical execution, you may observe that the RRF values obtained in your laboratory differ from those reported in the monograph. This variation can arise due to several factors such as changes in baseline stability, retention time shifts, peak width differences, detector sensitivity, or column interactions.

Before relying entirely on the monograph RRF values, it is essential to verify a few critical aspects:

i.Confirm the chemical structure of the impurity you are using matches exactly with the one defined in the monograph.

ii.heck the purity of your impurity standard and apply it while measuring actual impurity concentration.

iii.Ensure the sample preparation, instrument settings, and system suitability align with the monograph conditions as closely as possible.

If, after all checks, the observed RRF still differs, it is scientifically appropriate and often necessary to use the RRF value determined in your own study.

35.Blank Interference Near LOD/LOQ:

In analytical method validation, sensitivity is often pushed to its limits particularly during the determination of the Limit of Detection (LOD) and Limit of Quantitation (LOQ). At such low concentration levels, even minor interferences from blank injections can significantly affect the accuracy and reliability of results. These interferences may manifest as ghost peaks, elevated baseline noise, or unexpected responses that mimic the analyte signal, making it difficult to distinguish true analyte presence from background contamination.

Such interference is typically caused by impurities in the diluent, mobile phase, or reagents used during sample preparation. Additionally, contamination can arise from glassware, plastic containers, or poorly cleaned autosampler components. In some cases, even atmospheric contaminants or degraded solvents can introduce unwanted signals that interfere with blank readings.

To minimize these risks, it is crucial to evaluate all components of the analytical setup. High-purity reagents and solvents should be used consistently, and all glassware and containers must be thoroughly cleaned and, if necessary, pre-rinsed with diluent or mobile phase. Regular blank injections should be performed to monitor baseline integrity and detect any recurring background signals. If the interference persists despite all preventive measures, one must consider revising the LOQ to a practically achievable level where accuracy and precision are not compromised.

In rare but justified cases, blank subtraction may be applied to correct for baseline interference. However, this approach should only be considered if it is scientifically sound, thoroughly validated, and clearly documented in the method protocol. Analysts must exercise caution, as improper blank subtraction can mask genuine analyte signals or artificially inflate results.

36.Ambiguity in Acceptance Criteria:

One of the subtle yet significant challenges in analytical method validation is the use of vague or poorly defined acceptance criteria in the validation protocol. When terms like "approximately," "close to," or "near to" are used instead of precise numerical targets or ranges, it introduces ambiguity—leaving results open to subjective interpretation and potentially undermining the credibility of the validation.

Clear and measurable acceptance criteria are essential not only for ensuring consistency in execution but also for withstanding regulatory scrutiny. Parameters such as %RSD for precision, resolution between peaks, recovery ranges for accuracy, or linearity correlation coefficients should always be defined with explicit numerical limits. For instance, instead of stating "recovery should be near 100%," it is more appropriate to specify "recovery should be between 98.0% and 102.0%."

To prevent such ambiguity, it is crucial to align acceptance criteria with recognized regulatory standards and pharmacopeial guidelines wherever applicable. During the protocol drafting stage, the analytical team should engage in discussions with Quality Assurance (QA) and Regulatory Affairs teams to review and finalize these ranges. This collaborative approach ensures that the criteria are scientifically justified, practically achievable, and fully compliant with current expectations.

37.Not Capturing Method Changes or Deviations:

One of the often-overlooked pitfalls in analytical method validation is the failure to properly capture method changes or deviations that occur during the course of the study. Whether it's a change in injection volume, a column replaced due to performance issues, or a minor modification in sample preparation, every alteration no matter how small can potentially impact the outcome of the validation.

Ignoring or informally handling such changes can lead to discrepancies in data interpretation and weaken the scientific and regulatory standing of the validation. Regulatory agencies place a high value on traceability, and the absence of documented change management is often flagged as a data integrity concern.

To prevent this, a robust Change Control system must be integrated into the Quality Management System (QMS). Any method change should be formally recorded, justified, and subjected to a scientific impact assessment to determine whether the change affects method performance or validation outcomes. Similarly, any deviation such as failing to meet system suitability criteria or unexpected sample behavior should be thoroughly investigated and supported with documented Corrective and Preventive Actions (CAPA).

Furthermore, both changes and deviations should be clearly referenced in the final validation report. This transparency not only reinforces the credibility of the validation but also ensures that future reviewers whether internal or regulatory have a complete view of how the method was validated, challenged, and confirmed.

38.Failing to Identify Critical Validation Gaps:

One of the root causes of incomplete or unsuccessful method validations is the failure to identify critical gaps before the validation begins. Often, teams move directly into execution without thoroughly assessing whether all prerequisites, controls, and risk factors have been adequately addressed. This oversight can lead to missed parameters, unrealistic acceptance criteria, or inadequate documentation resulting in rework, delays, or regulatory observations.

To avoid this, it is essential to conduct a comprehensive gap assessment before initiating the validation. This assessment should review historical data from development studies, previous method versions, and even similar molecules or dosage forms. Any prior regulatory feedback or inspection findings should also be considered, as they offer valuable insight into what auditors and reviewers expect.

A structured and QA-approved validation checklist should be used to verify that all necessary elements such as system suitability criteria, solution stability data, and appropriate robustness testing are in place. Additionally, engaging cross-functional teams from Quality Assurance (QA), Regulatory Affairs (RA), and Manufacturing ensures that the method is not only scientifically sound but also aligned with practical and regulatory expectations.

39.Incomplete Validation Protocol or Report:

Even a well-performed method validation can fall short if the protocol or report lacks completeness and clarity. Missing ICH parameters, vague conclusions, or poorly linked raw data can create confusion during audits and weaken the credibility of the entire study.

To address this, standardized templates for both protocols and reports should be used covering all ICH parameters, system suitability criteria, raw data summaries, and final conclusions. Including a protocol-to-report traceability matrix helps ensure that every planned activity is accounted for and consistently reported.

Maintaining consistent terminology and structure between the protocol and the report is equally important for clarity. Lastly, all documents must undergo a thorough QA review before finalization to confirm scientific accuracy and regulatory compliance. A complete and well-documented validation package not only strengthens data integrity but also ensures audit readiness.

40.Discrepancy in Version-Controlled Documents:

Discrepancies in version-controlled documents such as using an outdated method version during validation can compromise the integrity of the entire study. These mismatches often go unnoticed until a QA review or audit, at which point they can raise serious concerns about data traceability and compliance.

To prevent such issues, it is essential to implement a centralized document control system where all method versions, protocols, and reports are uniquely identified and access is restricted to the current approved version. Before any validation activity begins, the team must verify that the method version in use matches the one referenced in the approved protocol.

During QA review, all documents including the protocol, raw data, and final report should be cross-referenced for version alignment. This ensures consistency, traceability, and confidence that the validation was conducted under the correct conditions. Proper version control is not just an administrative task it is a key component of good documentation practice and regulatory compliance.

41.Inadequate Sample Tracking During Validation:

Effective sample management is critical to the integrity of any analytical method validation.

Without proper tracking, there's a risk of mix-ups, mislabeling, or undocumented handling, all of which can compromise the reliability of results and raise red flags during audits.

To avoid such issues, assign a unique identification number to each validation sample including standards, placebos, spiked samples, and replicates. Every step, from sample preparation and storage to analysis, should be logged in detail. This can be managed using a Laboratory Information Management System (LIMS) or, where not available, manually maintained tracking sheets.

Additionally, establishing a clear chain of custody for each sample helps ensure complete traceability and accountability. Proper sample tracking not only supports data integrity but also demonstrates a strong quality culture and audit readiness.

42.Not Updating Standard Test Procedure (STP) After Method Changes or Validations:

A common oversight in analytical practice is the failure to update the Standard Test Procedure (STP) after post-validation changes or method refinements. Whether it's a change in the column type, buffer composition, calculation formula, or permitted variations in critical parameters like pH (±0.2) or column temperature (±5°C), these adjustments must be formally documented and reflected in the current version of the STP.

43.Statistical Tools Not Validated or Controlled:

Using unvalidated or uncontrolled tools like editable Excel sheets or unofficial calculators poses a significant risk to data integrity. Small errors in formulas, accidental edits, or lack of audit trails can lead to incorrect conclusions and non-compliance during regulatory audits.

To mitigate these risks, all statistical tools particularly Excel templates must be version-controlled, locked to prevent formula modifications, and formally validated for accuracy and reliability. Each template should undergo documented testing to confirm that calculations perform as intended and produce consistent results.

Where possible, it is advisable to use pre-approved calculation sheets with embedded formulas or transition to validated statistical software such as Minitab, JMP, or modules integrated within LIMS platforms. These tools offer enhanced control, traceability, and compliance with data integrity requirements, particularly those outlined under 21 CFR Part 11 and ALCOA+ principles.

44.Validation Being Treated as a Checklist Activity, not a Scientific Exercise:

Method validation should be more than just meeting regulatory checkboxes it must be approached as a scientific evaluation of method performance. When treated as a formality, critical insights into method behavior, robustness, and long-term usability are often missed, increasing the risk of failure during routine use or audits.

To shift this mindset, focus on understanding the "why" behind the "what." Encourage cross-functional teams (QA, RA, analysts) to interpret data critically, question unexpected outcomes, and explore method boundaries. Use real audit examples where superficial validations failed to highlight the consequences of a checklist approach.

Ultimately, treating validation as a thoughtful scientific exercise ensures stronger, more reliable methods and better preparedness for real-world application and regulatory scrutiny.

45.No Internal System for Continuous Method Performance Review:

A common gap in many QC laboratories is the absence of a structured system to monitor method performance after validation. Without ongoing oversight, gradual shifts in performance such as declining system suitability, increasing variability, or recurring deviationscan go unnoticed until they impact product quality or trigger regulatory findings.

To address this, implement Method Lifecycle Management (MLCM) practices that include regular trending of system suitability data, annual method performance reviews, and tracking of any investigations related to the method. Tools like control charts and dashboards can help visualize trends and quickly flag deviations or drifts.

Assigning a dedicated method owner ensures accountability for ongoing monitoring, timely improvements, and documentation of any changes. This proactive approach not only strengthens method robustness but also demonstrates a strong commitment to continuous quality improvement and regulatory compliance.

46.Pseudo Dose-Proportionate Formulation with Same Test and Standard Concentrations:

Let us understand formulation types, dose-proportionate and pseudo-dose proportionate.

Dose-Proportionate Formulation: A formulation in which all components including API and excipients are present in the same ratio across all strengths.

For example, if a 20 mg tablet contains 20 mg API and 80mg placebos, then a 40 mg tablet would contain 40 mg API and 160 mg placebo, and so on. In such cases, the composition remains proportionally identical, just scaled up or down. Dose proportionate formulation have same placebo:API ratios across strengths.

Pseudo Dose-Proportionate Formulation: A formulation where the API content increases with strength, but the excipient levels do not scale proportionally. Instead, certain excipients are kept constant or adjusted slightly, leading to varying placebo:API ratios across strengths. This is often done for manufacturability or stability purposes but requires careful analytical validation, especially for parameters sensitive to matrix composition.

Let us now consider pseudo dose – proportionate formulation of Telmisartan tablets in 20 mg, 40 mg, and 80 mg strengths, as per below table.

Strength	API (mg)	Placebo (mg)	Placebo:API Ratio
20 mg	20	80	4:1
40 mg	40	80	2:1
80 mg	80	80	1:1

The 20 mg strength has the highest Placebo:API ratio (4:1), which poses the greatest challenge in terms of method performance especially for recovery, interference, solution stability, filter compatibility, LOD/LOQ, and robustness. Here we are assuming same concentration of API in test solution across 3 strengths.

Let us assume 100 ppm as the test concentration across all strengths. Refer below table for more details.

Strength	Placebo (mg)	Telmisartan Conc. in Test Solution	Placebo Concentration
20 mg	80	100 ppm	400 ppm
40 mg	80	100 ppm	200 ppm
80 mg	80	100 ppm	100 ppm

Validation Strategy:

A. Precision: Precision should ideally be performed for all three strengths. However, a bracketing-based approach can be adopted. Perform precision on lowest strength (20 mg) and highest strength (80 mg). If both pass acceptance criteria, 40 mg strength may be waived as intermediate verification.

B. Accuracy: Accuracy should be performed on the strength with the highest Placebo:API ratio, which in this case is 20 mg.

C. Linearity: Linearity can be performed across entire analytical range with reference to any standard solution (as the concentration for standard solution across strengths is same).

D. Specificity, Robustness, Solution Stability, Filter Validation, LOD/LOQ, and Forced Degradation: All of these parameters should be evaluated using the strength with the highest Placebo:API ratio i.e., 20 mg strength. This is considered the worst-case formulation, making it the most suitable candidate to challenge method specificity and robustness.

47.Pseudo Dose-Proportionate Formulation with Different Test and Standard Concentrations:

In some cases, test and standard solution concentrations may vary based on the label strength of the dosage form.

Let us consider Telmisartan tablets in pseudo dose-proportionate formulations, with the following assumed test solution concentrations:

Strength	Placebo	Telmisartan Conc. in Test Solution	Placebo Concentration
20 mg	80 mg	100 ppm	400 ppm
40 mg	80 mg	200 ppm	400 ppm
80 mg	80 mg	400 ppm	400 ppm

This scenario introduces an added challenge in validation, as solution concentration vary across strengths.

Validation Strategy:

A. Precision: Precision must be performed for all three strengths. Bracketing (e.g., evaluating only 20 mg and 80 mg) is not applicable, since each test and standard solution has a different concentration. Precision data at each level ensures consistent performance of the method across the full dosing range.

B. Accuracy: Accuracy can be performed using the 80 mg strength for practicality, as it has the highest API concentration (400 ppm), representing a worst-case scenario. However, the accuracy range must still cover the full-strength spectrum, for example, 50% of the lowest test concentration- 50 ppm (w.r.t 20 mg strength) and 150% of the highest test concentration- 600 ppm (w.r.t 80 mg strength). This ensures the method's accuracy across all intended use concentrations.

C. Linearity: Linearity should span for example, from 50% of the lowest test concentration to 150% of the highest test concentration.

D. Specificity, Robustness, Solution Stability, Filter Validation, LOD/LOQ, and Forced Degradation: These can be performed on the 80 mg strength, as it includes the highest API level. Testing under these conditions ensures that the method is challenged for both analyte detectability and matrix interference. However, filter saturation study can be performed for lowest test concentration to check the saturation volume required with low API amount/concentration.

Key Points to Remember: When test and standard concentrations vary across the strengths, a strength-specific validation approach is required and mostly preferred.

Worst-case strength approach may be used (as explained above), but the method must be proven suitable across the entire working range. Regulatory bodies expect clear demonstration that the method is fit for purpose for each marketed strength when concentration and matrix both vary.

48.Dose-Proportionate Formulation with Same Test and Standard Concentration:

Let us now consider dose proportionate formulation of Telmisartan tablets in 20 mg, 40 mg, and 80 mg strengths, as per below table.

Strength	API (mg)	Placebo (mg)	Placebo:API Ratio
20 mg	20	80	4:1
40 mg	40	160	4:1
80 mg	80	320	4:1

Let us consider Telmisartan tablets in dose-proportionate formulations, with the following assumed test solution concentrations:

Strength	Placebo	Telmisartan Conc. in Test Solution	Placebo Concentration
20 mg	80 mg	100 ppm	400 ppm
40 mg	160 mg	100 ppm	400 ppm
80 mg	320 mg	100 ppm	400 ppm

When the formulation composition is dose-proportionate meaning the ratio of API to excipients remains the same across all strengths all validation parameters can be performed on any one strength. This is acceptable because the matrix and sample behavior are consistent, making results applicable across the entire range of strengths.

49. Dose-Proportionate Formulation with Different Test and Standard Concentration:

In certain analytical methods, even when a formulation is dose-proportionate (i.e., excipients and API are scaled uniformly across strengths), test and standard solution concentrations may still differ by strength. This typically occurs when assay solutions are prepared in direct proportion to label claim, resulting in different ppm levels for each strength.

Example: Consider a dose-proportionate formulation of Telmisartan tablets with the following test solution concentrations:

Strength	Placebo	Placebo: API ratio	Telmisartan Conc. in Test Solution	Placebo Concentration
20 mg	80 mg	4:1	100 ppm	400 ppm
40 mg	160 mg	4:1	200 ppm	800 ppm
80 mg	160 mg	4:1	400 ppm	1600 ppm

Even though the formulation is dose-proportionate, the varying test and standard concentrations introduce complexity in validation.

Validation Strategy:

A. Precision: Precision must be performed for all three strengths. Bracketing (e.g., evaluating only 20 mg and 80 mg) is not applicable, since each test and standard solution has a different concentration. Precision data at each level ensures consistent performance of the method across the full dosing range.

B. Accuracy: Accuracy can be performed using the 80 mg strength for practicality, as it has the highest API and Placebo concentration (API- 400 ppm, Placebo- 1600ppm), representing a worst-case scenario. However, the accuracy range must still cover the full-strength spectrum, for example, 50% of the lowest test concentration- 50 ppm (w.r.t 20 mg strength) and 150% of the highest test concentration- 600 ppm (w.r.t 80 mg strength). This ensures the method's accuracy across all intended use concentrations.

C. Linearity: Linearity should span for example, from 50% of the lowest test concentration to 150% of the highest test concentration.

D. Specificity, Robustness, Solution Stability, Filter Validation, LOD/LOQ, and Forced Degradation: These can be performed on the 80 mg strength, as it contains the highest API and placebo amount. Testing under these conditions ensures that the method is challenged for both analyte detectability and matrix interference. However, filter saturation study can be performed for lowest test concentration (20mg strength) to check the saturation volume required with low API amount/concentration.

Key Points to Remember: When test and standard concentrations vary across the strengths, a strength-specific validation approach is required and mostly preferred. Worst-case strength approach may be used (as explained above), but the method must be proven suitable across the entire working range. Regulatory bodies expect clear demonstration that the method is fit for purpose for each marketed strength when concentration and matrix both vary.

50. Same analytical method for different dosage forms:

If the analytical method is intended to be used across multiple dosage types (e.g., tablets, capsules), all validation parameters should be evaluated separately for each dosage type to account for potential differences in matrix or release characteristics.

51. Cross Specificity in Case of Combination Drug Products:

In combination drug products, establishing cross specificity is a critical part of method validation. This ensures that the analytical method for one active pharmaceutical ingredient (API) does not suffer interference from the co-formulated API or excipients. Let us consider example of Metformin HCl + Glimepiride Tablets.

Let's assume you have separate analytical methods for Metformin HCl and Glimepiride. To demonstrate specificity, the placebo used during validation must reflect the real formulation environment of each API.

- For Metformin HCl Method Validation: The placebo should include all excipients plus Glimepiride, but exclude Metformin HCl. This setup allows you to confirm that the Metformin HCl method does not detect or interfere with Glimepiride.
- For Glimepiride Method Validation: The placebo should include all excipients plus Metformin HCl, but exclude Glimepiride. This confirms the specificity of the Glimepiride method in the presence of Metformin HCl.

This approach helps ensure that each API is measured accurately and selectively in the presence of the other, the method is free from interference in assay, related substances (RS), dissolution, and other parameters, and the regulatory requirement for method specificity in complex formulations is met.

52.Placebo for Residual Solvents:

For residual solvent analysis, the placebo should be carefully designed to represent the actual formulation matrix without introducing any interference. It must include all excipients and API to closely mimic the sample's composition. However, it should not contain the specific residual solvents being analyzed. This approach ensures that any peaks observed during the chromatographic analysis can be confidently attributed to the target solvents and not to components of the formulation. Using such a placebo helps in accurately evaluating method specificity and detecting any potential matrix-related interferences.

53.A Precise Method May Not Be Accurate:

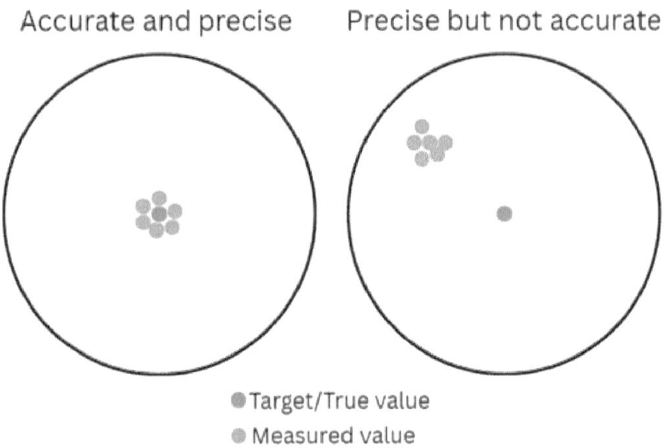

The image above beautifully illustrates a fundamental concept in analytical method validation the difference between accuracy and precision. In the first circle labeled "Accurate and Precise," the results (represented by gray dots) are tightly clustered around the dark dot target at the center, indicating that the method consistently produces results that are both close to one another and close to the true value. This is the ideal scenario for any analytical method, reflecting high reliability and correctness. In contrast, the second circle, "Precise but Not Accurate," shows a cluster of results that are consistent with each other but significantly offset from the true value. This means the method is repeatable (precise) but suffers from a systematic error that causes it to consistently miss the mark such as an incorrect calibration, mislabeling of standards, or a consistent dilution error. While such a method may initially seem acceptable due to its reproducibility, it fails to provide true results and can mislead decision-making. Therefore, during method validation, it is crucial to evaluate both precision and accuracy independently to ensure the method is not just consistently wrong, but genuinely reliable.

54.Understanding QL Requirement as per ICH Q3A and Q3B:

In the context of impurity profiling, the Quantitation Limit (QL) also known as the Limit of Quantitation (LOQ) is a critical parameter that determines the lowest concentration of an impurity that can be quantitatively measured with acceptable precision and accuracy. As per ICH guidelines Q3A (R2) and Q3B (R2), which govern impurities in drug substances and drug products respectively, the QL plays a vital role in defining the reporting threshold and qualification threshold for impurities.

Reporting threshold (Q3A(R2)	
Maximum Daily Dose[1]	Reporting Threshold[2,3]
≤ 2g/day	0.05%
> 2g/day	0.03%

Reporting threshold (Q3B(R2)	
Reporting Thresholds	
Maximum Daily Dose[1]	Threshold[2,3]
≤ 1 g	0.1%
> 1 g	0.05%

According to these guidelines, any impurity present in a drug substance or drug product above the reporting threshold (typically 0.05% or 0.03% depending on the maximum daily dose) must be quantified and reported individually. Hence, the analytical method must have a QL at or below this reporting threshold to be considered suitable. If the QL is higher than the reporting threshold, there is a risk that low-level impurities will remain undetected or unquantified, which compromises patient safety and regulatory compliance.

Importantly, this requirement should not be treated as an afterthought during method validation. Instead, the QL criteria must be actively considered during method development itself. Selecting inappropriate detection parameters, column chemistry, or sample concentration strategies can result in insufficient sensitivity, forcing a re-development or revalidation later in the process.

Conclusion:

Analytical method validation is a cornerstone of pharmaceutical quality assurance, ensuring that methods used for testing are scientifically sound, accurate, and compliant with regulatory expectations. However, as this chapter has illustrated in great detail, the path to a robust and reliable method is rarely free from obstacles. From unexpected response variations and mass balance discrepancies to practical limitations like unavailable impurity standards or low sample quantities each challenge represents a critical learning opportunity.

What sets successful laboratories apart is not the absence of these challenges, but their ability to identify, understand, and proactively address them. This chapter has emphasized the importance of root cause analysis, cross-functional collaboration, and scientific justification in overcoming real-world issues during method validation. The strategies presented are not just corrective they are preventive tools that can significantly enhance method robustness, data integrity, and audit readiness.

As pharmaceutical science continues to evolve with increasing complexity in formulations, detection technologies, and regulatory expectations it becomes even more important to adopt a risk-based and quality-by-design (QbD) approach to method validation. Relying on checklists alone is no longer sufficient; we must embrace a mindset of continuous improvement, critical thinking, and flexibility.

In closing, the insights and "way forward" strategies detailed in this chapter serve not only as solutions to common challenges but also as a guide to building a stronger analytical foundation one that ensures reliability, regulatory confidence, and above all, patient safety

www.ingramcontent.com/pod-product-compliance
Ingram Content Group UK Ltd.
Pitfield, Milton Keynes, MK11 3LW, UK
UKHW041318190726
13845UKWH00025B/356

9 789373 108056